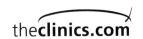

ENDOCRINOLOGY AND METABOLISM CLINICS OF NORTH AMERICA

Obesity: Brain–Gut and Inflammation Connection: Part I

GUEST EDITOR
Eddy Karnieli, MD

CONSULTING EDITOR
Derek LeRoith, MD, PhD

September 2008 • Volume 37 • Number 3

SAUNDERS

An Imprint of Elsevier, Inc.
PHILADELPHIA   LONDON   TORONTO   MONTREAL   SYDNEY   TOKYO

W.B. SAUNDERS COMPANY
A Division of Elsevier Inc.

1600 John F. Kennedy Boulevard • Suite 1800 • Philadelphia, Pennsylvania 19103-2899

http://www.theclinics.com

ENDOCRINOLOGY AND METABOLISM
CLINICS OF NORTH AMERICA
September 2008
Editor: Rachel Glover

Volume 37, Number 3
ISSN 0889-8529
ISBN-13: 978-1-4160-6291-2
ISBN-10: 1-4160-6291-2

Endocrinology and Metabolism Clinics of North America (ISSN 0889-8529) is published quarterly by Elsevier Inc., 360 Park Avenue South, New York, NY 10010-1710. Months of publication are March, June, September, and December. Business and editorial offices: 1600 John F. Kennedy Boulevard, Suite 1800, Philadelphia, PA 19103-2899. Customer Service Office: 6277 Sea Harbor Drive, Orlando, FL 32887-4800. Periodicals postage paid at New York, NY and additional mailing offices. Subscription prices are USD 220 per year for US individuals, USD 364 per year for US institutions, USD 113 per year for US students and residents, USD 276 per year for Canadian individuals, USD 437 per year for Canadian institutions, USD 301 per year for international individuals, USD 437 per year for international institutions and USD 157 per year for Canadian and foreign students/residents. To receive student/resident rate, orders must be accompanied by name of affiliated institution, date of term, and the *signature* of program/residency coordinator on institution letterhead. Orders will be billed at individual rate until proof of status is received. Foreign air speed delivery is included in all *Clinics* subscription prices. All prices are subject to change without notice. **POSTMASTER:** Send address changes to *Endocrinology and Metabolism Clinics of North America*, Elsevier Periodicals Customer Service, 6277 Sea Harbor Drive, Orlando, FL 32887-4800. **Customer Service: 1-800-654-2452 (US). From outside of the US: 1-407-563-6020. Fax: 1-407-363-9661. E-mail: JournalsCustomerService-usa@elsevier.com.**

Reprints. For copies of 100 or more, of articles in this publication, please contact the Commercial Rights Department, Elsevier Inc., 360 Park Avenue South, New York, NY 10010-1710; phone: (+1) 212-633-3812; fax: (+1) 212-462-1935; e-mail: reprints@elsevier.com.

Endocrinology and Metabolism Clinics of North America is covered in *MEDLINE/PubMed (Index Medicus), EMBASE/Excerpta Medica, Current Contents/Clinical Medicine, Current Contents/Life Sciences, Science Citation Index, ISI/BIOMED, BIOSIS, and Chemical Abstracts.*

Printed in the United States of America.

CONSULTING EDITOR

DEREK LEROITH, MD, PhD, Chief, Division of Endocrinology, Metabolism, and Bone Diseases, Mount Sinai School of Medicine, New York, New York

GUEST EDITOR

EDDY KARNIELI, MD, Director and Associate Professor, Institute of Endocrinology, Diabetes, Metabolism, Rambam Medical Center; and R.B. Rappaport Faculty of Medicine, Technion–Israel Institute of Technology, Haifa, Israel

CONTRIBUTORS

HENNING BECK-NIELSEN, MD, DMSc, Diabetes Research Center, Department of Endocrinology, Odense University Hospital, Odense, Dennmark

STEVE R. BLOOM, MA, MD, DSc, FRCPath, FRCP, FMedSci, Professor of Medicine, Department of Investigative Medicine, Imperial College London, Hammersmith Hospital, London, United Kingdom

GUENTHER BODEN, MD, Laura H. Carnell Professor of Medicine, Department of Medicine; and Chief, Division of Endocrinology/Diabetes/Metabolism, Temple University School of Medicine, Temple University Hospital, Philadelphia, Pennsylvania

MANU V. CHAKRAVARTHY, MD, PhD, Instructor in Medicine, Division of Endocrinology, Metabolism, and Lipid Research, Department of Medicine, Washington University School of Medicine, St. Louis, Missouri

EMILY JANE GALLAGHER, MRCPI, Division of Endocrinology, Diabetes, and Bone Diseases, Department of Medicine, Mount Sinai Medical Center, New York, New York

BARRY A. FRANKLIN, PhD, Director, Cardiac Rehabilitation and Exercise Laboratories, William Beaumont Hospital, Royal Oak, Michigan

REMCO FRANSSEN, MD, Department of Vascular Medicine, Academic Medical Center, Amsterdam, The Netherlands

NILS HALBERG, PhD, Touchstone Diabetes Center, Department of Internal Medicine, University of Texas Southwestern Medical Center, Dallas, Texas; Department of Biomedical Sciences, Faculty of Health Science, University of Copenhagen, Copenhagen, Dennmark

KURT HØJLUND, MD, PhD, Diabetes Research Center, Department of Endocrinology, Odense University Hospital, Odense, Dennmark

MICAELA IANTORNO, MD, Diabetes Unit, National Center for Complementary and Alternative Medicine, National Institutes of Health, Bethesda, Maryland

CHANNA N. JAYASENA, MA, MB BChir, MRCP, Clinical Research Fellow, Department of Investigative Medicine, Imperial College London, Hammersmith Hospital, London, United Kingdom

EDDY KARNIELI, MD, Director and Associate Professor, Institute of Endocrinology, Diabetes, Metabolism, Rambam Medical Center; and R.B. Rappaport Faculty of Medicine, Technion–Israel Institute of Technology, Haifa, Israel

JOHN J.P. KASTELEIN, MD, PhD, Department of Vascular Medicine, Academic Medical Center, Amsterdam, The Netherlands

L. ROMAYNE KURUKULASURIYA, MD, Assistant Professor of Clinical Medicine, Department of Internal Medicine; and Cosmopolitan International Diabetes and Endocrinology Center, University of Missouri-Columbia School of Medicine, Columbia, Missouri

DEREK LEROITH, MD, PhD, Chief, Division of Endocrinology, Diabetes, and Bone Diseases, Mount Sinai School of Medicine, New York, New York

GUIDO LASTRA, MD, Resident Physician in Internal Medicine, Department of Internal Medicine; and Cosmopolitan International Diabetes and Endocrinology Center, University of Missouri-Columbia School of Medicine, Columbia, Missouri

CAMILA MANRIQUE, MD, Resident Physician, Department of Internal Medicine; and Cosmopolitan International Diabetes and Endocrinology Center, University of Missouri-Columbia School of Medicine, Columbia, Missouri

PETER C. McCULLOUGH, MD, MPH, Consultant Cardiologist and Chief, Division of Nutrition and Preventative Medicine, William Beaumont Hospital, Royal Oak, Michigan

WENDY M. MILLER, MD, Medical Director, Weight Control Center, Division of Nutrition and Preventative Medicine, William Beaumont Hospital, Royal Oak, Michigan

MARTIN MOGENSEN, MSc, Institute of Sports Science and Clinical Biomechanics, University of Southern Dennmark, Odense, Dennmark

HOUSHANG MONAJEMI, MD, Department of Vascular Medicine, Academic Medical Center, Amsterdam, The Netherlands

RANGANATH MUNIYAPPA, MD, PhD, Diabetes Unit, National Center for Complementary and Alternative Medicine, National Institutes of Health, Bethesda, Maryland

ERIC D. PETERSON, MD, MPH, Duke Clinical Research Institute, Duke University School of Medicine, Durham, North Carolina

MICHAEL J. QUON, MD, PhD, Chief, Diabetes Unit, National Center for Complementary and Alternative Medicine, National Institutes of Health, Bethesda, Maryland

SAYALI A. RANADIVE, MD, Department of Pediatrics, Division of Endocrinology, University of California San Francisco, San Francisco, California

BABAK RAZANI, MD, PhD, Fellow in Cardiovascular Medicine, Cardiovascular Division, Department of Medicine, Washington University School of Medicine, St. Louis, Missouri

GERALD M. REAVEN, MD, Professor of Medicine (Active Emeritus), Division of Cardiovascular Medicine, Stanford University School of Medicine, Stanford Medical Center, Stanford, California

KENT SAHLIN, PhD, Institute of Sports Science and Clinical Biomechanics, University of Southern Dennmark, Odense, Dennmark; Swedish School of Sport and Health Sciences, Stockholm, Sweden

PHILIPP E. SCHERER, PhD, Touchstone Diabetes Center, Department of Internal Medicine; and Department of Cell Biology, University of Texas Southwestern Medical Center, Dallas, Texas

CLAY F. SEMENKOVICH, MD, Herbert S. Gasser Professor and Chief, Division of Endocrinology, Metabolism, and Lipid Research, Department of Medicine, Washington University School of Medicine, St. Louis, Missouri

JAMES R. SOWERS, MD, Professor of Medicine, Pharmacology, and Physiology; Thomas W. and Joan F. Burns Chair in Diabetes and Director of the Missouri University Diabetes and Cardiovascular Center, Department of Internal Medicine; Department of Medical Pharmacology and Physiology; Thomas W. Burns Center of Diabetes and Cardiovascular Research; and Harry S. Truman Veterans Affairs Medical Center, University of Missouri-Columbia School of Medicine, Columbia, Missouri

SAMEER STAS, MD, Assistant Professor of Clinical Medicine, Department of Internal Medicine; and Cosmopolitan International Diabetes and Endocrinology Center, University of Missouri-Columbia School of Medicine, Columbia, Missouri

ERIK S.G. STROES, MD, PhD, Department of Vascular Medicine, Academic Medical Center, Amsterdam, The Netherlands

CHRISTIAN VAISSE, MD, PhD, Department of Medicien and Diabetes Center, University of California San Francisco, San Francisco, California

INGRID WERNSTEDT-ASTERHOLM, PhD, Touchstone Diabetes Center, Department of Internal Medicine, University of Texas Southwestern Medical Center, Dallas, Texas

KERSTYN C. ZALESIN, MD, Department of Medicine, Division of Nutrition and Preventative Medicine, William Beaumont Hospital, Royal Oak, Michigan

CONTENTS

overall obesity, as estimated by body mass index, is comparable to that of abdominal obesity, as quantified by waist circumference.

and increased caloric expenditure, the development of methods to measure FFAs in small blood samples, and the development of efficient pharmacologic approaches to normalize increased plasma FFA levels.

Hypertension in Obesity

L. Romayne Kurukulasuriya, Sameer Stas, Guido Lastra, Camila Manrique, and James R. Sowers

Hypertension and obesity are major components of the cardiometabolic syndrome and are both on the rise worldwide, with enormous consequences on global health and the economy. The relationship between hypertension and obesity is multifaceted; the etiology is complex and it is not well elucidated. This article, reviews the current knowledge on obesity-related hypertension. Further understanding of the underlying mechanisms of this epidemic will be important in devising future treatment avenues.

Impact of Obesity on Cardiovascular Disease

Kerstyn C. Zalesin, Barry A. Franklin, Wendy M. Miller, Eric D. Peterson, and Peter A. McCullough

The epidemiology of cardiovacular disease risk factors is changing rapidly with the obesity pandemic. Obesity is independently associated with the risks for coronary heart disease, atrial fibrillation, and heart failure. Intra-abdominal obesity is also unique as a cardiovascular risk state in that it contributes to or directly causes most other modifiable risk factors, namely, hypertension, dysmetabolic syndrome, and type 2 diabetes mellitus. Obesity can also exacerbate cardiovascular disease through a variety of mechanisms including systemic inflammation, hypercoagulability, and activation of the sympathetic and renin-angiotensin systems. Thus, weight reduction is a key strategy for simultaneous improvement in global cardiovascular risk, with anticipated improvements in survival and quality of life.

An Integrated View of Insulin Resistance and Endothelial Dysfunction

Ranganath Muniyappa, Micaela Iantorno, and Michael J. Quon

Endothelial dysfunction and insulin resistance are frequently comorbid states. Vasodilator actions of insulin are mediated by phosphatidylinositol 3-kinase (PI3K)-dependent signaling pathways that stimulate production of nitric oxide from vascular endothelium. This helps to couple metabolic and hemodynamic homeostasis under healthy conditions. In pathologic states, shared causal factors, including glucotoxicity, lipotoxicity, and inflammation selectively impair PI3K-dependent insulin signaling pathways that contribute to reciprocal relationships between insulin resistance and endothelial dysfunction. This article discusses the implications of pathway-selective insulin resistance in vascular endothelium, interactions between endothelial dysfunction and insulin resistance, and therapeutic interventions that may simultaneously improve both metabolic and cardiovascular physiology in insulin-resistant conditions.

Insulin resistance in skeletal muscle is a major hallmark of type 2 diabetes mellitus (T2D) and obesity that is characterized by impaired insulin-mediated glucose transport and glycogen synthesis and by increased intramyocellular content of lipid metabolites. Several studies have provided evidence for mitochondrial dysfunction in skeletal muscle of type 2 diabetic and prediabetic subjects, primarily due to a lower content of mitochondria (mitochondrial biogenesis) and possibly to a reduced functional capacity per mitochondrion. This article discusses the latest advances in the understanding of the molecular mechanisms underlying insulin resistance in human skeletal muscle in T2D and obesity, with a focus on possible links between insulin resistance and mitochondrial dysfunction.

Human obesity has a strong genetic component. Most genes that influence an individual's predisposition to gain weight are not yet known. However, the study of extreme human obesity caused by single gene defects has provided a glimpse into the long-term regulation of body weight. These monogenic obesity disorders have confirmed that the hypothalamic leptin–melanocortin system is critical for energy balance in humans, because disruption of these pathways causes the most severe obesity phenotypes. Approximately 20 different genes and at least three different mechanisms have been implicated in monogenic causes of obesity; however, they account for fewer than 5% of all severe obesity cases. This finding suggests that the genetic basis for human obesity is likely to be extremely heterogeneous, with contributions from numerous genes acting by various, yet undiscovered, molecular mechanisms.

Adipose tissue contains many cell types. Among the more abundant are adipocytes, preadipocytes, immune cells, and endothelial cells. During times of excess caloric intake, these cells have to adjust and remodel to accommodate the increased demand for triglyceride storage. Based on a comprehensive analysis of the total adipose tissue secretome, this article focuses on three areas of adipokine biology: (1) How does the adipocyte interact with the extracellular matrix over the course of obestiy? (2) Does the adipocyte, per se, play a role in the innate immune response? (3) How is the angiogenic profile of adipose tissue linked to the development of insulin resistance? The authors present a comprehensive overview of all of the currently available secreted adipose tissue products that have been identified at the protein level.

A critical role for the gut in energy homeostasis has emerged. Gut hormones not only have a role in digestion but several of them have been found to modulate appetite in animals and humans. Current nonendocrine drugs for obesity are limited by their modest efficacies, and bariatric surgery is confined to use in severe cases. The discovery of important appetite-signaling pathways from the gut to the brain has led to the emergence of several gut hormone–derived drugs that are being investigated for clinical use. This article summarizes the physiology of the major gut hormones implicated in appetite regulation, and reviews clinical evidence that gives us insight into their potential as clinical treatments for obesity.

FORTHCOMING ISSUES

RECENT ISSUES

THE CLINICS ARE NOW AVAILABLE ONLINE!

Access your subscription at:
http://www.theclinics.com

ELSEVIER
SAUNDERS

Endocrinol Metab Clin N Am
37 (2008) xiii–xvi

ENDOCRINOLOGY
AND METABOLISM
CLINICS
OF NORTH AMERICA

Foreword

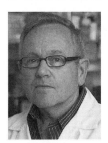

Derek LeRoith, MD, PhD
Consulting Editor

This is the first of two very informative issues on obesity that cover the etiology-related conditions with this growing problem that is a worldwide phenomenon.

The metabolic syndrome that includes obesity, hypertension, hyperlipidemia, and glucose intolerance has insulin resistance as the underlying cause and is commonly seen in patients with type-2 diabetes. As described in the article by Gallagher, LeRoith, and Karnieli, it is extremely common in both developed countries as well as in third world countries, and it is associated with visceral adiposity. Though the exact definitions of the metabolic syndrome differ slightly between various organizational and governing bodies, its existence and its relationship to type-2 diabetes are unequivocal. The article also presents the experimental evidence, upon which the insulin resistance is caused by the obesity and how the insulin resistance causes the hypertension, hyperlipidemia, and glucose intolerance.

Gerald Reaven, one of the investigators who described the metabolic syndrome (he originally named it syndrome "X"), describes the relationship between obesity and cardiovascular disease. He initially presents the relationship between abdominal obesity and reduced insulin-mediated glucose uptake into muscle. The resultant insulin resistance and hyperinsulinemia lead to increased risk factors for cardiovascular disease. Today, this cardio-metabolic syndrome is so common that major efforts are underway to attempt to reverse the abnormality, since heart attacks and strokes are the major causes of the high mortality rates in type-2 diabetic patients.

0889-8529/08/$ - see front matter © 2008 Elsevier Inc. All rights reserved.
doi:10.1016/j.ecl.2008.07.004   *endo.theclinics.com*

Razani, Chakravarthy, and Semenkovich describe the basic and clinical effects of insulin resistance on the cardiovascular system—how insulin resistance causes atherosclerosis by way of hyperlipidemia and inflammation. They also outline experimental evidence invoking NFκB, JNKinase, and oxidative stress in this process. They describe the various ways of preventing the atherosclerosis, such as angiotensin-converting enzyme inhibitors, angiotensin-II receptor blockers (ARBs), and statins, and present results of clinical trials that have utilized PPARα and PPARα agonists, but they point out that the latter trials have been rather disappointing.

Obesity and hyperlipidemia is another complication that is commonly appreciated in the medical community. The cardiovascular risk associated with obesity is mostly predicted by the hyperlipidemia, characterized by increased triglyceride levels, decreased high-density lipoproteins (HDL) levels, and a shift in low-density lipoproteins (LDL) to a more pro-atherogenic composition (small dense LDL). These features are covered in the article by Franssen, Monajemi, Stroes, and Kastelein. They describe how the classic concept of insulin resistance and lipolysis, with excess FFA release leading to hypertriglyceridemia, is still the central theme. However, newer concepts, such as the hypothalamic control of lipid metabolism, are undoubtedly important and may allow for the development of newer therapeutic agents.

Obesity is associated with increased free fatty acids, inflammation, and insulin resistance. Insulin resistance in adipocytes leads to increased lipolysis. One of the conundrums is what precedes and what the consequence is. Boden, in his scholarly article, describes how free fatty acids (FFAs) can induce or worsen insulin resistance at the cellular level in many metabolically important tissues, an effect called "lipotoxicity." He also describes how different medications, including fibrates, TZDs and the experimental agent Acipimox (a nicotinic analog), can reverse the situation, but points out that the insulin resistance, whether induced by FFAs or inflammation, is best reversed by weight loss.

Obesity-related hypertension has many causes, as outlined by Kurukulasuriya, Stas, Lastra, Manrique, and Sowers. These include well-known causes such as insulin resistance, activation of the renin-angiotensinogen-aldosterone system with renal sodium retention, and the sympathetic nervous system. More recent studies have demonstrated that adipocytokines, FFAs, and other molecules may cause endothelial dysfunction. More recently, the effect of sleep deprivation on obesity and, therefore, on hypertension has been described. Although the causes are being investigated, the need for intensive therapy is primary to prevent the cardiovascular and renal complications that result.

The relationship between obesity and cardiovascular disease is further explored in the article by Zalesin, Franklin, Miller, Peterson, and McCullough. They address the increased risk factors and increased cardiac disease in obese individuals that cause heart attacks, atrial fibrillation, and heart failure. Importantly, they describe the epidemic of obesity and the increased rates of hypertension, hyperlipidemia, and glucose intolerance in the pediatric population and the eventual increase in cardiovascular disease that is bound to result at younger ages.

Muniyappa, Iantorno, and Quon describe an integrated view of insulin resistance and endothelial function. The endothelium utilizes NO to affect vasodilation, a critical function in maintaining normal vasculature. NO production is also under the control of insulin action by way of the activation of Akt, and its downstream signaling pathway. Similar to the situation in classic metabolic tissues such as muscle, fat, and liver, insulin resistance in the endothelium involves inhibition of the insulin signaling cascade and reduced levels of NO, specifically in the endothelial cells. This effect may be secondary to inflammatory cytokines, FFAs, and other factors. Thus, insulin resistance and endothelium dysfunction in obesity and type-2 diabetes may be integrally related and therapies to overcome the resistance will improve both systems.

A fascinating new concept that has developed from recent studies is the role of skeletal muscle mitochondrial dysfunction in the cause of insulin resistance commonly associated with obesity and diabetes. Højlund, Mogensen, Sahlin, and Beck-Nielsen describe the defect and question whether it is of both genetic and environmental etiologies, since the alterations can often be detected prior to the onset of both obesity and diabetes. They point out, however, that exercise and diet (lifestyle changes) can partially reverse the defect, suggesting that environment is, at least partially, playing a role.

Ranadive and Vaisse cover the topic of monogenic causes of obesity. Though obesity in the general population is a polygenic disorder, monogenic disorders have helped to understand the disease. Leptin and leptin-receptor mutations have clearly established this pathway in control of appetite. Mutations in the proopiomelanocortin pathways and the melanocortin-4 receptor have extended our understanding of the condition. These single mutations that cause severe obesity represent less than 5% of the causes, but in animal and human studies have allowed the field to progress, and the signaling pathways involved have suggested new gene targets for therapy.

Until recently, the adipocyte was considered the tissue that stored triglyceride. Recent studies have demonstrated that the adipose tissue is an endocrine organ secreting a large number of adipocytokines and hormones; the exact number is still unclear. Halberg, Wernstedt, and Scherer describe exciting new information regarding adipocyte physiology. They discuss angiogenesis, the involvement of inflammation, and extracellular matrix in this tissue. Importantly, they present the information available on the adipocyte "secretome," an important component of the adipocytokine physiology.

As discussed by Jayasena and Bloom, there has been a fundamental change in our understanding of the role of gastrointestinal hormones that were considered factors primarily affecting the gastrointestinal function. Ghrelin is produced from the stomach and stimulates appetite, whereas cholecystokinin and other peptides inhibit appetite. Most importantly, the glucagon-like peptides (incretins) that are released from the intestinal tract affect insulin and glucagon secretion from the pancreas that may affect satiety have become the focus of the pharmaceutical industry and are being used for the treatment of obese type-2 diabetics.

The reader will undoubtedly find these articles of tremendous interest and should stimulate the desire to read the second issue on obesity that will cover, amongst other topics, the latest in therapeutics.

Derek LeRoith, MD, PhD
Division of Endocrinology, Metabolism, and Bone Diseases
Mount Sinai School of Medicine
One Gustave L. Levy Place
Box 1055, Altran 4-36
New York, NY 10029, USA

E-mail address: derek.leroith@mssm.edu

ELSEVIER
SAUNDERS

Endocrinol Metab Clin N Am
37 (2008) xvii–xviii

ENDOCRINOLOGY
AND METABOLISM
CLINICS
OF NORTH AMERICA

Preface

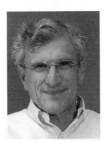

Eddy Karnieli, MD
Guest Editor

The growing prevalence of obesity worldwide is an increasing concern surrounding the rising rates of type-2 diabetes, cardiovascular disease, and the consequent health and financial implications for the population. The association between overweight/obesity and mortality has been well documented. The United States has the highest prevalance rates of obesity (body mass index [BMI] ≥ 30 kg/m^2) world wide, now exceeding 30%. Even more alarming is the fact that, in children and adolescents, overweight prevalence has tripled, leading to the expectation that by 2035 the prevalence of coronary heart disease will increase significantly compared to today's figures. A similar picture can be drawn for many of the counries in Europe and most of the developing countries in the world.

Not surprisingly, therefore, obesity is often described as an epidemic. Thus, it is essential to develop ways for preventing obesity while concomitantly devising efficient treatment strategies. The present issue of the *Endocrinology and Metabolism Clinics of North America* series is addressing this "call to action" in fighting obesity by encompassing the recent developments is obesity research from a genetic point of view to treatment options. The authors and the editors, in these articles, tried to balance the most recent and novel findings from the basic molecular aspects, such as the lessons that can be learned from monogenic obesity; to newly understood mechanisms of hormone secretion and action, such as gastrointestinal hormones that act on the hypothalamus and adipose-associated peptides and cytokines; to clinical applied protocols for therapy. We hope that the reader will benefit from this "translational medicine" approach and, as a result, the

doi:10.1016/j.ecl.2008.07.005
endo.theclinics.com

physician, scientist, and ultimately the patients will benefit from this issue, each in their point of need. That will be our token effort in fighting obesity.

Eddy Karnieli, MD
Institute of Endocrinology, Diabetes, and Metabolism
Rambam Medical Center
R.B. Rapaport Faculty of Medicine—Technion
12 Halia Street
Haifa 31096
Israel

E-mail address: eddy@tx.technion.ac.il

ELSEVIER
SAUNDERS

Endocrinol Metab Clin N Am
37 (2008) 559–579

ENDOCRINOLOGY
AND METABOLISM
CLINICS
OF NORTH AMERICA

The Metabolic Syndrome—from Insulin Resistance to Obesity and Diabetes

Emily Jane Gallagher, MRCPI[a],
Derek LeRoith, MD, PhD[a], Eddy Karnieli, MD[b],*

[a]Mount Sinai Medical Center, Department of Medicine,
Division of Endocrinology, Diabetes, and Bone Diseases,
One Gustave L. Levy Place, Box 1055, New York, NY 10029-6574, USA
[b]Institute of Endocrinology, Diabetes, and Metabolism, Rambam Medical Center and R.B.
Rapaport Faculty of Medicine–Technion, 12 Halia Street, Haifa 31096, Israel

The growing prevalence of obesity worldwide is increasing concern surrounding the rising rates of diabetes, coronary, and cerebrovascular disease with the consequent health and financial implications for the population [1]. The metabolic syndrome comprises an assembly of risk factors for developing diabetes and cardiovascular disease. Opinion varies with regard to the etiology of the metabolic syndrome and whether it should be defined as a syndrome of insulin resistance, the metabolic consequences of obesity, or risk factors for cardiovascular disease [2]. Some consider it not a to be a syndrome, but rather a collection of statistical correlations [3]. This article will try to unveil some of the molecular and physiologic mechanisms underlying the entities of insulin resistance and the metabolic syndrome. It will focus on their clinical relevance for the care of overweight and/or obese patients with or without diabetes as defined by the American Diabetes Association (ADA) criteria [4].

Historic overview

The metabolic syndrome has undergone a host of incarnations in the medical literature since the clustering of metabolic risk factors for coronary artery disease, diabetes, and hypertension was described as "Syndrome X" by Reaven in 1988 [5]. The initial factors described by Reaven included impaired

* Corresponding author.
E-mail address: eddy@tx.technion.ac.il (E. Karnieli).

glucose tolerance (IGT), hyperinsulinemia, elevated triglycerides (TG), and reduced high-density lipoprotein cholesterol (HDLc). Subsequently, hyperuricemia and raised plasminogen activator inhibitor 1 (PAI-1) were suggested as components of the same syndrome [5,6]. Obesity was not included in Reaven's definition of Syndrome X, as he suggested that insulin resistance, rather than obesity, was the unifying feature. The core components of what we now call the metabolic syndrome: obesity, insulin resistance, dyslipidemia, and hypertension have remained since the World Health Organization (WHO) produced its definition in 1998. WHO published criteria to define the metabolic syndrome in an attempt to harmonize reporting of prevalence through epidemiologic studies. The criteria included a measure of insulin resistance, by a hyperinsulinemic euglycemic clamp, impaired fasting glucose (IFG), impaired glucose tolerance (IGT) or diabetes, obesity (BMI >30 kg/m^2), hypertension ($\geq 140/90$ mm Hg), and microalbuminuria [7]. Critics of the WHO definition highlighted the impracticality of performing hyperinsulinemic clamp studies in epidemiologic research. They also pointed out that rather than measuring the waist-to-hip ratio, waist circumference measurement was more convenient and had a comparable correlation to obesity. In addition, some believed that microalbuminuria should not be included at all given the insufficient evidence of a close correlation with insulin resistance [3]. These opinions lead to the second definition in 1999, from the European Group for the Study of Insulin Resistance (EGIR). They renamed the syndrome, "insulin resistance syndrome" and excluded subjects with diabetes because of excessive complexities in measuring insulin resistance in these individuals. Insulin resistance remained an essential component, defined as a fasting insulin level above the 75th percentile for the population. Two of these other elements (criteria associated with increased risk of coronary artery disease from the Second Joint Task Force of European and other Societies on Coronary Prevention) were also required: obesity defined as waist circumference 94 cm (37 inches) or more for men and 80 cm (32 inches) or more for women, hypertension remained defined as 140/90 mm Hg or higher, and dyslipidemia with TG 180 mg/dL (2.0 mmol/L) or more, and/or HDLc less than 39 mg/dL (1.01 mmol/L) [3]. In 2001, The National Cholesterol Education Program (NCEP) Adult Treatment Panel III (ATP III) changed the focus to cardiovascular risk factors and away from relying on measures of insulin resistance and possible etiologies; therefore, the title "The Metabolic Syndrome" was reassigned. The criteria were any three of the following: obesity (waist circumference ≥ 102 cm [40 inches] in males and ≥ 88 cm [35 inches] in females, based on the 1998 National Institutes of Health [NIH] obesity clinical guidelines), hypertension ($\geq 130/85$ mm Hg based on Joint National Committee guidelines), fasting glucose more than 110 mg/dL (6.1 mmol/L, including diabetes), TG 150 mg/dL (1.69 mmol/L) or more, and HDLc less than 40 mg/dL (1.03 mmol/L) in men or less than 50 mg/dL (1.3 mmol/L) in women [8]. Waist circumference was not a required element as the NCEP/ATP III wished to include certain individuals and ethnic groups that have metabolic and blood pressure abnormalities associated with elevated cardiovascular risk, but do not meet the criteria for abdominal obesity. Subsequently, in 2003, the American Association of Clinical Endocrinologists (AACE) modified the ATP III criteria and renamed the disorder "Insulin Resistance Syndrome." The AACE did not set out stringent criteria to define the syndrome, but described it as a group of abnormalities associated with insulin resistance, including glucose intolerance (but not diabetes), abnormalities in uric acid metabolism, dyslipidemia (consistent with NCEP/ATP III criteria), hemodynamic changes, prothrombotic factors, markers of inflammation, endothelial dysfunction and elevated blood pressure (as NCEP/ATP III). This consensus also endeavored to identify individuals at increased risk of developing the insulin resistance syndrome in the future: BMI greater than 25 kg/m^2 (or waist circumference > 40 inches in men and 35 inches in women), known cardiovascular disease, hypertension, polycystic ovarian syndrome (PCOS), nonalcoholic fatty liver disease (NAFLD), or acanthosis nigricans; family history of type 2 diabetes (T2DM), hypertension, or cardiovascular disease; history of gestational diabetes or glucose intolerance; non-Caucasian ethnicity; sedentary lifestyle; and age older than 40 years [9]. In parallel, the International Diabetes Federation (IDF) aimed to create a straightforward, clinically useful definition, to provide worldwide conformity for epidemiologic studies and identify those at greatest risk of developing diabetes and cardiovascular disease. To this end, the IDF proposed a new consensus definition of the metabolic syndrome in 2005. Obesity (BMI > 30 kg/m^2 or if ≤ 30 kg/m^2 by ethnic-specific waist circumference measurements) was a prerequisite factor, as they felt it was a central etiologic component of the syndrome. Two of four other factors were also required: TG 150 mg/dL or higher, HDLc less than 40 mg/dL in men or less than 50 mg/dL in women, systolic blood pressure 130 mm Hg or higher or diastolic blood pressure 85 mm Hg or higher, fasting glucose more than 100 mg/dL (5.6 mmol/L, 2003 ADA definition of IFG [10]) including diabetes, and those with a previous diagnosis of or treatment for any of these conditions [11].

Definitions

In this *Clinics of North America* series, we follow the 2005 American Heart Association (AHA)/National Heart, Lung and Blood Institute (NHLBI) criteria as shown in Table 1. The revised definition is based on the ATP III criteria, requires three of the five factors listed in Table 1 [12] and primarily aims to diagnose those patients at increased risk of type 2 diabetes and cardiovascular disease. When using these criteria, the reader should take into account the updated differences relating to waist circumference measures by ethnic origin (as suggested by the IDF) as well as the

Table 1
Criteria for diagnosis of the metabolic syndrome (American Heart Association/National Heart, Lung and Blood Institute) 2005

Any three of the following criteria	Parameter
Elevated waist circumference	≥ 102 cm (≥ 40 inches) in men
	≥ 88 cm (≥ 35 inches) in women
Elevated triglycerides	≥ 150 mg/dL (1.7 mmol/L)
Reduced HDLc	<40 mg/dL (1.03 mmol/L) in men
	<50 mg/dL (1.3 mmol/L) in women
Elevated blood pressure	≥ 130 mm Hg systolic blood pressure
	OR
	≥ 85 mm Hg diastolic blood pressure
Elevated fasting glucose	≥ 100 mg/dL (≥ 5.6 mmol/L)

International Diabetes Foundation ethnic-specific values for waist circumference: Europoids: male ≥ 94 cm, female ≥ 80 cm; South Asians: male ≥ 90 cm, female ≥ 80 cm; Japanese: male ≥ 90 cm, female ≥ 80 cm. Ethnic south and central Americans use South Asian criteria until more specific criteria are available; sub-Saharan Africans, eastern Mediterranean, and Middle Eastern (Arab) populations use Europoid data at present.

Data from Grundy S, Cleeman J, Daniels S, et al. Diagnosis and management of the metabolic syndrome: an American Heart Association/National Heart, Lung, and Blood Institute scientific statement. Circulation 2005;112(17):2735–52.

revised criterion for impaired fasting glucose indicating those individuals at greater risk of developing the metabolic syndrome [9,10,12].

Comparing the AHA/NHLBI to the IDF definition of the metabolic syndrome, blood pressure, lipid, and glucose ranges are the same; however, in contrast to the IDF, the AHA/NHLBI have not made obesity essential to the diagnosis but draw attention to the increased risk of insulin resistance and the metabolic syndrome in certain ethnic groups (ie, populations from South Asia, China, Japan, and other Asian countries) with only moderate increases in waist circumference. The IDF waist circumference cut-off values that define obesity for Europoids are 8 cm less for both males and females than those measurements in the AHA/NHLBI criteria, which were based on the National Health and Nutrition Examination Survey (NHANES) [11,12]. The waist circumference cut-off measurements in the AHA/NHLBI definition approximate a BMI of 29.8 kg/m^2 in males and 24.9 kg/m^2 in females [12,13].

It is likely that the definitions of the metabolic syndrome will continue to develop. Which definition is most useful will depend on its ability to predict cardiovascular outcomes in prospective studies.

Prevalence

Reported rates of prevalence vary widely with the criteria used, age of the population, gender, ethnic group, prevalence of obesity in the background population, and environment. Based on the NHANES 1999–2002, it is estimated that 34.6% of the US population meet the ATP III criteria for the metabolic syndrome. There is minimal gender difference: 34.4% of males and 34.5% of females. An increased prevalence has been shown with advancing age [14–16].

Worldwide, prevalence rates of the metabolic syndrome were found to be similar irrespective of which set of criteria was applied, however different individuals were identified using different criteria [17]. The ATP III and IDF criteria similarly classified 92.9% of individuals in the NHANES. The IDF (with the lower waist circumference cut-off points) increased the overall age-adjusted prevalence estimate to 39.1% (40.7% in males and 37.1% in females) [18]. However, concordance rates vary widely between studies. Both the Dallas Heart Study and the NHANES demonstrated the lowest concordance rate among Hispanic males. The PROCAM study from Germany, along with other European population studies, revealed low concordance rates [19]. Other European population studies have shown large differences in estimated prevalence [20,21]. In a northern Mexican population study the IDF criteria classified 94.4% of females as having obesity by waist circumference measurements (≥ 80 cm), which may suggest the waist circumference cut-off levels are inappropriately low for this population [22]. Of particular interest, the IDF criteria underestimate the metabolic syndrome prevalence in Asian populations, for example in Korea and China, as many individuals in these regions have metabolic risk factors without significant obesity [23,24].

The NHANES study showed that with both the ATP III and IDF criteria, in males, the highest prevalence of the metabolic syndrome is in whites at 35% (IDF 42.6%). The lowest was in African American males, 21.6% (IDF 24.2%) despite the higher overall prevalence of hypertension and diabetes in this group. Mexican American women had the highest overall prevalence 37.8% (IDF 39.2%). White and African American women had similar prevalence, 33.7% and 33.8% respectively (36.9% and 35.8% by IDF) [18]. The NHANES group had insufficient numbers of other ethnic groups to calculate their prevalence rates. Apart from the Mexican American population, other studies have shown that American Indians, Hawaiian, Filipino, and Polynesian populations have a higher incidence than those of European descent [15,25–28].

Rural populations tend to have lower prevalence rates than urban populations, which have been demonstrated in multiple ethnic groups and studies of migrations to western society [22,29]. Western diet appears to bring with it increased risk of the metabolic syndrome particularly in Chinese, Indian, and Middle Eastern populations [30–32]. Arab populations living in the United States have been shown to have higher prevalence than those living in the Middle East [22,29–33].

Low cardiorespiratory fitness in some studies correlates significantly with incidence of the metabolic syndrome in both men and women. In a Swedish study of healthy volunteers over age 60, metabolic syndrome prevalence was 24% and 19% in men and women, respectively. The adjusted odds ratio for having the metabolic syndrome in the high leisure-time physical activity group was 0.33, that of the low physical activity group [34]. A study of volunteers in Dallas, TX, with an age range of 20–80 years yielded similar results, showing a hazard ratio of 0.47 in men and 0.37 in the physically active women [35].

Prognosis

Equal to, if not exceeding, the importance of clinically practical definitions of the metabolic syndrome is having criteria that are pertinent for predicting the development of type 2 diabetes and cardiovascular disease. In the United States in 2003, the prevalence of cardiovascular disease was 34.2% and was a contributing or underlying cause of death in 37.3% of cases, which equates to 1 in every 2.7 deaths or 2500 deaths each day and a cost of $403.1 billion [36]. Data from the NHANES II show that combined, preexisting cardiovascular disease and diabetes carry the greatest hazard for mortality from coronary artery disease (hazard ratio [HR] 6.25) and cardiovascular disease (HR 5.26) [37]. Diabetes alone carries a HR of 2.87 for coronary artery disease mortality and 2.42 for all cardiovascular disease mortality [37]. Independent of the traditional Framingham risk factors (age, smoking, total cholesterol, HDLc levels, and systolic blood pressure), some researchers have found that the metabolic syndrome is associated with an increased probability of cardiovascular disease and conveys a higher risk than the Framingham risk score of developing type 2 diabetes [38–45]. However, the Framingham investigators report little or no increase in the predictive power for coronary heart disease by adding abdominal obesity, triglycerides, or fasting glucose to their 10-year risk algorithm (Fig. 1) [46,47]. Debate surrounds which definition is the best predictor of diabetes, cardiovascular disease, and mortality [24,48,49].

Three recent meta-analyses of prospective studies investigating the metabolic syndrome as a significant risk for cardiovascular disease and mortality show increased relative risk of both events [50–52]. One study demonstrated a relative risk of diabetes of 2.99 [50] and all three analyses revealed more moderate increases in risk for cardiovascular events ranging from 1.53 to 2.7. All-cause mortality risk was estimated to be between 1.37 and 1.60 for those with the metabolic syndrome, depending on the criteria employed [50,51]. This greater probability of cardiovascular events and mortality has been shown to exist with the metabolic syndrome both in the presence and absence of diabetes; however, as in the NHANES II, the presence of diabetes, along with the metabolic syndrome, significantly increases this risk (HR 1.56 without diabetes, 1.82 with diabetes) [37,39,53]. The increased risk of cardiovascular disease with the metabolic syndrome does not appear to be explained entirely by insulin resistance. In studies that calculate insulin resistance by the homeostasis model assessment of insulin resistance

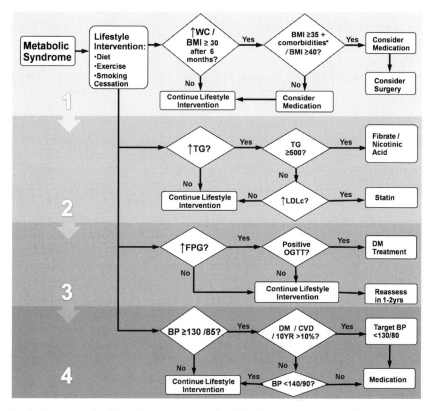

Fig. 1. Four-step algorithm for management of modifiable aspects of the metabolic syndrome. ↑WC, Waist Circumference >102 cm (men), >88 cm women; BMI, Body Mass Index in kg/m^2; ↑TG, Elevated triglycerides; ↑LDLc, Elevated low-density lipoprotein cholesterol (see text); ↑FPG, Elevated fasting plasma glucose (>100 mg/dL); Positive OGTT, Oral glucose tolerance test (75 g) with 2-hour glucose of ≥200 mg/dL; DM, diabetes mellitus; BP, blood pressure: CVD, cardiovascular disease; 10YR, 10-year risk of CAD calculated by Framingham risk score. *Age >45years (male), >55years (female), cigarette smoking, dyslipidemia, hypertension, IFG, IGT, type 2 diabetes, family history of premature CVD in first-degree relative (male <55 years, female <65 years). (*Data from* Grundy SM, Brewer Jr HB, Cleeman JI, et al. Definition of metabolic syndrome: Report of the National Heart, Lung, and Blood Institute/American Heart Association Conference on scientific issues related to definition. Circulation 2004;109(3):433–8.)

(HOMA-IR), the predictive power of the metabolic syndrome for diabetes and cardiovascular disease development has been demonstrated to be independent of the HOMA-IR [39–41]. There is also conflict regarding whether the metabolic syndrome as a whole confers a greater risk of cardiovascular disease and diabetes than its individual components [49,53–55]. In the Atherosclerosis Risk in Communities (ARIC) study, hypertension and low HDLc were found to be the strongest predictors of coronary heart disease; the metabolic syndrome as a whole was not found to have a greater prediction power than these individual elements [53].

Pathogenesis

Whether the metabolic syndrome is an assortment of unrelated risk factors or allied traits attributable to a common mechanism is a matter of ongoing debate [56,57]. Although risk factors for the metabolic syndrome have been identified, the etiology remains incompletely understood [9,12]. As initially proposed by Reaven, it appears that insulin resistance is likely to be a significant link between the components of the metabolic syndrome [5,58]. Indeed, as mentioned previously, the metabolic syndrome is also known as the insulin resistance syndrome [3,9]. Many lifestyle, molecular, and genetic contributors [59] leading to the metabolic syndrome have been described; these include obesity and disorders of adipose tissue; physical inactivity; diet; insulin receptor and signaling anomalies [60,61]; inflammatory cascades; mitochondrial dysfunction [62]; molecules of immunologic, hepatic, or vascular origin (including adiponectin, leptin, PAI-1, resistin, angiotensinogen); endocannabinoid receptors; nuclear receptors; hormones; and polygenic variability in individuals and ethnic groups. Here, we will summarize how some of these factors contribute to the abnormalities within the metabolic syndrome.

In response to glucose stimulation, pancreatic β cells release insulin, leading to suppression of hepatic gluconeogenesis and increased glucose uptake and metabolism by the muscle and adipose tissue. Glucose transport into cells is mediated by glucose transporters (GLUT). One of the most important glucose transporters, GLUT4, is regulated by insulin. In response to insulin, GLUT4 is mobilized from intracellular storage vesicles and fuses to the cellular membrane to internalize glucose (see review [63]). This is the major rate-controlling step in insulin mediated glucose uptake and muscle glycogen synthesis [60,64,65]. GLUT4 cellular concentration in adipocytes is decreased with advancing age, obesity, and type 2 diabetes [60]. In skeletal muscle of obese and diabetic humans, GLUT4 is not decreased, but rather dysfunctional [66]. Exercise and adiponectin appear to increase the expression of GLUT4, coincident with insulin sensitivity. With insulin resistance, there is an initial loss of the immediate postprandial (first phase) response to insulin, leading to postprandial hyperglycemia. Subsequently, there is an exaggerated second-phase insulin response, which over time causes chronic hyperinsulinemia [59]. The resulting chronic hyperinsulinemia leads to resistance to the action of insulin (as further detailed) [1,67,68].

At a cellular level, insulin binds to the insulin receptor (IR) activating the tyrosine kinase pathway. This pathway stimulates the phosphorylation of receptor substrates and adaptor proteins, including insulin receptor substrates 1 and 2 (IRS1, IRS2), Gab1, Shc, and APS on selected tyrosine residues and these form docking sites for further downstream effectors [69,70]. There are then two major pathways in insulin-mediated activities: one is initiated by phosphatidylinositol 3-kinase (PI3K) and is the major channel of the metabolic effects of insulin; second is that downstream of mitogen-activated protein (MAP) kinase signaling, mostly involved in growth and mitogenesis [69]. Within the PI3K pathway, tyrosine-phosphorylated IRSs recruit and interact with the regulatory p85 subunit of PI3K, resulting in synthesis of phosphatidylinositol 3,4,5 phosphate (PIP3). Downstream kinases PDK (phosphoinositide dependent kinase) and Akt, bind to PIP3 and this results in their activation. Akt is known to mediate the effects of insulin on glucose transport and storage, protein synthesis, and prevention of lipid degradation. Some of these metabolic effects are mediated through Akt phosphorylation of FOXO (forkhead box class O) transcription factors [61,71]. FOXO1 plays a key role in hepatic gluconeogenesis. When phosphorylated it is sequestered in the cytoplasm and prevented from activating gluconeogenic genes [72,73]. It has also been shown in vitro to repress the transcription of peroxisome proliferator activated-receptor (PPAR)γ promoter genes [73]. PPARγ is one of a family of nuclear receptors, also including PPARα and PPARβ/d, which are key transcription factors involved in the regulation of glucose and lipid metabolism, along with insulin sensitivity. PPARγ is found in insulin-responsive tissues, whereas PPARα is expressed in hepatocytes, cardiac myocytes, and enterocytes, and PPARβ/d is ubiquitous. While PPARγ represses GLUT4 transcription [71,74], its thiazoledinedione synthetic ligands enhance insulin sensitivity, probably by dismissal of co-repressor complexes, switching them with co-activator complexes [75,76] while concomitantly detaching PPARγ/RXR dimer from its DNA binding site on the GLUT4 gene promoter [76]. This, along with serine phosphorylation of IRS (and prevention of tyrosine phosphorylation) by hyperinsulinemia, cytokines (ie, tumor necrosis factor alpha [TNFα]), decreased PI3K activity and genetic defects (ie, Akt2) have been shown in vitro, in mouse models, and in humans to induce insulin resistance [70,77]. The result of deficits in the insulin-signaling pathway is increased nuclear activity of FOXO1 with greater expression of gluconeogenic genes, as well as induction of lipogenic transcription factor sterol regulatory element binding protein 1c (SREBPIc) and elevated expression of lipogenic genes and a rise in VLDL secretion [60,78].

Obesity has an important role in insulin resistance [2]. Adipose tissue is not simply a storehouse for fat, but has been shown to be an endocrine organ producing many factors, including interleukin (IL)-6, TNFα, resistin, lipoprotein lipase, acylation stimulation protein, cholesteryl-ester protein, retinol binding protein-4 (RBP4), estrogens, leptin, angiotensinogen, adiponectin, insulin like growth factor-1 (IGF-1), and monobutyrin [79]. In this series of *Clinics of North America*, other articles will further discuss the adipose cell as an endocrine system as well as the mechanisms through which adipose tissue leads to insulin resistance.

Visceral adiposity is independently associated with insulin resistance; lower HDLc levels; higher apolipoprotein B, RBP4, and triglyceride levels; smaller LDLc particles; aortic stiffness; coronary calcification; and hypertension [79–81]. Obesity has been shown to contribute to the metabolic syndrome by increasing nonesterified fatty acids (NEFA) and production of inflammatory cytokines that result in insulin resistance, dyslipidemia, hypertension, and production of prothrombotic factors.

NEFA are fatty acids derived from lipolysis of adipose tissue triglycerides that are usually a source of energy in the fasting state. In obese subjects, NEFA levels are increased despite higher levels of insulin. In skeletal muscle, excess NEFA contribute to insulin resistance by increasing levels of diacylglycerol (DAG), which lead to serine phosphorylation of IRS, thereby inhibiting normal insulin signaling. In the liver, NEFA cause insulin resistance in a similar manner, leading to increased gluconeogenesis and accentuation of hyperglycemia by increasing hepatic glucose output resulting in nonalcoholic fatty liver disease (NAFLD). They also contribute to increased VLDL production and secretion by the liver, with increased triglycerides, apolipoprotein B (Apo-B), and small LDLc particles. In addition, NEFA lead to a decreased level of HDLc by increasing the hepatic exchange of VLDL for HDL along with increasing hepatic lipase, which degrades HDL. Other abnormalities associated with elevated levels of NEFA are endothelial dysfunction, beta cell apoptosis, and increased PAI-1 [2,60]. In another article the role of fatty acids in obesity and insulin resistance will be further described.

Inflammatory cytokines such as TNFα and IL-1β are produced by macrophages in adipose tissue. They trigger proinflammatory cytokines c-jun N terminal kinase (JNK) and inhibitor of κB kinase β/nuclear factor κB (IKKβ/NF-κB) through classical receptor-mediated mechanisms. JNK leads to phosphorylation of c-jun compartment of activator protein complex 1 (APC1) transcription factor, which leads to serine phosphorylation of IRS, leading to impaired insulin signaling. JNK and IKKβ/NF-κB also, directly or indirectly, activate proinflammatory genes, leading to a self-perpetuating cycle of up-regulation of inflammatory cytokines and inadequate utilization of body energy. TNFα has also been shown to decrease endothelial nitric oxide synthase (eNOS), causing decreased expression of mitochondrial oxidative phosphorylation genes, leading to increased oxidative cellular stress, with the accumulation of reactive oxygen species (ROS), as well as increased endoplasmic reticulum stress and decreased half-life of nitric oxide (NO). Decreased expression of PPARγ co-activator 1α (PGC1α), an inducible co-regulator of nuclear receptors involved in the control of mitochondrial biogenesis and function, has also been found in subjects with insulin resistance and type 2 diabetes. These responses to cellular stress further increase IKKβ/NF-κB and thus the inflammatory process and well as PAI-1 [2,60,62,69]. A perceived energy deficit may occur with obesity, because of decreased hepatic ATP, possibly because of impaired mitochondrial function, leading to central appetite stimulation. It is also associated with decreased exercise capacity and increased fatigability, possibly because of mitochondrial dysfunction [82]. The role of mitochondria in obesity and diabetes is also reviewed in this issue of the journal.

Retinol binding protein 4 (RBP4) is the transporter for vitamin A (retinol) in the blood. Serum levels and expression of RBP4 in adipose tissue were found to be increased in mice with adipose-specific knockout for GLUT4 [83]. As mentioned above, decreased GLUT4 expression is a common feature of obesity, insulin resistance, and type 2 diabetes [60]. These mice develop impaired insulin action in the muscle, liver, and adipose tissue [84]. Injecting RBP4 into mice or transgenic overexpression of RBP4 leading to increased concentrations caused impaired insulin signaling and increased expression of the gluconeogenic enzyme phosphoenolpyruvate carboxylase in the liver [83]. Analogous to this, RPB4 knockout mice developed increased insulin sensitivity and glucose tolerance [83]. These findings led to interest in the possible causal role of RBP4 in insulin resistance. In humans, higher levels of RBP4 are found with obesity, type 2 diabetes, impaired glucose tolerance, and those with a strong family history of type 2 diabetes [85]. RBP4 is correlated with insulin resistance and has been shown in some studies to correlate more specifically with insulin resistance than leptin, adiponectin, IL-6, or C-reactive protein (CRP) [81,85]. As RBP4 is the main transport protein for vitamin A, it has been postulated that the synthetic retinoid, fenretinide could lower RBP4 levels and improve insulin sensitivity, although this has yet to be determined [85].

Hypertension is about 6 times more frequent in obese than in lean subjects. According to the NHANES III, hypertension is present in 15% of males and females with a BMI 25 kg/m^2 or less, and 42% of males and 38% of females with a BMI greater than 30 kg/m^2 [79,86]. The mechanism behind hypertension is hypothesized to be a combination of the direct hemodynamic effects of obesity on cardiac output, which is increased, and normal or increased peripheral vascular resistance (PVR). The increased PVR is thought to be a result of sympathetic overactivity, volume expansion from the antinatiuretic effects of insulin, and increased angiotensinogen II and proinflammatory cytokine IL-6 with associated increased oxidative stress, leading to decreased NO and endothelial dysfunction [79,80,87]. PPARγ has been shown to be a major regulator of many of these components in adipocytes [87]. Weight loss improves hypertension in 50% of subjects [79]. Further consideration on the relationship between obesity and hypertension is also detailed in this issue.

Other factors involved in the metabolic abnormalities associated with obesity and cardiovascular risk include leptin, adiponectin, resistin, and adipocyte fatty acid binding protein (A-FABP). The absence of leptin leads to extreme obesity, as demonstrated in the ob/ob mice and humans with congenital leptin deficiency [88,89]. Most obese individuals will however have elevated leptin levels with resistance to its appetite-suppressing effects [90]. It is also linked to marked insulin resistance, but has mixed consequences on other cardiovascular abnormalities [80]. Leptin appears to work in adipocytes and augments the expression of PGC1α gene, which has been shown to increase mitochondrial biogenesis and potentially increased mitochondrial oxidation [62]. Adiponectin is an anti-inflammatory adipokine produced by adipocytes. Its expression is affected by insulin, glucocorticoids, β-adrenergic agonists, and TNFα. It is decreased in obesity and increased in lean persons. It appears to have a direct anti-atherogenic affect via its anti-inflammatory properties (reducing production of proin-flammatory and increasing anti-inflammatory cytokines) or via its insulin sensitizing action. Adiponectin receptors 1 and 2 (Adipo R1 and adipo R2) are expressed in macrophages and modulated by PPAR ligands; adipo R2 is a more predominant receptor and is induced by PPAR α and PPARγ in primary and THP-1 macrophages. There is some evidence that adiponec-tin may in fact be a proinflammatory agent, but desensitizes macrophages to itself and other inflammatory stimuli; there is ongoing investigation into its mechanism of action [91,92]. Resistin, a hormone produced by adipocytes, appears to oppose the action of insulin; however, its functional significance in humans is not as yet known [2]. A-FABP is a cytosolic protein present in mature adipocytes, macrophages, and in the bloodstream. Elevated levels correspond with the features of the metabolic syndrome. Recently, subjects from the Nurses Health study and Health Professionals follow-up study [93] have been found to carry a functional genetic variant of A-FABP gene, resulting in decreased adipose tissue A-FABP expression, associated with reduced triglycerides and lower incidence of type 2 diabetes and coronary artery disease. Its proatherogenic activity is believed to be mediated by its direct affect in macrophages. A-FABP decreases PPARγ activity and cho-lesterol efflux in macrophages, thus leading to the formation of foam cells. A-FABP correlates with CRP levels. Its levels are inversely related to those of adiponectin [94].

Recently, the cannabinoid system has received much interest because of its effects of cardiometabolic parameters and potential for pharmacologic manipulation. Two cannabinoid receptors (CB1 and CB2) have been iden-tified to date. CB1 is found in the central nervous system (CNS), notably in the cerebral cortex, hypothalamus, reward circuits (nucleus accumbens and amygdala), and anterior pituitary [95]. It is also found in white adipose tissue, enteric nervous system, hepatocytes, and skeletal muscle myocytes [96,97]. The ligands for CB1 and CB2 are anandamide and 2-arachidonyl-glycerol (2-AG). The receptor is a G-protein coupled receptor, the activa-tion of which leads to activation of inward-rectifying potassium (Kir) channels in the CNS and inhibition of voltage-gated calcium channels. The expression of CB1 and CB2 is down-regulated by glucocorticoids, lep-tin, and dopamine and up-regulated by glutamate [96]. Activation of CB1 receptors has been shown to have central effects on appetite stimulation as well as increasing hepatic lipogenesis (via increase in lipoprotein lipase and SREBP1c), increasing adipocyte tissue accumulation and decreasing muscle glucose uptake. Increased activation is also associated with decreased adiponectin levels. CB2 appears to be more prevalent in the immune system [96,97]. Antagonists of this endocannabinoid system have been shown to suppress appetite, induce weight loss, improve dyslipidemia, and improve glucose utilization [98]. At least one such drug (Rimonabant) has been approved for therapy in Europe [95,96].

There appears to be a role of glucocorticoids, sex hormones, and growth hormone (GH) in the development of the metabolic syndrome. Adipocytes express the enzyme 11β-hydroxysteroid dehydrogenase (11β-HSD), which converts inactive cortisone to active cortisol, resulting in locally enhanced cellular glucocorticoid levels. The enzyme is particularly elevated in visceral adipose tissue from obese individuals [99]. Sex steroids have been implicated in the regulation of adiponectin expression/secretion. Testosterone has been shown to selectively inhibit high molecular weight adiponectin, believed to be associated with the higher risk of insulin resistance in men than women. Low adiponectin levels have been associated with development of the metabolic syndrome in postmenopausal women [80]. Growth hormone deficiency has also been related to an increased risk of metabolic syndrome [100].

Clinical approach to a patient with the metabolic syndrome

Aggressive intervention to reduce the risk of cardiovascular disease and type 2 diabetes is recommended in individuals with the metabolic syndrome; therefore, long-term intervention and monitoring by their primary care physician is warranted. As an underlying mechanism has yet to be elucidated, treating the individual components is necessary at this time.

Identifying patients of having metabolic abnormalities and thus at high risk for CVD and diabetes is important. Overall, the metabolic syndrome is highest among Mexican American females [14]; however, it is worth noting that certain ethnic groups such as Southern Asian groups may have metabolic abnormalities without abdominal obesity [29,30]. It is recommended to monitor blood pressure, pulse rate, fasting glucose and insulin levels, lipid profile, and liver and kidney function tests together with body weight, height, and waist circumference. In certain individuals, a glucose tolerance test will be warranted as suggested by the ADA guidelines. Establishing a risk category for coronary artery disease can be done using an online risk calculator based on the Framingham heart study (http://hp2010. nhlbihin.net/atpiii/calculator.asp?usertype=prof) [101]. As the Framingham heart study was based on a middle-aged white population, with a minority of individuals with diabetes, it should be used with a degree of caution in other ethnic groups, who may have a higher population prevalence of coronary disease and in those with diabetes.

The primary management is a healthy lifestyle. The Diabetes Prevention Program showed that lifestyle intervention reduced the incidence of metabolic syndrome by 41% compared with placebo [102]. Weight loss of the order of 7% to 10% body weight over 6 to 12 months is recommended [103]. This should be achieved through moderate calorie restriction

(500–1000 kcal/day deficit), physical activity of ideally 30 to 60 minutes daily, supplemented by an increase in daily lifestyle activities. In the Diabetes Prevention Program and Finnish Diabetes Prevention Study, weight loss contributed to a 58% reduction in the development of diabetes [104,105]. Exercise is also associated with improvement in dyslipidemia independent of weight loss [106]. Exercise enhances the expression and translocation of GLUT4 and improves insulin sensitivity [107,108]. The composition of the diet should be altered to contain less than 200 mg/day of cholesterol, less than 7% saturated fat, with total fat of 25% to 35% of calories, low simple sugars, and increased intake of fruits, vegetables, and whole grains [12]. Smoking cessation should be implemented in all individuals with the metabolic syndrome. Low dose of aspirin is recommended in all cases of moderate to high risk of cardiovascular disease [12].

For those in whom lifestyle change is not sufficient, pharmacotherapy is available for treatment of obesity, dyslipidemia, and hyperglycemia. Pharmacologic treatment for obesity includes sibutramine, a serotonin norepinephrine reuptake inhibitor; orlistat, which is an inhibitor of intestinal lipase; rimonabant, which is an endocannabinoid receptor-1 antagonist; and metformin, which reduces hepatic glucose production. Metformin was shown to induce weight loss and was associated with a 31% decreased incidence of diabetes when compared with placebo in the Diabetes Prevention Program [104,109]. It is worthy to note that some of the above-mentioned drugs have not yet been approved for the treatment of metabolic syndrome or prevention of diabetes. Individuals with morbid obesity (BMI >40 kg/m^2 or >35 kg/m^2 with major comorbidities) can be candidates for bariatric surgery or laparoscopic gastric banding [110]. The treatments of obesity are discussed in other chapters in this issue.

Drug therapy for dyslipidemia is very successful with the use of HMG Co-A reductase inhibitors (statins), niacin, fibrates, ezetimibe (with statins), and fish oils. LDLc lowering is the primary therapeutic target (<100 mg/dL [2.6 mmol/L] with a history of cardiovascular disease or diabetes and possibly <70 mg/dL [1.8 mmol/L] in the presence of both) with statins as the primary pharmaceutical treatment. The second target in lipid manipulation is to target the non-HDL cholesterol (30 mg/dL above the LDLc goal) [111]. Presently, niacin is effective for HDLc raising as well as for lowering triglycerides and LDLc, however causes significant flushing. Fibrates act via the PPARα receptor and are more effective for lowering triglycerides but do not have the beneficial effects on HDLc or LDLc. The risk of myositis and rhabdomyolysis with statins is greater with gemfibrozil, which inhibits the glucouronidation of statins, therefore increasing the plasma levels of all except for fluvastatin [112]. Fenofibrate does not have this interaction and is preferred for combination therapy with statins. Omega-3 polyunsaturated fatty acids in fish oil lower triglycerides also by activating the PPARα receptor. Doses of 3000 mg of eicosapentaenoic acid (EPA) and docosahexaenoic acid (DHA) are required.

The 7th Joint National Committee guidelines require the blood pressure to be recorded as an average of two or more properly seated blood pressure measurements (with the patient on a chair with feet flat on the floor and the arm at the same level as the heart and a blood pressure cuff covering 80% of the upper arm) taken at two or more office visits. Treatment with lifestyle modification is first recommended, which if fails (blood pressure >140/90 or 130/80 in those with diabetes or chronic kidney disease) should be followed by addition of medication. First-line medication would be a thiazide diuretic in uncomplicated cases; angiotensin-converting enzyme (ACE) inhibitors or angiotensin receptor blockers (ARBs) in those with diabetes, congestive cardiac failure, or chronic kidney disease; and possibly beta blockers in those with angina [113]. Prevention of the development of diabetes in those with impaired fasting glucose has been studied in the Diabetes Prevention Program, Finnish Diabetes Prevention Study, and the DREAM trial [104,105,114]. The ADA currently recommends lifestyle modification rather than medication (metformin or thiazoledinediones) for the prevention of diabetes in view of the cost and potential side-effects, including possible cardiovascular risk associated with medication [4,115]. In those with diabetes, current guidelines include a target HbA1c of <7% aiming toward 6% (reference range 4%–6%), blood pressure goal of lower than 130/80 mm Hg, LDLc less than <100 mg/dL, triglycerides <150 mg/dL, and HDLc >40 mg/dL in men and >50 mg/dL in women [4].

Summary

In today's society with the escalating levels of obesity, diabetes, and cardiovascular disease, the metabolic syndrome is receiving considerable attention and is the subject of much controversy. Greater insight into the mechanism(s) behind the syndrome may improve our understanding of how to prevent and best manage this complex condition.

References

[1] Roth J, Qiang X, Marban SL, et al. The obesity pandemic: where have we been and where are we going? Obes Res 2004;12(Suppl 2):88S–101S.

[2] Grundy SM. Obesity, metabolic syndrome, and cardiovascular disease. J Clin Endocrinol Metab 2004;89(6):2595–600.

[3] Balkau B, Charles MA. Comment on the provisional report from the WHO consultation. European group for the study of insulin resistance (EGIR). Diabet Med 1999;16(5):442–3.

[4] American Diabetes Association. Standards of medical care in diabetes–2008. Diabetes Care 2008;31(Suppl 1):S12–54.

[5] Reaven GM. Banting lecture 1988. Role of insulin resistance in human disease. Diabetes 1988;37(12):1595–607.

[6] Reaven GM. Role of insulin resistance in human disease (syndrome X): an expanded definition. Annu Rev Med 1993;44:121–31.

[7] Alberti K, Zimmet P. Definition, diagnosis and classification of diabetes mellitus and its complications. Part 1: diagnosis and classification of diabetes mellitus. Provisional report of a WHO consultation. Diabet Med 1998;15:539–53.

[8] Expert Panel on Detection, Evaluation, and Treatment of High Blood Cholesterol in Adults. Executive summary of the third report of the National Cholesterol Education Program (NCEP) expert panel on detection, evaluation, and treatment of high blood cholesterol in adults (Adult Treatment Panel III). J Am Med Assoc 2001;285(19):2486–97.

[9] Einhorn D, Reaven GM, Cobin RH, et al. American college of endocrinology position statement on the insulin resistance syndrome. Endocr Pract 2003;9(3):237–52.

[10] Report of the expert committee on the diagnosis and classification of diabetes mellitus. Diabetes Care 2003;26(Suppl 1):S5–20.

[11] Alberti KG, Zimmet P, Shaw J. The metabolic syndrome—a new worldwide definition. Lancet 2005;366(9491):1059–62.

[12] Grundy S, Cleeman J, Daniels S, et al. Diagnosis and management of the metabolic syndrome: an American Heart Association/National Heart, Lung, and Blood Institute scientific statement. Circulation 2005;112(17):2735–52.

[13] Ford ES. The metabolic syndrome and mortality from cardiovascular disease and all-causes: findings from the National Health and Nutrition Examination Survey II mortality study. Atherosclerosis 2004;173(2):307–12.

[14] Ford ES, Giles WH, Dietz WH. Prevalence of the metabolic syndrome among US adults: findings from the third National Health and Nutrition Examination Survey. J Am Med Assoc 2002;287(3):356–9.

[15] Maggi S, Noale M, Gallina P, et al. Metabolic syndrome, diabetes, and cardiovascular disease in an elderly Caucasian cohort: the Italian longitudinal study on aging. J Gerontol A Biol Sci Med Sci 2006;61(5):505–10.

[16] Patel A, Huang KC, Janus ED, et al. Is a single definition of the metabolic syndrome appropriate? A comparative study of the USA and Asia. Atherosclerosis 2006;184(1):225–32.

[17] Cameron AJ, Shaw JE, Zimmet PZ. The metabolic syndrome: prevalence in worldwide populations. Endocrinol Metab Clin North Am 2004;33(2):351–75, table of contents.

[18] Ford ES. Prevalence of the metabolic syndrome defined by the International Diabetes Federation among adults in the US. Diabetes Care 2005;28(11):2745–9.

[19] Assmann G, Guerra R, Fox G, et al. Harmonizing the definition of the metabolic syndrome: comparison of the criteria of the Adult Treatment Panel III and the International Diabetes Federation in United States American and European populations. Am J Cardiol 2007;99(4):541–8.

[20] Adams RJ, Appleton S, Wilson DH, et al. Population comparison of two clinical approaches to the metabolic syndrome: implications of the new International Diabetes Federation consensus definition. Diabetes Care 2005;28(11):2777–9.

[21] Athyros VG, Ganotakis ES, Elisaf M, et al. The prevalence of the metabolic syndrome using the national cholesterol educational program and International Diabetes Federation definitions. Curr Med Res Opin 2005;21(8):1157–9.

[22] Lorenzo C, Serrano-Rios M, Martinez-Larrad MT, et al. Geographic variations of the International Diabetes Federation and the National Cholesterol Education Program-Adult Treatment Panel III definitions of the metabolic syndrome in non diabetic subjects. Diabetes Care 2006;29(3):685–91.

[23] Yoon Y, Lee E, Park C, et al. The new definition of metabolic syndrome by the International Diabetes Federation is less likely to identify metabolically abnormal but non-obese individuals than the definition by the revised national cholesterol education program: the Korea NHANES study. Int J Obes (Lond) 2007;31(3):528–34.

[24] Tong P, Kong A, So W, et al. The usefulness of the International Diabetes Federation and the National Cholesterol Education Program's Adult Treatment Panel III definitions of the metabolic syndrome in predicting coronary heart disease in subjects with type 2 diabetes. Diabetes Care 2007;30(5):1206–11.

[25] Mancia G, Bombelli M, Corrao G, et al. Metabolic syndrome in the Pressioni Arteriose Monitorate e Loro Associazioni (PAMELA) study: daily life blood pressure, cardiac damage, and prognosis. Hypertension 2007;49(1):40–7.

[26] Welty TK, Lee ET, Yeh J, et al. Cardiovascular disease risk factors among American Indians: the strong heart study. Am J Epidemiol. 1995;142(3):269–87.

[27] Araneta MRG, Wingard DL, Barrett-Connor E. Type 2 diabetes and metabolic syndrome in Filipina-American women: a high-risk nonobese population. Diabetes Care 2002;25(3): 494–9.

[28] Simmons D, Thompson CF. Prevalence of the metabolic syndrome among adult New Zealanders of Polynesian and European descent. Diabetes Care 2004;27(12):3002–4.

[29] Feng Y, Hong X, Li Z, et al. Prevalence of metabolic syndrome and its relation to body composition in a chinese rural population. Obesity 2006;14(11):2089–98.

[30] Thomas GN, Ho SY, Janus ED, et al. The US National Cholesterol Education Programme Adult Treatment Panel III (NCEP ATP III) prevalence of the metabolic syndrome in a Chinese population. Diabetes Res Clin Pract 2005;67(3):251–7.

[31] McKeigue PM, Ferrie JE, Pierpoint T, et al. Association of early-onset coronary heart disease in South Asian men with glucose intolerance and hyperinsulinemia. Circulation 1993;87(1):152–61.

[32] Whincup PH, Gilg JA, Papacosta O, et al. Early evidence of ethnic differences in cardiovascular risk: cross sectional comparison of British South Asian and white children. BMJ 2002; 324(7338):635–40.

[33] Al-Lawati JA, Mohammed AJ, Al-Hinai HQ, et al. Prevalence of the metabolic syndrome among Omani adults. Diabetes Care 2003;26(6):1781–5.

[34] Halldina M, Rosella M, de Fairea U, et al. The metabolic syndrome: prevalence and association to leisure-time and work-related physical activity in 60-year-old men and women. Nutr Metab Cardiovasc Dis 2007;17(5):349–57.

[35] LaMonte MJ, Barlow CE, Jurca R, et al. Cardiorespiratory fitness is inversely associated with the incidence of metabolic syndrome: a prospective study of men and women. Circulation 2005;112(4):505–12.

[36] Thom T, Haase N, Rosamond W, et al. Heart disease and stroke statistics—2006 update: a report from the American Heart Association Statistics Committee and Stroke Statistics Subcommittee. Circulation 2006;113(6):e85–151.

[37] Malik S, Wong ND, Franklin SS, et al. Impact of the metabolic syndrome on mortality from coronary heart disease, cardiovascular disease, and all causes in United States adults. Circulation 2004;110(10):1245–50.

[38] Girman CJ, Rhodes T, Mercuri M, et al. The metabolic syndrome and risk of major coronary events in the Scandinavian Simvastatin Survival Study (4S) and the Air Force/Texas Coronary Atherosclerosis Prevention Study (AFCAPS/TexCAPS). Am J Cardiol 2004; 93(2):136–41.

[39] Saely CH, Aczel S, Marte T, et al. The metabolic syndrome, insulin resistance, and cardiovascular risk in diabetic and nondiabetic patients. J Clin Endocrinol Metab 2005;90(10): 5698–703.

[40] Rutter MK, Meigs JB, Sullivan LM, et al. Insulin resistance, the metabolic syndrome, and incident cardiovascular events in the Framingham offspring study. Diabetes 2005;54(11): 3252–7.

[41] Jeppesen J, Hansen TW, Rasmussen S, et al. Insulin resistance, the metabolic syndrome, and risk of incident cardiovascular disease: a population-based study. J Am Coll Cardiol 2007;49(21):2112–9.

[42] Eberly LE, Prineas R, Cohen JD, et al. Metabolic syndrome: risk factor distribution and 18-year mortality in the multiple risk factor intervention trial. Diabetes Care 2006;29(1):123–30.

[43] de Simone G, Devereux RB, Chinali M, et al. Prognostic impact of metabolic syndrome by different definitions in a population with high prevalence of obesity and diabetes: the strong heart study. Diabetes Care 2007;30(7):1851–6.

[44] Anderson KM, Wilson PW, Odell PM, et al. An updated coronary risk profile. A statement for health professionals. Circulation 1991;83(1):356–62.

[45] Wannamethee SG, Shaper AG, Lennon L, et al. Metabolic syndrome vs Framingham risk score for prediction of coronary heart disease, stroke, and type 2 diabetes mellitus. Arch Intern Med 2005;165(22):2644–50.

[46] Grundy SM, Brewer HB Jr, Cleeman JI, et al. For the conference p: definition of metabolic syndrome: report of the National Heart, Lung, and Blood Institute/American Heart Association conference on scientific issues related to definition. Circulation 2004;109(3):433–8.

[47] Wilson PW. Estimating cardiovascular disease risk and the metabolic syndrome: a Framingham view. Endocrinol Metab Clin North Am 2004;33(3):467–81, v.

[48] Lorenzo C, Williams K, Hunt KJ, et al. The National Cholesterol Education Program-Adult Treatment Panel III, International Diabetes Federation, and World Health Organization definitions of the metabolic syndrome as predictors of incident cardiovascular disease and diabetes. Diabetes Care 2007;30(1):8–13.

[49] Wang JJ, Ruotsalainen S, Moilanen L, et al. The metabolic syndrome predicts cardiovascular mortality: a 13-year follow-up study in elderly non-diabetic Finns. Eur Heart J 2007;28(7):857–64.

[50] Ford ES. Risks for all-cause mortality, cardiovascular disease, and diabetes associated with the metabolic syndrome: a summary of the evidence. Diabetes Care 2005;28(7):1769–78.

[51] Gami AS, Witt BJ, Howard DE, et al. Metabolic syndrome and risk of incident cardiovascular events and death: a systematic review and meta-analysis of longitudinal studies. J Am Coll Cardiol 2007;49(4):403–14.

[52] Galassi A, Reynolds K, He J. Metabolic syndrome and risk of cardiovascular disease: a meta-analysis. Am J Med 2006;119(10):812–9.

[53] McNeill AM, Rosamond WD, Girman CJ, et al. The metabolic syndrome and 11-year risk of incident cardiovascular disease in the Atherosclerosis Risk in Communities study. Diabetes Care 2005;28(2):385–90.

[54] Monami M, Lambertucci L, Ungar A, et al. Is the third component of metabolic syndrome really predictive of outcomes in type 2 diabetic patients? Diabetes Care 2006;29(11):2515–7.

[55] Sundstrom J, Riserus U, Byberg L, et al. Clinical value of the metabolic syndrome for long-term prediction of total and cardiovascular mortality: prospective, population-based cohort study. BMJ 2006;332(7546):878–82.

[56] Kahn R, Buse J, Ferrannini E, et al. The metabolic syndrome: time for a critical appraisal: joint statement from the American Diabetes Association and the European Association for the Study of Diabetes. Diabetes Care 2005;28:2289–304.

[57] Iribarren C, Go AS, Husson G, et al. Metabolic syndrome and early-onset coronary artery disease: is the whole greater than its parts? J Am Coll Cardiol 2006;48(9):1800–7.

[58] Smith DO, LeRoith D. Insulin resistance syndrome, pre-diabetes, and the prevention of type 2 diabetes mellitus. Clin Cornerstone 2004;6(2):7–16.

[59] LeRoith D. Beta-cell dysfunction and insulin resistance in type 2 diabetes: role of metabolic and genetic abnormalities. Am J Med 2002;113(Suppl 6A):3S–11S.

[60] Armoni M, Harel C, Karnieli E. Transcriptional regulation of the GLUT4 gene: from PPAR-gamma and FOXO1 to FFA and inflammation. Trends Endocrinol Metab 2007;18(3):100–7.

[61] Taniguchi CM, Emanuelli B, Kahn CR. Critical nodes in signalling pathways: insights into insulin action. Nat Rev Mol Cell Biol 2006;7(2):85–96.

[62] Nisoli E, Clementi E, Carruba MO, et al. Defective mitochondrial biogenesis: a hallmark of the high cardiovascular risk in the metabolic syndrome? Circ Res 2007;100(6):795–806.

[63] Larance M, Ramm G, James DE. The GLUT4 code. Mol Endocrinol 2008;22:226–33.

[64] Karnieli E, Armoni M. Transcriptional regulation of the insulin-responsive glucose transporter GLUT4 gene: from physiology to pathology. Am J Physiol Endocrinol Metab 2008, in press.

[65] Charron MJ, Katz EB. Metabolic and therapeutic lessons from genetic manipulation of GLUT4. Mol Cell Biochem 1998;182(1–2):143–52.

[66] Kahn BB, Flier JS. Obesity and insulin resistance. J Clin Invest 2000;106(4):473–81.

[67] Del Prato S. Loss of early insulin secretion leads to postprandial hyperglycaemia. Diabetologia 2003;46(Suppl 1):M2–8.

[68] Minokoshi Y, Kahn CR, Kahn BB. Tissue-specific ablation of the glut4 glucose transporter or the insulin receptor challenges assumptions about insulin action and glucose homeostasis. J Biol Chem 2003;278(36):33609–12.

[69] Liang CP, Han S, Senokuchi T, et al. The macrophage at the crossroads of insulin resistance and atherosclerosis. Circ Res 2007;100(11):1546–55.

[70] Paz K, Hemi R, LeRoith D, et al. A molecular basis for insulin resistance. Elevated serine/threonine phosphorylation of IRS-1 and IRS-2 inhibits their binding to the juxtamembrane region of the insulin receptor and impairs their ability to undergo insulin-induced tyrosine phosphorylation. J Biol Chem 1997;272(47):29911–8.

[71] Armoni M, Harel C, Karni S, et al. FOXO1 represses peroxisome proliferator-activated receptor-{gamma}1 and -{gamma}2 gene promoters in primary adipocytes: a novel paradigm to increase insulin sensitivity. J Biol Chem 2006;281(29):19881–91.

[72] Nakae J, Biggs WH III, Kitamura T, et al. Regulation of insulin action and pancreatic beta-cell function by mutated alleles of the gene encoding forkhead transcription factor FOXO1. Nat Genet 2002;32(2):245–53.

[73] Puigserver P, Rhee J, Donovan J, et al. Insulin-regulated hepatic gluconeogenesis through FOXO1-PGC-1alpha interaction. Nature 2003;423(6939):550–5.

[74] Armoni M, Kritz N, Harel C, et al. Peroxisome proliferator-activated receptor-gamma represses GLUT4 promoter activity in primary adipocytes, and rosiglitazone alleviates this effect. J Biol Chem 2003;278(33):30614–23.

[75] Yki-Jarvinen H. Thiazolidinediones. N Engl J Med 2004;351(11):1106–18.

[76] Guan H-P, Ishizuka T, Chui PC, et al. Corepressors selectively control the transcriptional activity of PPAR{gamma} in adipocytes. Genes Dev 2005;19(4):453–61.

[77] George S, Rochford JJ, Wolfrum C, et al. A family with severe insulin resistance and diabetes due to a mutation in AKT2. Science 2004;304(5675):1325–8.

[78] Pegorier JP, Le May C, Girard J. Control of gene expression by fatty acids. J Nutr 2004; 134(9):2444S–9S.

[79] Poirier P, Giles TD, Bray GA, et al. Obesity and cardiovascular disease: pathophysiology, evaluation, and effect of weight loss: an update of the 1997 American Heart Association scientific statement on obesity and heart disease from the Obesity Committee of the Council on Nutrition, Physical Activity, and Metabolism. Circulation 2006; 113(6):898–918.

[80] Hutley L, Prins JB. Fat as an endocrine organ: relationship to the metabolic syndrome. Am J Med Sci 2005;330(6):280–9.

[81] Kloting N, Graham TE, Berndt J, et al. Serum retinol-binding protein is more highly expressed in visceral than in subcutaneous adipose tissue and is a marker of intra-abdominal fat mass. Cell Metab 2007;6(1):79–87.

[82] Khayat ZA, Patel N, Klip A. Exercise- and insulin-stimulated muscle glucose transport: distinct mechanisms of regulation. Can J Appl Physiol 2002;27(2):129–51.

[83] Yang Q, Graham TE, Mody N, et al. Serum retinol binding protein 4 contributes to insulin resistance in obesity and type 2 diabetes. Nature 2005;436(7049):356–62.

[84] Abel ED, Peroni O, Kim JK, et al. Adipose-selective targeting of the GLUT4 gene impairs insulin action in muscle and liver. Nature 2001;409(6821):729–33.

[85] Graham TE, Yang Q, Bluher M, et al. Retinol-binding protein 4 and insulin resistance in lean, obese, and diabetic subjects. N Engl J Med 2006;354(24):2552–63.

[86] Brown CD, Higgins M, Donato KA, et al. Body mass index and the prevalence of hypertension and dyslipidemia. Obes Res 2000;8(9):605–19.

[87] Sharma AM, Staels B. Review: peroxisome proliferator-activated receptor gamma and adipose tissue—understanding obesity-related changes in regulation of lipid and glucose metabolism. J Clin Endocrinol Metab 2007;92(2):386–95.

[88] Zhang Y, Proenca R, Maffei M, et al. Positional cloning of the mouse obese gene and its human homologue. Nature 1994;372(6505):425–32.

[89] Farooqi IS, Jebb SA, Langmack G, et al. Effects of recombinant leptin therapy in a child with congenital leptin deficiency. N Engl J Med 1999;341(12):879–84.

[90] Maffei M, Fei H, Lee GH, et al. Increased expression in adipocytes of ob RNA in mice with lesions of the hypothalamus and with mutations at the db locus. Proc Natl Acad Sci U S A 1995;92(15):6957–60.

[91] Kim C-H, Pennisi P, Zhao H, et al. MKR mice are resistant to the metabolic actions of both insulin and adiponectin: discordance between insulin resistance and adiponectin responsiveness. Am J Physiol Endocrinol Metab 2006;291(2):E298–305.

[92] Tsatsanis C, Zacharioudaki V, Androulidaki A, et al. Peripheral factors in the metabolic syndrome: the pivotal role of adiponectin. Ann N Y Acad Sci 2006;1083:185–95.

[93] Tuncman G, Erbay E, Hom X, et al. A genetic variant at the fatty acid-binding protein aP2 locus reduces the risk for hypertriglyceridemia, type 2 diabetes, and cardiovascular disease. Proc Natl Acad Sci USA 2006;103:6970–5.

[94] Xu A, Tso AW, Cheung BM, et al. Circulating adipocyte-fatty acid binding protein levels predict the development of the metabolic syndrome: a 5-year prospective study. Circulation 2007;115(12):1537–43.

[95] Matias I, Vergoni AV, Petrosino S, et al. Regulation of hypothalamic endocannabinoid levels by neuropeptides and hormones involved in food intake and metabolism: insulin and melanocortins. Neuropharmacology 2008;54(1):206–12.

[96] Cota D. CB1 receptors: emerging evidence for central and peripheral mechanisms that regulate energy balance, metabolism, and cardiovascular health. Diabetes Metab Res Rev 2007;23(7):507–17.

[97] Woods SC. The endocannabinoid system: mechanisms behind metabolic homeostasis and imbalance. Am J Med 2007;120(2 Suppl 1):S9–17 [discussion S29–32].

[98] Kakafika AI, Mikhailidis DP, Karagiannis A, et al. The role of endocannabinoid system blockade in the treatment of the metabolic syndrome. J Clin Pharmacol 2007;47(5):642–52.

[99] Walker BR, Andrew R. Tissue production of cortisol by 11beta-hydroxysteroid dehydrogenase type 1 and metabolic disease. Ann N Y Acad Sci 2006;1083:165–84.

[100] van der Klaauw AA, Biermasz NR, Feskens EJ, et al. The prevalence of the metabolic syndrome is increased in patients with GH deficiency, irrespective of long-term substitution with recombinant human GH. Eur J Endocrinol 2007;156(4):455–62.

[101] Wilson PW, D'Agostino RB, Levy D, et al. Prediction of coronary heart disease using risk factor categories. Circulation 1998;97(18):1837–47.

[102] Orchard TJ, Temprosa M, Goldberg R, et al. The effect of metformin and intensive lifestyle intervention on the metabolic syndrome: the diabetes prevention program randomized trial. Ann Intern Med 2005;142(8):611–9.

[103] Expert Panel on the Identification, Evaluation and Treatment of Overweight in Adults. Clinical guidelines on the identification, evaluation, and treatment of overweight and obesity in adults: executive summary. Am J Clin Nutr 1998;68(4):899–917.

[104] Knowler W, Barrett-Connor E, Fowler S, et al. Reduction in the incidence of type 2 diabetes with lifestyle intervention or metformin. N Engl J Med 2002;346(6):393–403.

[105] Tuomilehto J, Lindstrom J, Eriksson JG, et al. Prevention of type 2 diabetes mellitus by changes in lifestyle among subjects with impaired glucose tolerance. N Engl J Med 2001;344(18):1343–50.

[106] Kraus WE, Houmard JA, Duscha BD, et al. Effects of the amount and intensity of exercise on plasma lipoproteins. N Engl J Med 2002;347(19):1483–92.

[107] Kim HJ, Lee JS, Kim CK. Effect of exercise training on muscle glucose transporter 4 protein and intramuscular lipid content in elderly men with impaired glucose tolerance. Eur J Appl Physiol 2004;93(3):353–8.

[108] Goodyear LJ, Kahn BB. Exercise, glucose transport, and insulin sensitivity. Annu Rev Med 1998;49(1):235–61.

[109] Pi-Sunyer FX. Use of lifestyle changes, treatment plans, and drug therapy in controlling cardiovascular and metabolic risk factors. Obesity 2006;14(Suppl 3):135S–42S.

[110] Elder KA, Wolfe BM. Bariatric surgery: a review of procedures and outcomes. Gastroenterology 2007;132(6):2253–71.

[111] National Cholesterol Education Program (NCEP) Expert Panel on Detection, Evaluation, and Treatment of High Blood Cholesterol in Adults (Adult Treatment Panel III). Third report of the National Cholesterol Education Program (NCEP) Expert Panel on Detection, Evaluation, and Treatment of High Blood Cholesterol in Adults (Adult Treatment Panel III) final report. Circulation 2002;106(25):3143–421.

[112] Bottorff MB. Statin safety and drug interactions: clinical implications. The American Journal of Cardiology 2006;97(8 Suppl 1):S27–31.

[113] Chobanian AV, Bakris GL, Black HR, et al. Seventh report of the Joint National Committee on Prevention, Detection, Evaluation, and Treatment of High Blood Pressure. Hypertension 2003;42(6):1206–52.

[114] DREAM Trial Investigators, Gerstein HC, Yusuf S, et al. Effect of rosiglitazone on the frequency of diabetes in patients with impaired glucose tolerance or impaired fasting glucose: a randomised controlled trial. Lancet 2006;368(9541):1096–105.

[115] Nissen SE, Wolski K. Effect of rosiglitazone on the risk of myocardial infarction and death from cardiovascular causes. N Engl J Med 2007;356(24):2457–71.

ELSEVIER
SAUNDERS

Endocrinol Metab Clin N Am
37 (2008) 581–601

ENDOCRINOLOGY
AND METABOLISM
CLINICS
OF NORTH AMERICA

Insulin Resistance: the Link Between Obesity and Cardiovascular Disease

Gerald M. Reaven, MD

*Division of Cardiovascular Medicine, Stanford University School of Medicine, Falk CVRC,
Stanford Medical Center, 300 Pasteur Drive, Stanford, CA 94305, USA*

One need not be an epidemiologist to recognize the fact that the prevalence of overweight/obesity is increasing rapidly in the United States, and by simply strolling down the streets of any city, going to the movies, attending a ballgame, and so forth, the magnitude of this problem (no pun intended) is identified. The impact of the "obesity epidemic" has also been chronicled in probably every magazine published in this country, and hardly a month goes by without this dilemma occupying prominent space in some newspaper.

The fact that more and more Americans are overweight has been well documented in the medical literature [1,2], as has the association between overweight/obesity and mortality [3–7]. The relationship between obesity and excess mortality is consistent with evidence that these individuals are at increased risk of essential hypertension, type 2 diabetes mellitus (2DM), and cardiovascular disease (CVD) [8–10]. In light of these findings, it is not surprising that a "call to action" has been issued to health care professionals to begin addressing the harmful effects of the increase in adiposity and the decrease in physical activity that seem to characterize the United States population [11].

In view of the apparent consensus over the adverse impact of obesity on important clinical syndromes and overall morality, a recent study's conclusion that the magnitude of the impact of the increase in prevalence of overweight/obesity on excess death may not be as great as is feared was unexpected [12]. In this report, moderately obese participants (body mass index [BMI] 30.0 kg/m^2 to <35.0 kg/m^2) in the National Health and Nutrition Examination Survey (NHANES) demonstrated only modestly increased mortality compared with individuals whose BMI was 18.5 kg/m^2 to <25.0 kg/m^2, with increased relative risk statistically significant

E-mail address: greaven@cvmed.stanford.edu

0889-8529/08/$ - see front matter © 2008 Elsevier Inc. All rights reserved.
doi:10.1016/j.ecl.2008.06.005   *endo.theclinics.com*

in NHANES I but not in NHANES II or III [12]. The investigators did not contest the view that being obese increases the likelihood of developing a number of serious clinical syndromes but suggested that the association between obesity and mortality may have decreased over time because of improvements in public health or medical care for obesity-related conditions. Indeed, analysis of trends in CVD risk factors shows decreases in the prevalence of hypercholesterolemia and high blood pressure and a stable prevalence of diabetes despite increasing prevalence of obesity [13].

There is no simple way to reconcile these conflicting views of the impact that obesity has on mortality, and doing so is not the goal of this article. Such conflicting views, however, open the door to propose a somewhat different approach to the relationship between obesity and disease, and in particular, the relationship between excess adiposity and CVD. Specifically, it is argued that (1) resistance to insulin action (and associated abnormalities) is the link between obesity and CVD; and (2) overweight/obese individuals differ in terms of their degree of insulin resistance and, therefore, their risk of CVD.

Fitness versus fatness

Although there is general agreement that overweight/obese individuals tend to be sedentary, relatively little attention is paid to the impact that variations in physical activity might have on the putative relationships among obesity, metabolic abnormalities, and disease. The result is that the adverse health-related consequences of being overweight are exaggerated and the deleterious effects of decreases in physical activity receive much less attention.

Relationship between insulin-mediated glucose uptake and fitness

Rosenthal and colleagues [14] quantified insulin-mediated glucose uptake (IMGU) by using the hyperinsulinemic, euglycemic clamp technique and physical fitness by measuring maximal aerobic capacity ($\dot{V}o_2max$) in 33 apparently healthy individuals of Caucasian ancestry and found the two variables to be highly correlated ($r = 0.63$, $P < .001$). This relationship was independent of age and obesity; it was also noted that the higher the $\dot{V}o_2max$, the lower the plasma glucose and insulin responses during an oral glucose tolerance test ($P < .05$).

Essentially similar findings were noted in a study of 55 nondiabetic, apparently healthy Pima Indians [15]. The values of IMGU varied considerably in these subjects, and it was estimated that differences in maximal oxygen uptake appeared to make an independent contribution of approximately 20% to the variations in IMGU seen in this population. The results of a subsequent study of 55 Pima Indians and 35 Caucasians also indicated that differences in $\dot{V}o_2max$ were significantly related to IMGU and pointed out that differences in $\dot{V}o_2max$ and estimates of adiposity, taken together, could account for approximately 50% of the variation in measures of IMGU, with each making independent contributions of approximately 25% [16].

The existence of a positive relationship between degree of physical fitness and insulin sensitivity in cross-sectional studies of apparently healthy individuals is not surprising in view of the substantial evidence of the beneficial effects of training on improving insulin sensitivity [17–19].

The convergence of the facts that overweight/obese individuals tend to be less physically active and that decreased activity is associated with insulin resistance supports the notion that the adverse impact of obesity may, at least partly, be due to obesity-related sedentary lifestyle, rather than obesity, per se. This distinction may be scientifically the case, but it could also be argued that this issue is somewhat irrelevant, and the relative importance of the untoward effects of obesity versus those of fitness is beside the point; pragmatically, both are bad. It could also be well argued that not truly understanding the problem makes devising solutions infinitely more difficult.

Impact of variations in adiposity versus activity level on clinical outcome

Efforts have been made to evaluate the relative importance of obesity and inactivity to increasing risk of CVD and 2DM [20–24]. In some cases, measures of obesity appeared to incur greater risk [21,24], and in other cases, level of activity seemed to be the more important risk factor [20], whereas in some instances, the contribution seemed to be approximately the same [22,23]. A good example of this last finding is the study by Sullivan and colleagues [23] that evaluated data collected from 2000 to 2002 by the Medical Expenditure Panel Survey on 68,500 adults. These investigators found that the likelihood of developing diabetes, diabetes plus heart disease, diabetes plus hypertension, and diabetes plus hyperlipidemia was lowest in those who had a normal BMI and increased progressively with degree of obesity. Within each specific obesity category, however, the likelihood of developing all of these morbidities was higher in those individuals classified as being inactive. For example, in individuals who had a normal BMI (<25.0 kg/m^2), the odds ratio for developing 2DM was 1.52 (1.25–1.86) when inactive to active individuals were compared; the odds ratio of 1.65 (1.40–1.96) for active overweight individuals (BMI = 25.0–29.9 kg/m^2) did not increase compared with inactive individuals who had normal weight (BMI <25.0 kg/m^2). As a result of their analysis, Sullivan and colleagues [23] concluded, "both physical inactivity and obesity seem to be strongly and independently associated with diabetes and diabetes-related comorbidities."

Obesity and insulin resistance

Relationship between obesity and insulin-mediated glucose uptake

It has been known for more than 30 years that obesity is associated with a decrease in IMGU [25]. Despite this long history, however, the relationship between obesity and insulin resistance remains controversial at several levels. Indeed, it is frequently assumed that obesity is essentially synonymous with insulin resistance and associated metabolic abnormalities. If this were not the case, it would be difficult to understand the genesis of the concept of a metabolically obese, normal-weight individual [26]. This notion is obviously based on the belief that the natural state of the obese individual is to be insulin resistant and metabolically abnormal and that these findings rarely occur in nonobese persons. Perhaps the strongest evidence that insulin resistance is not a simple function of overweight/obesity comes from the report from the European Group for the Study of Insulin Resistance [27]: the results of euglycemic, hyperinsulinemic clamp studies in 1146 nondiabetic, normotensive volunteers showed that only approximately 25% of the obese volunteers were classified as being insulin resistant with the criteria used.

Although not the major focus of their study, these investigators also pointed out that waist circumference (WC) and ratio of waist-to-hip girth were not related to insulin sensitivity after adjustments for age, sex, and BMI [27]. This observation seems to have been overlooked in the emphasis on the importance of the role played by abdominal obesity in the development of insulin resistance and CVD. For example, the criteria published by the Adult Treatment Panel III (ATP III) [28] for the diagnosis of the metabolic syndrome included obesity as one of the components, but an individual could not be considered obese unless he or she exceeded an arbitrary value of WC. The importance of abdominal obesity reached its apotheosis with the publication of the International Diabetes Federation definition of the metabolic syndrome [29]. Not only is an abnormal WC the only criterion with which to define obesity but an abnormal WC is also the one essential ingredient that must be present to make a diagnosis of the metabolic syndrome.

Relationship between overall (body mass index) or abdominal obesity (waist circumference) and insulin resistance

The apparent hegemony of abdominal (WC) compared with overall (BMI) obesity in the association with insulin resistance seemed somewhat surprising in light of the fact that BMI and WC are so closely related. For example, measurements obtained from approximately 15,000 participants in the NHANES indicated that the correlation coefficient between BMI and WC was greater than 0.9, irrespective of the age, sex, and ethnicity of the groups evaluated [30].

Given these data, we have made an effort to evaluate the magnitude of the relationship between BMI and WC to a specific measure of IMGU. For this purpose, IMGU was quantified with the insulin suppression test (IST). The IST was introduced and validated some years ago [31,32] and, in its current form, involves the continuous infusion for 180 minutes of octreotide, insulin, and glucose [33]. Under these conditions, endogenous insulin secretion is inhibited, as is the secretion of all other hormones that modulate glucose uptake. Steady-state plasma insulin (SSPI) and steady-state plasma glucose (SSPG) concentrations are reached 90 to 120 minutes after the start of the infusion, and blood is drawn for measurement of plasma insulin and glucose concentrations every 10 minutes during the last 30 minutes of the continuous infusion. These four values are averaged and used to determine the SSPI and SSPG concentrations observed during that study. Because the SSPI concentrations at the end of the infusion are similar in all individuals and because the glucose infusion rate during the infusion is also identical, the SSPG concentrations provide a direct estimate of the ability of the same amount of insulin to promote glucose disposal in the person being studied: the higher the SSPG concentration, the more insulin resistant the individual. It should be emphasized that quantification of insulin action with the IST and the hyperinsulinemic, euglycemic clamp technique yields results that are highly correlated ($r > 0.9$) in normal subjects and in patients who have 2DM, both obese and nonobese [32].

The relationship between BMI or WC and SSPG concentration was examined in 330 apparently healthy individuals [34]; the results of this analysis are shown in Fig. 1. It is clear from these data that there was no difference in the magnitude of the correlation coefficient between BMI and SSPG ($r = 0.58$, $P < .001$) compared with that between WC and SSPG ($r = 0.57$, $P < .001$). Furthermore, the best-fit lines describing the relationship between the specific adiposity measures and SSPG concentrations were also not different ($P = .90$). It is also clear that there are many obese individuals, whether defined by an abnormal BMI or by WC, who are insulin sensitive (low SSPG concentrations).

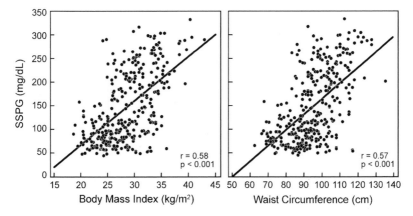

Fig. 1. Relationship between SSPG concentration and BMI (*left panel*) and WC (*right panel*). (*From* Farin HMF, Abbasi F, Reaven GM. Body mass index and waist circumference both contribute to differences in insulin-mediated glucose disposal in nondiabetic adults. Am J Clin Nutr 2006;83:47–51; with permission.)

The fact that BMI and WC are significantly related to measures of IMGU has been shown by other groups, but the putative superiority of WC is based on the argument that the relationship between WC and insulin sensitivity remains significant when adjusted for differences in BMI; however, and for unclear reasons, the converse is rarely attempted—that is, determining whether the relationship between BMI and insulin sensitivity remains significant when adjusted for differences in WC. Our attempt to address this issue is illustrated in Figs. 2 and 3 [34]. Fig. 2 displays the impact of differences in WC classification on SSPG concentration when participants are subdivided based on BMI category. These data show that 96% of individuals who had a normal BMI also had a normal WC, and that 93% of those within the obese BMI category were abdominally obese. Thus, a valid comparison of the impact of differences in WC on IMGU within a given BMI category was limited to those who had a BMI between 25 kg/m^2 and 29.9 kg/m^2, and the results show that abdominally obese individuals had significantly higher ($P < .05$) SSPG concentrations than those who had a normal WC.

The data in Fig. 3 illustrate the alternative analysis, that is, the impact of differences in BMI category when the same population is subdivided on the basis of being abdominally obese (abnormal WC) or not (normal WC). Similar to the results in Fig. 2, only 6% of those in the normal WC group were obese by BMI criteria, and only 2% of the 179 persons classified as abdominally obese had a normal BMI. Consequently, within the normal

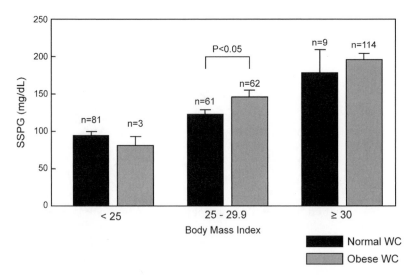

Fig. 2. Comparison of SSPG concentrations as a function of WC classification in subjects stratified by BMI category. (*From* Farin HMF, Abbasi F, Reaven GM. Body mass index and waist circumference both contribute to differences in insulin-mediated glucose disposal in nondiabetic adults. Am J Clin Nutr 2006;83:47–51; with permission.)

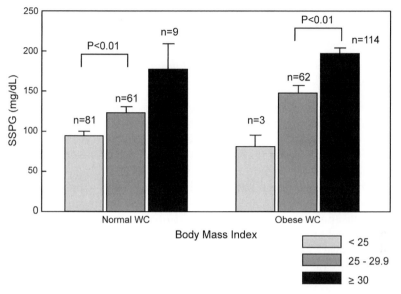

Fig. 3. Comparison of SSPG concentrations as a function of BMI category in subjects stratified by WC classification. (*From* Farin HMF, Abbasi F, Reaven GM. Body mass index and waist circumference both contribute to differences in insulin-mediated glucose disposal in nondiabetic adults. Am J Clin Nutr 2006;83:47–51; with permission.)

WC group, we could only compare the SSPG concentrations of individuals who were normal or overweight by BMI criteria. Likewise, in the abdominally obese group, the comparison was limited to those whose BMI classified them as being overweight or obese. These comparisons show that irrespective of WC classification, the greater the BMI, the higher the SSPG concentration. Thus, among those who had a normal WC, the mean SSPG concentration of overweight subjects (123 ± 7 mg/dL) was significantly greater ($P < .01$) than that of normal-weight individuals (94 ± 5 mg/dL). The magnitude of the effect on IMGU due to differences in BMI was even greater in abdominally obese participants, with significantly higher ($P < .01$) SSPG concentrations in those who had an obese BMI (197 ± 7 mg/dL) compared with individuals whose BMI classified them as being overweight (147 ± 9 mg/dL).

The results in Figs. 1–3 are based on measurements made in 330 apparently healthy individuals and provide evidence at the simplest level that there is an extremely close relationship between the two indices of obesity: it is rare for an individual classified as being obese to have a normal WC and rare for someone who is of normal weight to have abdominal adiposity (an abnormal WC). Furthermore, the relationship to a quantitative measure of IMGU is essentially identical, irrespective of which index of adiposity is used (WC or BMI), and that in either instance, there are substantial numbers of individuals who have excess adiposity who are not insulin resistant, just as there are persons who have a normal WC or BMI who are insulin resistant.

Relationship between visceral obesity and insulin-mediated glucose uptake

The evidence presented to this point has demonstrated that measurements of BMI and WC are closely related and are associated with a specific measure of IMGU to an identical degree. These conclusions are at odds with the conventional wisdom that overweight/obesity is synonymous with insulin resistance and the notion, codified by the ATP III [28] and the International Diabetes Federation [29], that abdominal obesity is the source of all metabolic evil. One possible explanation for this discrepant view of the central role (pun intended) of abdominal obesity in the genesis of insulin resistance and its consequences is the failure to take into consideration the importance of visceral obesity.

The results of 21 studies attempting to define the relative magnitude of the relationship between IMGU and various estimates of adiposity in non-diabetic subjects are provided in Table 1 [35–55]. The studies are listed in chronologic order, and the following inclusion criteria were used to construct the table: imaging techniques had to be used to determine the magnitude of the various fat depots; IMGU had to be quantified with a reasonably specific method (studies using surrogate estimates of IMGU were not included); and the experimental data had to be available before the use of arbitrary "adjustments" or multiple regression analysis. Table 1 provides a comprehensive list of studies that meet these criteria; the omission of any published study that would have been appropriately included was inadvertent. In-depth analysis of the possible impact of differences in the experimental populations, the imaging techniques used in each study, and the specific methods used to quantify IMGU are not possible within the context of this presentation.

The results of this analysis are presented in Table 1, and it should be noted that the correlation coefficients (r values) between visceral fat (VF) and IMGU are certainly no better than the r values between IMGU and BMI or WC seen in Fig. 1. Indeed, r values between IMGU and VF varied from 0.33 to 0.6 in 20 of the 25 measurements in Table 1, with differences in VF accounting for approximately 25% of the variability in IMGU in most instances.

Although total fat (TF) was not quantified as often as VF, the magnitude of the relationship between IMGU and TF seemed to be comparable to that between IMGU and VF.

The emphasis in the analysis of these studies was a comparison of the relationship between IMGU and subcutaneous abdominal fat (SF) with that between IMGU and VF. Although the magnitude of the relationship with IMGU was reasonably comparable with VF or SF, there were two

Table 1
Correlation coefficients (r values) between insulin-mediated glucose uptake and body fat distribution in nondiabetic subjects

Study	Population	Visceral fat	Subcutaneous abdominal fat	Total fat
Abate et al, 1995 [35]	39 men	−0.51	−0.62	−0.61
Cefalu et al, 1995 [36]	60 subjects	−0.50	−0.50	−0.57
Macor et al, 1997 [37]	26 obese subjects	−0.56	—	−0.54
Goodpaster et al, 1997 [38]	54 subjects	−0.52	−0.61	−0.58
Banerji et al, 1999 [39]	20 Southeast Asian men	−0.59	−0.54	−0.56
Kelley et al, 2000 [40]	47 men	−0.61	−0.53	—
Sites et al, 2000 [41]	27 postmenopausal women	−0.39	−0.43	−0.30
Brochu et al, 2001 [42]	44 obese postmenopausal women	−0.40	−0.17	—
Goran et al, 2001 [43]	68 Caucasian children	−0.59	−0.70	−0.68
	51 African American children	−0.43	−0.47	−0.52
Rendell et al, 2001 [44]	55 postmenopausal women	−0.49	0.43	—
Purnell et al, 2001 [45]	48 subjects	−0.58	−0.41	—
Raji et al, 2001 [46]	24 subjects	−0.55	−0.47	−0.61
Ross et al, 2002 [47]	89 obese men	−0.41	—	—
Ross et al, 2002 [48]	40 obese premenopausal women	−0.34	−0.06	—
Cnop et al, 2002 [49]	174 subjects	−0.69	−0.57	—
Cruz et al, 2002 [50]	32 Hispanic children	−0.44	−0.46	−0.46
Gan et al, 2003 [51]	39 men	−0.71	—	—
Tulloch-Reid et al, 2004 [52]	44 African American men	−0.57	−0.57	—
	35 African American women	−0.50	−0.67	—
Rattarasarn et al, 2004 [53]	11 Thai women	−0.60	−0.47	−0.38
	11 Thai men	−0.54	−0.45	−0.80
Raji et al, 2004 [54]	40 Southeast Asian/ Caucasian subjects	−0.33	−0.45	−0.46
	25 Southeast Asian subjects	−0.55	−0.46	−0.54
Bush et al, 2005 [55]	150 African American/ Caucasian children	−0.33	−0.38	−0.54

examples in which the values were discrepant [42,48]. In the remaining 20 available comparisons, the r values between IMGU and VF or SF did not vary a great deal, being somewhat higher with VF in nine studies, higher with SF in nine studies, and identical on two occasions.

Given the information in Figs. 1–3 and Table 1, the basis for the "conventional wisdom" that abdominal obesity, and in particular visceral obesity, has a uniquely adverse effect on IMGU is not self-evident. Most likely, it is the widespread use of multiple regression analysis to decide which variable is an "independent" predictor of IMGU that is responsible for this belief. Although this approach may provide useful information, it is understood that it presents problems when closely related variables are entered into the model being used. Because all measures of adiposity are highly correlated, it is not clear what the biologic significance is of the results of multivariate analysis that indicate that only one measure is an "independent" predictor of IMGU. In any event, the data presented to this point make it legitimate to at least question the notion of a uniquely close relationship between IMGU and WC or VF, in contrast to the relationship between IMGU and BMI, SF, or TF. Indeed, this conclusion should not be too surprising in view of the results of a study showing that "independent of age and sex, the combination of BMI and WC explained a greater variance in nonabdominal, abdominal, subcutaneous and visceral fat than either BMI or WC alone" [56].

Obesity, insulin resistance, and cardiovascular disease risk

Body mass index and waist circumference as predictors of cardiovascular disease risk

The discussion to this point has focused on the relationship between adiposity and insulin resistance. Although this issue is clearly important, it is necessary to also consider how these variables interact in increasing the risk of adverse clinical outcomes. More specifically, what are the relationships among obesity, insulin resistance, and CVD risk? For example, WC and BMI may be related to insulin resistance to a similar degree, but what is their impact on the abnormalities related to insulin resistance that are more closely related to the risk of clinical disease? We recently addressed this latter question in 261 apparently healthy adults who were divided into two groups based on having a normal or abnormal WC using ATP III criteria [28] or into three groups based on their BMI: normal weight (<25.0 kg/m^2), overweight (25.0 to <30.0 kg/m^2), or obese (≥ 30.0 kg/m^2). Table 2 compares the SSPG, plasma glucose, triglyceride (TG), and total cholesterol, low-density lipoprotein cholesterol (LDL-C), and high-density lipoprotein cholesterol (HDL-C) concentrations of the nonobese (normal WC) and abdominally obese (obese WC) subgroups. These data show that abdominally obese individuals had significantly higher SSPG, glucose, and TG concentrations than their normal WC counterparts; however, there were no significant differences in the total cholesterol, LDL-C, or HDL-C concentrations between the nonobese and abdominally obese groups.

Changes in insulin sensitivity and CVD risk factors as a function of differences in BMI are presented in Table 3. By one-way analysis of variance it can be seen that every variable measured differed as a function of BMI group. Furthermore, all of the CVD risk factors were significantly different when normal-weight individuals (BMI <25.0 kg/m^2) were compared with obese subjects (BMI 30.0–35.0 kg/m^2). It should also be noted that SSPG concentrations of all three BMI groups were different from each other.

Results in Tables 2 and 3 show that insulin sensitivity and related metabolic CVD risk factors worsened as a function of increased obesity whether

Table 2
Metabolic variables in 261 apparently healthy individuals classified by waist circumference

| Variables | WC | | P |
	Normal (n = 128)	Obese (n = 133)	
SSPG (mg/dL)	107 ± 5	174 ± 6	<.001
Glucose (mg/dL)	92 ± 1	98 ± 1	<.001
Triglyceride (mg/dL)	128 ± 10	163 ± 9	.01
Total cholesterol (mg/dL)	193 ± 3	201 ± 3	.09
LDL-C (mg/dL)	118 ± 3	124 ± 3	.14
HDL-C (mg/dL)	52 ± 1	49 ± 1	.13

Data are expressed as mean ± SEM; statistical significance by Student *t* test.

Abbreviations: HDL-C = high-density lipoprotein cholesterol; LDL-C = low-density lipoprotein cholesterol.

Data from Farin HFM, Abbasi F, Reaven GM. Comparison of body mass index versus waist circumference with the metabolic changes that increase the risk of cardiovascular disease in insulin-resistant individuals. Am J Cardiol 2006;98:1053–6.

BMI or WC was used as the index of excess adiposity. To further asses the clinical relevance of using BMI or WC to identify individuals at increased CVD risk, we compared all of the experimental variables in individuals classified as being overweight/obese by BMI criteria or abdominally obese on the basis of their WC values. The metabolic characteristics of the subjects identified by the two different obesity criteria were then compared. Comparison of the two groups in Table 4 shows that more individuals met criteria for being overweight/obese (n = 193) than were classified as abdominally obese (n = 133). It can also be seen that the values for all of the CVD risk factors measured were comparable, irrespective of whether BMI or WC was used to classify the groups. Thus, if the goal is to have normal

Table 3
Metabolic variables in the 261 apparently healthy individuals classified by body mass index

| Variables | BMI (kg/m²) | | | P |
	<25 (n = 68)	25–29.9 (n = 106)	≥30 (n = 87)	
SSPG (mg/dL)*	91 ± 5	132 ± 6	192 ± 8	<.001
Glucose (mg/dL)**	91 ± 1	95 ± 1	98 ± 1	<.001
TG (mg/dL)**	98 ± 7	154 ± 12	173 ± 12	<.001
Total cholesterol (mg/dL)**	186 ± 4	201 ± 4	201 ± 4	.03
LDL-C (mg/dL)**	111 ± 3	124 ± 3	126 ± 4	.01
HDL-C (mg/dL)**	56 ± 2	50 ± 1	47 ± 1	<.001

Data are expressed as mean ± SEM; statistical significance by analysis of variance.

*P < .001 for pairwise comparisons of BMI groups <25 versus 25–29.9, <25 versus ≥30, and 25–29.9 versus ≥30; **P < .05 for pairwise comparisons of BMI groups <25 versus 25–29.9 and <25 versus ≥30.

Data from Farin HFM, Abbasi F, Reaven GM. Comparison of body mass index versus waist circumference with the metabolic changes that increase the risk of cardiovascular disease in insulin-resistant individuals. Am J Cardiol 2006;98:1053–6.

Table 4
Metabolic variables in 261 apparently healthy individuals classified as overweight/obese or abdominally obese

Variables	Overweight/obese[a] (n = 193)	Abdominally obese[b] (n = 133)
SSPG (mg/dL)	159 ± 5	174 ± 6
Glucose (mg/dL)	96 ± 1	98 ± 1
TG (mg/dL)	163 ± 8	163 ± 9
Total cholesterol (mg/dL)	200 ± 3	201 ± 3
LDL-C (mg/dL)	123 ± 3	124 ± 3
HDL-C (mg/dL)	49 ± 1	49 ± 1

[a] BMI ≥ 25.0 kg/m^2.

[b] WC > 88 cm for women, > 102 cm for men.

Data from Farin HFM, Abbasi F, Reaven GM. Comparison of body mass index versus waist circumference with the metabolic changes that increase the risk of cardiovascular disease in insulin-resistant individuals. Am J Cardiol 2006;98:1053–6.

and abnormal values for classifying individuals as being obese and therefore at increased risk to develop adverse outcomes, it seems that applying criteria for an abnormal BMI or an abnormal WC identifies populations at comparable CVD risk.

Variability of cardiovascular disease risk in equally obese, apparently healthy individuals

Because it is apparent that not all overweight/obese individuals are insulin resistant, the question then becomes what proportion of this population displays the metabolic abnormalities associated with the defect in insulin action [57,58]. In several relatively small studies, we presented evidence that a significant proportion of obese individuals are insulin sensitive and do not demonstrate the panoply of CVD risk factors that equally obese insulin-resistant individuals do [59–65]. More recently, we compared a number of CVD risk factors in 211 obese individuals [64] who were divided into three groups based on their SSPG concentration (ie, their degree of insulin resistance). SSPG concentrations (mean ± SD) increased progressively from 81 ± 26 mg/dL, to 166 ± 25 mg/dL, and to 247 ± 29 mg/dL, going from the most insulin-sensitive to the most insulin-resistant tertile. BMI values also tended to increase in parallel with the higher SSPG concentrations, with values of 31.7 kg/m^2, 32.0 kg/m^2, and 32.5 kg/m^2 in SSPG tertiles 1, 2, and 3, respectively.

Table 5 presents the comparison of multiple metabolic variables in the three SSPG tertiles, adjusted for any differences in age, sex, and BMI. For the purposes of this analysis, impaired fasting glucose and impaired glucose tolerance were as defined by the American Diabetes Association [66]. In the most general sense, it is apparent that the values of every risk factor measured were accentuated as a function of the degree of insulin

Table 5

Comparison of cardiovascular and diabetes risk factors in obese individuals as a function of steady-state plasma glucose tertile

Risk factor	Tertile 1 (n = 70)	Tertile 2 (n = 70)	Tertile 3 (n = 71)	P^d	P for trend[e]
Systolic blood pressure (mm Hg)	123 (18)	130 (17)	139 (20)[a,b]	<.001	<.001
Diastolic blood pressure (mm Hg)	75 (10)	78 (12)	83 (3)[a]	<.001	<.001
TG (mg/dL)	114 (51)	156 (66)[c]	198 (105)[a,b]	<.001	<.001
HDL-C (mg/dL)	50 (13)	47 (13)	41 (9)[a,b]	<.001	<.001
LDL-C (mg/dL)	123 (38)	134 (33)	123 (29)	.88	.77
Fasting plasma glucose (mg/dL)	95 (11)	99 (10)	103 (11)[a]	<.001	<.001
2-h plasma glucose during OGTT (mg/dL)	104 (19)	124 (35)[c]	139 (39)[a]	<.001	<.001
% Impaired fasting glucose	29%	46%	68%[a,b]	<.001	<.001
% Impaired glucose tolerance	1%	29%[c]	46%[a,b]	<.001	<.001

Data are expressed as mean (SD).

Abbreviation: OGTT, oral glucose tolerance test.

[a] $P < .05$ for tertile 3 versus tertile 1.

[b] $P < .05$ for tertile 3 versus tertile 2.

[c] $P < .05$ for tertile 2 versus tertile 1.

[d] Analysis of covariance, adjusted for age, BMI, and sex.

[e] P for trend analyzed by way of general linear model for continuous variables and Cochran-Armitage test for categoric variables.

resistance, with the exception of LDL-C concentration. Regarding every other variable, the comparison of the three SSPG groups showed that they were all worse when comparing tertile 3 (the most insulin-resistant group) to tertile 1 (the most insulin-sensitive group), and most of the values in tertile 3 were also significantly different from those in tertile 2 (the intermediate group).

There are many clinical implications of these findings, but at least two points are worth emphasizing. All of the values of the subjects in SSPG tertile 1 indicate that the risk for CVD (or 2DM for that matter) in the most insulin-sensitive third of this obese population is markedly attenuated. In dramatic contrast are the findings in the most insulin-resistant third of this obese population, in which the level of risk is clearly greatly magnified. Perhaps the most striking example of the disparity in metabolic abnormalities in obese individuals is a prevalence of impaired glucose tolerance of 1% in the most insulin-sensitive third compared with a 46% in the most insulin-resistant tertile. These findings clearly point out that not all obese individuals are insulin resistant and that approximately one third of them are at reduced risk to develop CVD.

Effects of weight loss on cardiovascular disease risk

Insulin resistance and the metabolic benefits of weight loss

The biologic implications of the findings in Table 5 are substantial and require consideration of the clinical approach to weight loss in overweight/obese individuals. At the simplest level, the most insulin-sensitive third of an apparently healthy group of obese individuals was at greatly decreased risk of CVD and 2DM compared with the most insulin-resistant third of this population. Are the metabolic benefits of weight loss similar in these two groups? The answer, not surprisingly, is no, and whereas obese insulin-resistant individuals become more insulin sensitive (lower SSPG concentrations) and have an improvement in all CVD risk factors associated with insulin resistance, there is essentially no change in insulin sensitivity and related CVD risk factors when insulin-sensitive obese individuals lose the same amount of weight [59–65]. Given this information, it seems mandatory to reconsider how health care professionals approach the overweight/obese individual. At the most elementary, it is necessary to cease thinking of overweight/obesity as a cosmetic issue and focus on its importance as increasing the risk of serious clinical syndromes. When that is realized, it also becomes necessary to stop thinking of obese individuals as an undifferentiated group of subjects that is at equal risk for adverse clinical outcomes and to realize that it is the insulin-resistant subset of these individuals who are at greatest health risk. The obvious corollary to this is the necessity to identify those overweight/obese individuals who are insulin resistant and initiate an aggressive weight loss program aimed at improving their insulin sensitivity and associated CVD risk factors.

How to identify the overweight/obese individual at greatest cardiovascular disease risk

Based on the data in Table 5, it could be argued that the first step in the clinical approach to overweight/obese individuals should be to identify the subset of overweight/obese individuals that is insulin resistant. As simple as this may seem at first glance, it is not clear whether it is necessary or attainable. For example, although being insulin resistant may increase the risk of developing the CVD risk factors listed in Table 5, it is not clear whether it is insulin resistance per se or the CVD risk factors associated with the defect in insulin action that are the culprit to be focused on. Therefore, simply measuring fasting plasma glucose, TG, LDL-C, and HDL-C concentrations provides an enormous degree of insight into those individuals who are insulin resistant (and thereby at greatest CVD risk) and who will benefit the most from weight loss.

Parenthetically, and of particular relevance to 2DM, it would be prudent to include a measurement of plasma glucose concentration 120 minutes after a 75-g oral glucose load as part of a health care evaluation in overweight/obese individuals. Conversely, patients who have values for these measurements that resemble those seen in the most insulin-sensitive tertile in Table 5 are at greatly reduced risk to develop CVD or 2DM and will gain little metabolic benefit from weight loss.

In addition to understanding that insulin resistance, by itself and in the absence of its associated metabolic abnormalities, may not increase risk of CVD, it should also be understood that although insulin-resistant individuals are more likely to be glucose intolerant, dyslipidemic, and hypertensive, these abnormalities do not necessarily always develop. Thus, at a clinical level, it is more important to know whether the potential adverse consequences of being insulin resistant are present, rather than whether or not a given individual can be classified as being insulin resistant. For example, results of studies in 490 apparently healthy individuals [67] showed that values of IMGU vary more than sixfold, without any obvious cut-point in the values of SSPG concentration that provides an objective way to define a person as being insulin resistant or insulin sensitive. In our two relatively small prospective studies, however, we showed that the third of an apparently healthy population that has the highest SSPG concentrations (the most insulin resistant) is at significantly greater risk to develop the adverse clinical outcomes related to the defect in insulin action [68,69].

Despite the complexity of trying to relate insulin resistance per se to clinical outcome, there seems to be a desire among health care professionals to "know" whether a subject is or is not insulin resistant. Even if it was possible to come up with a clear definition of who is or is not insulin resistant, the techniques necessary to determine this are not possible within the context of the clinical practice of medicine. As a consequence, an effort has been made to use surrogate markers of insulin resistance, with an emphasis on plasma insulin concentrations. Although nondiabetic insulin-resistant individuals tend to be hyperinsulinemic, there are two basic problems with the use of plasma insulin concentrations as a clinical tool to classify an individual as being insulin resistant. At the simplest level, there is no standardized clinical assay to measure plasma insulin concentration, making it essentially impossible to come up with a specific value that can be applied that will have meaning beyond the specific methodology used.

In addition to the technical problem related to the measurement of plasma insulin concentration, there remains the issue of how closely related insulin concentration is to a specific measure of IMGU. The best surrogate estimate of IMGU is the plasma insulin response to a 75-g oral glucose challenge, with a correlation coefficient (r value) of approximately 0.8 [67], accounting for approximately two thirds of the variability in IMGU. The correlation drops to an r value of approximately 0.6 when the fasting plasma insulin concentration is used instead of the response to oral glucose [67], thereby accounting for no more than one third of the variability in IMGU. Furthermore, surrogate estimates of IMGU based on combining concentrations of fasting plasma glucose with fasting insulin (ie, the homeostasis model assessment of insulin resistance or the quantitative insulin sensitivity check index) provide essentially the same information as the fasting plasma insulin concentration [67,70,71].

Following hyperinsulinemia, hypertriglyceridemia is the metabolic abnormality most closely related to differences in IMGU [63]. For example, in a recent analysis of 449 apparently healthy individuals, we found that the correlation coefficient between SSPG and TG concentrations was 0.57, which was not that different from the r value of 0.6 between SSPG and fasting plasma insulin concentrations in the same population [72]. There was also an inverse relationship ($r = -0.40$) between SSPG and HDL-C concentrations, and the plasma concentration ratio of TG to HDL-C was as closely related ($r = 0.6$) to SSPG concentration as was fasting plasma insulin concentration. Because a high TG concentration and a low HDL-C concentration are known to increase CVD risk [73–76], the use of the TG/HDL-C concentration ratio could provide the means to identify insulin-resistant subjects who also display the characteristic dyslipidemia associated with the defect in insulin action. In pursuit of this issue, we applied receiver operating characteristic curves to 258 apparently healthy overweight/obese individuals [63] and found that a plasma TG concentration greater than 130 mg/dL and a TG/HDL-C concentration ratio greater than 3.0 were relatively comparable in their ability to identify overweight/obese individuals classified (based on their SSPG concentration) as being insulin resistant. If BMI were the only criterion to initiate an intensive program of weight loss, then 258 individuals would be started; however, only 129 individuals were identified as insulin resistant and would benefit metabolically in response to weight loss. In contrast, only 125 of the 258 had the increase in TG concentration suggesting that they were insulin resistant, and in this instance, 87 would derive substantial metabolic benefit from weight loss. Essentially similar findings were obtained using the TG/HDL-C concentration ratio. Thus, if the goal is to reserve more aggressive attempts at weight loss for those overweight/individuals who are insulin resistant and at greater risk for CVD, then the use of these dyslipidemic markers appears to be of some clinical benefit by reducing the number of subjects identified for this purpose and ensuring that the individuals chosen would gain substantial clinical benefit from successful weight loss.

Summary

There seems to be general agreement that the prevalence of obesity is increasing in the United States [1,2] and that we are in the midst of an obesity epidemic [11]. The disease-related implications of this epidemic have received an enormous amount of publicity in the popular media, but public awareness of the untoward effects of excess weight has not led to an effective approach to dealing with the dilemma. The gravity of the problem is accentuated in light of the report that only approximately 50% of physicians polled provided weight loss counseling [77].

Given the importance of excess adiposity as increasing the risk of CVD, 2DM, and hypertension [8–10] and the combination of an increase in the prevalence of overweight/obesity and a health care system unprepared to deal with this situation, it is essential that considerable thought be given as to how to best address this dilemma. In this context, it must be emphasized that CVD, 2DM, and hypertension are characterized by resistance to insulin-mediated glucose disposal [57,58] and that insulin resistance and the compensatory hyperinsulinemia associated with insulin resistance have been shown to be independent predictors of all three clinical syndromes [68,69,78]. It has also been apparent for many years that overweight/obese individuals tend to be insulin resistant and become more insulin sensitive with weight loss [25]. In light of these observations, it seems reasonable to suggest that insulin resistance is the link between overweight/obesity and the adverse clinical syndromes related to excess adiposity. The evidence summarized in this review shows that the more overweight an individual, the more likely he or she is insulin resistant and at increased risk to develop all the abnormalities associated with this defect in insulin action. Not all overweight/obese individuals are insulin resistant, however, any more than all insulin-resistant individuals are overweight/obese. More important, there is compelling evidence that CVD risk factors are present to a significantly greater degree in the subset of overweight/obese individuals that is also insulin resistant. Not surprisingly, we have also demonstrated that an improvement in CVD risk factors with weight loss occurs to a significantly greater degree in those overweight/obese individuals who are also insulin resistant at baseline. In view of the ineffectiveness of current clinical approaches to weight loss, it seems necessary to recognize that not all overweight/obese individuals are at equal risk to develop CVD and that it is clinically useful to identify those at highest risk. The simplest way to achieve this task seems to be focusing on the CVD risk factors that are highly associated with insulin resistance/hyperinsulinemia. If this is done, then intense efforts at weight control can be brought to bear on those who not only need it the most but also have the most to gain by losing weight.

References

[1] Flegal KM, Carroll MD, Ogden CL, et al. Prevalence and trends in obesity among US adults, 1999–2000. JAMA 2002;288:1723–7.
[2] Hedley AA, Ogden CL, Johnson CL, et al. Prevalence of overweight and obesity among US children, adolescents, and adults, 1999–2002. JAMA 2004;291:2847–50.
[3] Allison DB, Fontaine KR, Manson JE, et al. Annual deaths attributable to obesity in the United States. JAMA 1999;282:1530–8.
[4] Fontaine KR, Redden DT, Wang C, et al. Years of life lost due to obesity. JAMA 2003;289: 187–93.

[5] Hu FB, Willett WC, Li T, et al. Adiposity as compared with physical activity in predicting mortality among women. N Engl J Med 2004;351:2964–703.

[6] Calle EE, Thun MJ, Petrelli JM, et al. Body-mass index and mortality in a prospective cohort of US adults. N Engl J Med 1999;341:1097–105.

[7] Yan LL, Daviglus ML, Liu K, et al. Midlife body mass index and hospitalization and mortality in older age. JAMA 2006;295:190–8.

[8] West KM, Kalbfleisch JM. Influence of nutritional factors on prevalence of diabetes. Diabetes 1971;20:99–108.

[9] Havlik RJ, Hubert HB, Fabsitz RR, et al. Weight and hypertension. Ann Intern Med 1983; 98:855–9.

[10] Wilson PW, D'Agostino RB, Sullivan L, et al. Overweight and obesity as determinants of cardiovascular risk: the Framingham experience. Arch Intern Med 2002;162:1867–72.

[11] Manson JE, Skerrett PJ, Greenland P, et al. The escalating pandemics of obesity and sedentary lifestyle. Arch Intern Med 2004;164:249–58.

[12] Flegal KM, Graubard BI, Williamson DF, et al. Excess deaths associated with underweight, overweight, and obesity. JAMA 2005;293:1861–7.

[13] Gregg EW, Cheng YJ, Cadwell BL, et al. Secular trends in cardiovascular disease risk factors according to body mass index in US adults. JAMA 2005;293:1868–74.

[14] Rosenthal M, Haskell WL, Solomon R, et al. Demonstration of a relationship between level of physical training and insulin-stimulated glucose utilization in normal humans. Diabetes 1983;32:408–11.

[15] Bogardus C, Lillioja S, Mott D, et al. Relationship between obesity and maximal-insulin stimulated glucose uptake in vivo and in vitro in Pima Indians. J Clin Invest 1984;73:800–5.

[16] Bogardus C, Lillioja S, Mott DM, et al. Relationship between degree of obesity and in vivo insulin action in man. Am J Physiol 1985;248:E286–91.

[17] Soman VR, Koivisto VA, Deibert D, et al. Increased insulin sensitivity and insulin binding to monocytes after physical training. N Engl J Med 1978;301:1200–4.

[18] Koivisto VA, Yki-Jarvinen H, DeFronzo RA. Physical training and insulin sensitivity. Diabetes Metab Rev 1986;445–81.

[19] Goodyear LJ, Kahn BB. Exercise, glucose transport, and insulin sensitivity. Annu Rev Med 1998;49:235–61.

[20] Wessel TR, Arant CB, Olson MB, et al. Relationship of physical fitness vs body mass index with coronary artery disease and cardiovascular events in women. JAMA 2004;292:1179–87.

[21] Weinstein AR, Sesso HD, Lee IM, et al. Relationship of physical activity vs body mass index with type 2 diabetes in women. JAMA 2004;292:1188–94.

[22] Li TY, Rana JS, Manson JE, et al. Obesity as compared with physical activity in predicting risk of coronary heart disease in women. Circulation 2006;31:499–506.

[23] Sullivan PW, Morrato EH, Ghushchyan V, et al. Obesity, inactivity, and the prevalence of diabetes and diabetes-related cardiovascular comorbidities in the U.S., 2000–2002. Diabetes Care 2005;28:1599–603.

[24] Rana JS, Li TY, Manson JE, et al. Adiposity compared with physical inactivity and risk of type 2 diabetes in women. Diabetes Care 2007;30:53–8.

[25] Olefsky JM, Reaven GM, Farquhar JW. Effects of weight reduction on obesity: studies of carbohydrate and lipid metabolism. J Clin Invest 1974;53:64–76.

[26] Ruderman NB, Schneider SH, Berchtold P. The "metabolically-obese," normal weight individual. Am J Clin Nutr 1981;1617–21.

[27] Ferrannini E, Natali A, Bell P, et al. Insulin resistance and hypersecretion in obesity. J Clin Invest 1997;100:1166–73.

[28] Executive summary of the third report of the National Cholesterol Education Program (NCEP) Expert Panel on Detection, Evaluation, and Treatment of High Blood Cholesterol in Adults (Adult Treatment Panel III). JAMA 2002;285:2486–97.

[29] Alberti KG, Zimmet P, Shaw J, for the IDF Epidemiology Task Force Consensus Group. The metastatic syndrome—a new worldwide definition. Lancet 2004;366:1059–61.

[30] Ford ES, Mokdad AH, Giles WH. Trends in waist circumference among U.S. adults. Obes Res 2003;11:1223–31.

[31] Pei D, Jones CN, Bhargava R, et al. Evaluation of octreotide to assess insulin-mediated glucose disposal by the insulin suppression test. Diabetologia 1994;37:843–5.

[32] Shen S-W, Reaven GM, Farquhar JW. Comparison of impedance to insulin mediated glucose uptake in normal and diabetic subjects. J Clin Invest 1970;49:2151–60.

[33] Greenfield MS, Doberne L, Kraemer FB, et al. Assessment of insulin resistance with the insulin suppression test and the euglycemic clamp. Diabetes 1981;30:387–92.

[34] Farin HM, Abbasi F, Reaven GM. Body mass index and waist circumference both contribute to differences in insulin-mediated glucose disposal in nondiabetic adults. Am J Clin Nutr 2006;83:47–51.

[35] Abate N, Garg A, Peshock RM, et al. Relationships of generalized and regional adiposity to insulin sensitivity in man. J Clin Invest 1995;96:88–98.

[36] Cefalu WT, Wang ZQ, Werbgel S, et al. Contribution of visceral fat to the insulin resistance of aging. Metabolism 1995;44:954–9.

[37] Macor C, Ruggeri A, Mazzonetto P, et al. Visceral adipose tissue impairs insulin secretion and sensitivity, but not energy expenditure in obesity. Metabolism 1997;46:123–9.

[38] Goodpaster BH, Thaete JA, Simoneau JA, et al. Subcutaneous abdominal fat and thigh muscle composition predict insulin sensitivity independently of visceral fat. Diabetes 1997; 46:1579–85.

[39] Banerji MA, Faridi N, Atluri R, et al. Body composition, visceral fat, leptin and insulin resistance in Asian Indian men. J Clin Endocrinol Metab 1999;84:137–44.

[40] Kelley DE, Thaete FL, Troost F, et al. Subdivisions of subcutaneous abdominal tissue and insulin resistance. Am J Physiol Endocrinol Metab 2000;278:E941–8.

[41] Sites CK, Calles-Escandon J, Brochu M, et al. Relation of regional fat distribution to insulin sensitivity in postmenopausal women. Fertil Steril 2000;73:61–5.

[42] Brochu M, Starling RD, Tchernof A, et al. Visceral adipose tissue is an independent correlate of glucose disposal in older postmenopausal women. J Clin Endocrinol Metab 2001;85: 2378–84.

[43] Goran MI, Bergman RN, Gower BA. Influence of total vs. visceral fat on insulin action and secretion in African American and white children. Obes Res 2001;423–31.

[44] Rendell M, Hulthen UL, Tornquist C, et al. Relationship between abdominal fat compartments and glucose and lipid metabolism in early postmenopausal women. J Clin Endocrinol Metab 2001;86:744–9.

[45] Purnell JQ, Kahn SE, Schwartz RS, et al. Relationship of insulin sensitivity and apoB levels to intra-abdominal fat in subjects with combined hyperlipidemia. Arterioscler Thromb Vasc Biol 2001;21:567–72.

[46] Raji A, Seeley EW, Arky RA, et al. Body fat distribution and insulin resistance in healthy Asian Indians and Caucasians. J Clin Endocrinol Metab 2001;86:5366–71.

[47] Ross R, Aru J, Freman J, et al. Abdominal obesity and insulin resistance in obese men. Am J Physiol Endocrinol Metab 2002;282:E657–63.

[48] Ross R, Freeman J, Hudson R, et al. Abdominal obesity, muscle composition and insulin resistant in premenopausal women. J Clin Endocrinol Metab 2002;87:5044–51.

[49] Cnop M, Landchild MJ, Vidal J, et al. The concurrent accumulation of intra-abdominal and subcutaneous fat explains the association between insulin resistance and plasma leptin concentrations. Diabetes 2002;51:1005–15.

[50] Cruz ML, Bergman RN, Goran MI. Unique effect of visceral fat on insulin sensitivity in obese Hispanic children with a family history of type 2 diabetes. Diabetes Care 2002;25: 1631–6.

[51] Gan SK, Krikeos AD, Poynten AM, et al. Insulin action, regional fat, and myocyte lipid; altered relationships with increased adiposity. Obes Res 2003;11:1295–305.

[52] Tulloch-Reid MK, Hanson RL, Sebring NG, et al. Both subcutaneous and visceral adipose tissues correlate highly with insulin resistance in African Americans. Obes Res 2004;1352–9.

[53] Rattarasarn C, Leelawattan R, Soonthornpun S, et al. Gender differences of regional abdominal fat distribution and their relationships with insulin sensitivity in healthy and glucose-intolerant Thais. J Clin Endocrinol Metab 2004;89:6266–70.

[54] Raji A, Gerhard-Herman MD, Warren M, et al. Insulin resistance and vascular dysfunction in nondiabetic Asian Indians. J Clin Endocrinol Metab 2004;89:3965–72.

[55] Bush NC, Darnell BE, Oster RA, et al. Adiponectin is lower among African Americans and is independently related to insulin sensitivity in children and adolescents. Diabetes 2005;54: 2772–8.

[56] Janssen I, Heymsfield SB, Allison DB, et al. Body mass index and waist circumference independently contribute to the prediction of nonabdominal, abdominal, subcutaneous, and visceral fat. Am J Clin Nutr 2002;75:683–8.

[57] Reaven GM. Role of insulin resistance in human disease. Diabetes 1988;37:1595–607.

[58] Reaven GM. The insulin resistance syndrome. Curr Atheroscler Rep 2003;5:364–71.

[59] McLaughlin T, Abbasi F, Carantoni M, et al. Differences in insulin resistance do not predict weight loss in response to hypocaloric diets in healthy obese women. J Clin Endocrinol Metab 1999;84:578–81.

[60] Jones CN, Abbas F, Carantoni M, et al. Roles of insulin resistance and obesity in regulation of plasma insulin concentrations. Am J Physiol Endocrinol Metab 2000;278:E501–8.

[61] McLaughlin T, Abbasi F, Kim H-S, et al. Relationship between insulin resistance, weight loss, and coronary heart disease risk in healthy, obese women. Metabolism 2001;50:795–800.

[62] McLaughlin T, Abbasi F, Lamendola C, et al. Differentiation between obesity and insulin resistance in the association with C-reactive protein. Circulation 2002;106:2908–12.

[63] McLaughlin T, Abbasi F, Cheal K, et al. Use of metabolic markers to identify overweight individuals who are insulin resistant. Ann Intern Med 2003;139:802–9.

[64] McLaughlin T, Abbasi F, Lamendola C, et al. Heterogeneity in the prevalence of risk factors for cardiovascular disease and type 2 diabetes in obese individuals: effect of differences in insulin sensitivity. Arch Intern Med 2007;167:642–8.

[65] McLaughlin T, Stuhlinger M, Lamendola C, et al. Plasma asymmetric dimethylarginine concentrations are elevated in obese insulin resistant women and fall with weight loss. J Clin Endocrinol Metab 2006;91:1896–900.

[66] Genuth S, Alberti KG, Bennett P, et al. Follow-up report on the diagnosis of diabetes mellitus. Diabetes Care 2003;26:3160–7.

[67] Yeni-Komshian H, Carantoni M, Abbasi F, et al. Relationship between several surrogate estimates of insulin resistance and quantification of insulin-mediated glucose disposal in 490 healthy, nondiabetic volunteers. Diabetes Care 2000;23:171–5.

[68] Yip J, Facchini FS, Reaven GM. Resistance to insulin-mediated glucose disposal as a predictor of cardiovascular disease. J Clin Endocrinol Metab 1998;83:2773–6.

[69] Facchini FS, Hua N, Abbasi F, et al. Insulin resistance as a predictor of age- related diseases. J Clin Endocrinol Metab 2001;86:3574–8.

[70] Abbasi F, Reaven GM. Evaluation of the quantitative insulin sensitivity check index as an estimate of insulin sensitivity in humans. Metabolism 2002;51:235–7.

[71] Kim SH, Abbasi F, Reaven GM. Impact of degree of obesity on surrogate estimates of insulin resistance. Diabetes Care 2004;27:1998–2002.

[72] McLaughlin T, Reaven G, Abbasi F, et al. Is there a simple way to identify insulin-resistant individuals at increased risk of cardiovascular disease? Am J Cardiol 2005;96:399–404.

[73] Miller GJ, Miller NE. Plasma high-density-lipoprotein concentration and development of ischaemic heart disease. Lancet 1975;1:16–9.

[74] Carlson LA, Bottiger LE, Ahfeldt PE. Risk factors for myocardial infarction in the Stockholm prospective study: a 14-year follow-up focusing on the role of plasma triglycerides and cholesterol. Acta Med Scand 1979;206:351–60.

[75] Castelli WP, Garrison RJ, Wilson PW, et al. Incidence of coronary heart disease and lipoprotein cholesterol levels: the Framingham Study. JAMA 1986;256:2385–7.

[76] Hokanson JE, Austin MA. Plasma triglyceride level in a risk factor for cardiovascular disease independent of high-density lipoprotein cholesterol level: a meta-analysis of population-based prospective studies. J Cardiovasc Risk 1996;3:213–9.

[77] Galuska DA, Will JC, Serdula MK, et al. Are health care professionals advising obese patients to lose weight? JAMA 1999;282:1576–8.

[78] Zavaroni I, Bonini L, Gasparini P, et al. Hyperinsulinemia in a normal population as a predictor of non-insulin-dependent diabetes mellitus, hypertension, and coronary heart disease: the Barilla factory revisited. Metabolism 1999;48:989–94.

ELSEVIER
SAUNDERS

Endocrinol Metab Clin N Am
37 (2008) 603–621

ENDOCRINOLOGY
AND METABOLISM
CLINICS
OF NORTH AMERICA

Insulin Resistance and Atherosclerosis

Babak Razani, MD, PhD[a],
Manu V. Chakravarthy, MD, PhD[b],
Clay F. Semenkovich, MD[b],*

[a]Cardiovascular Division, Department of Medicine, Washington University
School of Medicine, Campus Box 8127, 660 South Euclid Avenue,
St. Louis, MO 63110, USA
[b]Division of Endocrinology, Metabolism, and Lipid Research,
Department of Medicine, Washington University School of Medicine,
Campus Box 8127, 660 South Euclid Avenue, St. Louis, MO 63110, USA

The term "insulin resistance" has existed in the medical vernacular nearly as long as the clinical use of insulin itself. In fact, the first report of a patient resistant to the effects of insulin was published in 1924, only 2 years after 14-year-old Leonard Thompson became the first human to be successfully treated with insulin [1,2]. Although the early medical literature is replete with such examples, the etiology of this resistance was imprecise purification, varied absorption, and immune-mediated clearance of impure/canine insulin. In the modern era, insulin resistance most commonly denotes a condition in which there is an insufficient peripheral (eg, muscle, liver, and adipose) tissue response to a given quantity of insulin. The progression of such a subnormal response is usually insidious, with affected individuals living subclinically for years with glucose levels nearly normal as a result of hypersecretion of insulin. In the subset of individuals with both chronic insulin resistance and pancreatic beta cell failure, glucose levels become sufficiently elevated to fulfill the diagnostic criteria for type 2 diabetes mellitus, the end-stage of the insulin resistance spectrum.

Although impaired glucose tolerance and hyperglycemia are classical manifestations of insulin resistance and type 2 diabetes, many patients present with several associated signs and laboratory abnormalities (ie, abdominal obesity, elevated blood pressure, elevated triglycerides, and low high-density

This work was supported by Grants HL083762 and DK076729 from the National Institutes of Health.

* Corresponding author.

E-mail address: csemenko@wustl.edu (C.F. Semenkovich).

lipoprotein [HDL] cholesterol). Insulin resistance is thought to play a role in the association of these metabolic phenotypes; indeed, such clustering of phenotypes has been termed the insulin resistance syndrome or the metabolic syndrome. The National Cholesterol Education Program's Adult Treatment Panel III (ATPIII) and the World Health Organization (WHO) have rigorously defined the components of the metabolic syndrome in recently published/updated criteria [3–5].

One of the most devastating complications of long-standing insulin resistance and its associated metabolic derangements is progressive macrovascular pathology (namely atherosclerosis). Atherosclerosis remains the major cause of morbidity and mortality among diabetic patients. Diabetic patients have higher rates of coronary artery disease (CAD) and myocardial infarctions (MIs) than nondiabetic patients with similar risk factor profiles [6–8]. Diabetic patients without a prior MI have a similar mortality risk to nondiabetic individuals with a prior MI [6,9]. Revealing results from such large studies prompted the most recent ATPIII guidelines to designate diabetes as a coronary disease equivalent [3].

Although hyperglycemia is a hallmark of diabetes, it is not clear that elevated glucose levels alone contribute in a major way to cardiovascular disease (CVD) progression. Indeed, diabetic patients without the metabolic syndrome have less CVD than nondiabetic patients with the metabolic syndrome [10]. It is becoming increasingly clear that metabolic derangements associated with insulin resistance are important contributors to atherogenesis (Fig. 1). Regardless of which criteria are used to define this syndrome, afflicted patients are at approximately two- to fourfold increased risk for

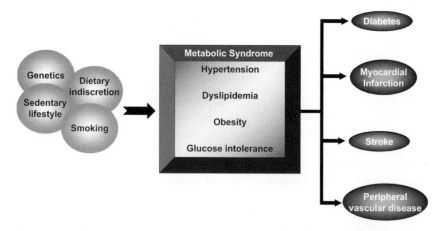

Fig. 1. The central role of insulin resistance in vascular disease. Multiple environmental and genetic factors contribute to the formation of the insulin resistance phenotype (also known as the "metabolic syndrome"), marked by hypertension, dyslipidemia, obesity, and glucose intolerance. These risk factors in turn contribute to initiation and progression of type 2 diabetes and the macrovascular diseases (ie, myocardial infarctions, strokes, and peripheral vascular disease).

CVD mortality [11]. Furthermore, there is a graded risk depending on the number of risk factors present [12].

The wealth of evidence in the past few decades points to a striking relation between insulin resistance and atherosclerosis. With this background, the goal of this review is threefold: (1) to provide an overview of the currently used treatment strategies to reduce CVD mortality in insulin-resistant patients, (2) to establish a framework for further defining the role of insulin resistance in vascular disease, and (3) to summarize preclinical data that may lead to future therapeutics.

Prevention of cardiovascular disease in insulin resistance (current approaches)

Current primary prevention treatment modalities in patients with the metabolic syndrome and/or diabetes rely on risk factor modification (ie, reduction of hyperlipidemia, hypertension, obesity, and lifestyle changes). Although beyond the focus of this review, a few treatment options are especially worthy of mention. Beginning in the 1990s, large clinical trials demonstrated the enormous clinical utility of two classes of drugs, statins and angiotensin-converting enzyme inhibitors (ACEi)/angiotensin receptor blockers (ARB), in diminishing the cardiovascular morbidity and mortality of insulin-resistant/diabetic patients.

The first large secondary prevention (ie, patients with a prior MI) trial to demonstrate the CV benefits of statins (in this case simvastatin) was the 4S trial [13]. This was followed by West of Scotland Coronary Prevention Study (WOSCOPS), the first large primary prevention trial to demonstrate statin benefits in patients with no known CVD but including many with metabolic profiles resembling incipient insulin resistance [14]. These findings have been corroborated by numerous other trials showing the utility of statins as a class in different patient subgroups. One of the most surprising statin trials was the Heart Protection Study, a comparison of simvastatin versus placebo in a cohort of approximately 20,000 patients with known CVD or diabetes mellitus (DM) [15]. In addition to showing similar CV mortality benefits as prior studies, this trial also clearly demonstrated that patients with the lowest category of low-density lipoprotein (LDL) cholesterol levels (<116 mg/dL) derived benefits from statin therapy that was comparable to benefits in statin-treated hypercholesterolemic patients. In this regard, there is accumulating evidence that statins are more than simply cholesterol-lowering agents, having beneficial effects on endothelial dysfunction, inflammation, and the coagulation cascade, as well as platelet function (reviewed in [16]).

It has been known for some time that inhibition of the renin-angiotensin system is critical for reducing CV mortality and improving cardiac function in patients with left ventricular dysfunction/ischemic cardiomyopathy [17,18]. What remained unclear was whether ACEi and ARBs would be effective in patients with high-risk features (including known vascular disease and diabetes) without overt heart failure. The Heart Outcomes Prevention Evaluation (HOPE) and Losartan Intervention for Endpoint Reduction (LIFE) trials were two large randomized studies designed to address the effectiveness of the ACEi ramipril and the ARB losartan, respectively, in such patients [19,20]. The significant decrease in CV mortality observed with treatment in these trials has elevated this class of drugs to first-line agents in the treatment of hypertension in diabetic patients, even in the absence of heart failure.

Is modulation of insulin resistance beneficial for cardiovascular disease prevention?

As described above, the classical approach to the treatment of insulin resistance and diabetes is risk-factor modification (ie, directed treatment of the most skewed parameters of the disorders). Despite clear successes with this approach, it represents a reaction to long-standing metabolic derangements rather than treatment for a potentially unifying process, such as insulin resistance. Thiazolidinediones are a class of drugs known to improve insulin resistance that were found to act by binding to Peroxisome-Proliferator-Activated Receptor gamma (PPARγ), a discovery providing a new mechanistic approach to diabetes treatment [21]. PPARs are ligand-activated nuclear receptors of which PPARγ is one subtype. As PPARγ is highly expressed in adipose tissue where it is involved in lipid homeostasis (especially fatty acid uptake/storage), it stood to reason its activation might enhance insulin sensitivity by directing toxic-free fatty acids away from other insulin-dependent organs and into adipose tissue. This hypothesis was supported by some studies in humans focusing on glucose metabolism. Although trogilitazone, the first thiazolidinedione to be approved for clinical use, was withdrawn because of hepatotoxicity, the continued success of other members of this class of drugs, rosiglitazone and pioglitazone, was heralded by some as a revolution in diabetes and insulin-resistance management [22].

Although not supported by disease-related outcome data, the use of thiazolidinediones in diabetic subjects was expected to not only improve surrogate end points such as glycemic control but also end points such as macrovascular events. The utility of these agents came under scrutiny when a meta-analysis of rosiglitazone trials showed increased CV mortality [23]. Although pioglitazone faired better in the 5,238-patient Prospective Pioglitazone Clinical Trial in Macrovascular Events (PROACTIVE) study (non-significant reduction in CV events) [24] and a follow-up meta-analysis (a statistically significant decrease in death, MI, and strokes) [25], concerns over the lack of prospective outcomes data with thiazolidinediones and the known increased risk of volume overload/heart failure with these drugs [26] have raised doubts about this class of therapeutic agents.

Despite the current controversy about thiazolidinediones, an understanding of the molecular underpinnings driving insulin resistance and their relation to atherosclerosis is pivotal in the development of rational drug design.

There are several aspects of insulin resistance that are actively being pursued in hopes of better understanding atherosclerotic events.

Insulin resistance and proatherogenic lipids

Despite the traditional focus on LDL and CVD risk, a portion of the connection between blunted insulin signaling, abnormal lipid metabolism, and atherosclerosis appears to be mediated by aberrations in triglyceride/very low-density lipoprotein and HDL levels instead of LDL [27]. Derangements in adipocyte and hepatocyte function play a central role in these abnormalities [28,29].

Insulin resistance reduces the ability of adipose tissue to clear/store circulating lipids, in part because of reduced lipoprotein lipase enzyme activity. Abnormal adipocyte insulin signaling also results in inappropriate lipolysis even during times of nutrient excess. The result is paradoxical elevations in serum triglycerides as well as circulating free fatty acids (FFA). In conjunction with elevations in apolipoprotein B (apoB) (thought to be due to post-translational stabilization of the protein) and enhanced lipogenesis by the liver, increases in apoB-containing/triglyceride-rich lipids (primarily present as VLDL particles) are a hallmark of patients with insulin resistance [30,31].

Several trials have demonstrated the CV risks associated with the hypertriglyceridemia of insulin resistance. Hypertriglyceridemia has the strongest correlation with CVD among the five components of the metabolic syndrome [32]. Although the significance of fasting triglycerides (as an independent factor) with respect to CV events has been a matter of debate [27], elevated non-fasting triglycerides, a state classically associated with insulin resistance as described above, significantly elevates CV mortality risk [33,34].

Insulin resistance can also have adverse consequences on LDL and HDL metabolism. Although elevations in LDL cholesterol levels are not a hallmark of insulin resistance/diabetes, the composition and possibly proatherogenic function of LDL is affected. The hypertriglyceridemia/VLDL excess brought on by insulin resistance expedites cholesteryl ester transfer protein (CETP)-mediated exchange of LDL cholesteryl ester for VLDL triglyceride. In turn, the newly acquired LDL triglyceride undergoes lipolysis by hepatic and lipoprotein lipase, resulting in LDL particles that are smaller in size, more dense, and depleted of their usual cholesteryl ester content [35,36]. A similar mechanism involving CETP-mediated exchange of lipids also occurs between VLDL and HDL; however, in addition to the eventual creation of small/dense particles, HDL clearance is also enhanced with the end result being low levels of dysfunctional HDL particles [37,38].

The role of insulin resistance in inflammatory signaling and atherosclerosis

An obvious connection between insulin resistance and atherosclerosis is derived from observations that obesity and insulin resistance often occur in concert with significant increases in inflammatory mediators [39,40]. Athero-sclerosis acts in many ways like an inflammatory condition with prominent cellular infiltration and robust cytokine expression [41]. One of the first links between obesity, insulin resistance, and inflammation was the demonstration that mouse adipose tissue can produce tumor necrosis factor alpha (TNFα), its production is proportional to the degree of obesity, and neutralization of the TNF-receptor can significantly decrease obesity-induced insulin resis-tance [42]. Numerous subsequent studies have debunked the initial view of the adipocyte as a stagnant lipid storage entity; adipose tissue is now known to be an active secretory organ, dynamically producing a variety of proinflam-matory mediators such as TNFα, interleukin (IL)-1, IL-6, monocyte chemo-attractant protein (MCP)-1, and type 1 plasminogen activator inhibitor (PAI-1), factors traditionally associated with inflammatory cells [43]. Similar to TNFα the production of these "adipokines" is a function of the health of the tissue and under conditions of nutrient excess, obesity, and progressive insulin resistance, there is substantial proinflammatory adipokine production [44–48]. A substantial body of work has shown that these inflammatory me-diators perpetuate the insulin resistance phenotype and result in deleterious effects on the vasculature (reviewed in Ref. [43]). A detailed review of the ef-fects of proatherogenic signaling including the role of protein kinase C (PKC) has recently appeared [49], but two of the major pathways likely to be clini-cally relevant to vascular disease in insulin resistance involve the Nuclear Factor kappa B (NF-κB) and c-Jun N-terminal kinase (JNK) cascades.

NF-κB signaling and atherogenesis

A central mediator of inflammatory signaling in the vasculature of an insulin-resistant individual is the NF-κB family of nuclear transcription factors (Fig. 2). The classical and most prominent member of this family is a heterodimer of the p65/RelA and p50 proteins. In the cytoplasm, this dimer is bound to IκB proteins in an inactive state [50]. The arrival of extra-cellular signals (including several of the cytokines described above including TNFα and IL-1), stimulates the membrane-associated IκB kinase (IKK) to serine-phosphorylate IκB, thus facilitating its proteosomal degradation and liberating NF-κB to undergo nuclear translocation and set into motion a potent feed-forward production of proinflammatory transcripts [51,52]. A global survey of such NF-κB targets, as has been performed by both individual target gene assessment and more broad expression profiling ap-proaches, reveals striking proatherogenic features. Broad categories include mononuclear cell chemoattractants, vascular adhesion molecules, mediators of chemotaxis, inducers of the monocyte to macrophage differentiation pro-gram, stimulators of smooth muscle cell proliferation, angiogenic factors, and amplification of proteases involved in the breakdown of the intercellular matrix, spanning the entire gamut of mediators required for plaque forma-tion, progression, and destabilization [53].

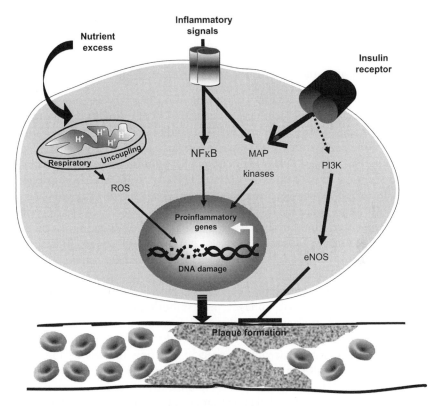

Fig. 2. Critical proatherogenic signaling events at the vasculature in the setting of insulin resistance. The secretion of proinflammatory mediators initiated by systemic insulin resistance stimulate several intracellular signaling cascades, of which NFκB and JNK (a member of the MAP kinase family) are prominent examples; these potent inducers of proinflammatory genes create a feedforward cycle of signaling that provokes several aspects of atherogenesis. In addition, insulin resistance also selectively interferes with PI-3-kinase-mediated insulin receptor signaling, in turn suppressing eNOS activity in favor of the proproliferative/proatherogenic MAP kinases. Finally, states of nutrient excess dysregulate mitochondrial energy balance thus promoting respiratory uncoupling and the generation of reactive oxygen species (ROS); this can wreak havoc on the integrity of the genome and blunt vascular defenses against atherogenesis.

Although the potential for cytokine-mediated vascular damage is evident, attempts at studying the NF-κB pathway with mouse models have produced contradictory results. For example, genetic targeting of p55, one of two TNFα receptors and the predominant mediator of inflammation actually protects mice against atherosclerosis [54]. Furthermore, a partial macrophage-specific deletion of IKK2 leading to an approximately 50% reduction in NF-κB activation increases the extent and the complexity of atherosclerotic lesions in mice [55] while bone marrow reconstitution experiments with NF-κB1-null macrophages in mice fed a high-fat diet leads to decreased atheromatous plaque formation but an increased cellular infiltration [56]. These confounding results point to the tremendous complexity of the inflammatory response and our current inability to tease out such nuances with available technologies.

JNK signaling and atherosclerosis

JNK is a member of the mitogen-activated protein (MAP) kinase family (which also includes extracellular signal-related kinase [ERK1/2], big MAP kinase [BMK1], and p38 MAP kinase) (reviewed in Ref. [57]). Although these serine/threonine kinases are responsive to a variety of stimuli, JNK signaling is potently activated by mediators of inflammatory and stress responses including cytokines and environmental stresses. Upon activation, JNK can phosphorylate a host of transcription factors, including the one for which it is named (c-Jun component of the AP-1 transcription factor), thereby triggering robust gene expression. Similar to NF-κB signaling, cytokine-induced JNK signaling fuels a feed-forward cycle of proinflammatory/proatherogenic factor production including TNFα, IL-2, matrix metalloproteinases, and adhesion molecules [58–60].

Initial data suggesting a role for JNK in atherosclerosis were based on observations that the macrophages and smooth muscle cells of human and animal model atheromatous plaques had prominently activated JNK signaling [61,62]. Further evidence was provided by Ricci and colleagues [63] by creating mice with macrophage-specific ablation of two of the JNK family members, JNK1 and JNK2, in an ApoE-null background. Interestingly, only the JNK2(−/−) mice had significantly reduced atherosclerotic burden; this was because of defective foam cell formation proposed to occur via reduced uptake of modified LDL.

Direct effects of insulin resistance on the vasculature and atherogenesis

One of the early events in the pathophysiology of atherosclerosis appears to be endothelial dysfunction, a state of blunted vasodilatory capacity and reduced ability to protect against platelet aggregation, blood cell adhesion, and smooth muscle proliferation. A pivotal factor involved in vascular health is nitric oxide (NO), which is dynamically controlled by signaling processes [64,65]. As patients with either the metabolic syndrome or diabetes have impaired NO-mediated vasodilation [66–68], insulin resistance may have direct pathogenic effects on the vasculature. Insulin is a major stimulus for NO-mediated vasodilation [69].

In many tissues, including the vasculature, insulin effects can be generally divided into two pathways, involving either PI-3-kinase/Akt or MAP kinase signaling. Upon ligand binding, the insulin receptor activates a signaling cascade involving insulin receptor substrate (IRS) adapter molecules, PI-3-kinase, and Akt, subsequently leading in the endothelium to the phosphorylation/activation of endothelial nitric oxide synthase, a process independent of classical calcium-based eNOS signaling [70,71]. In contradistinction, the growth factor functions of insulin occur via its MAP kinase–dependent arm and are more involved with cellular migration, vascular smooth muscle cell proliferation, and prothrombotic states [72]. During insulin-resistant states, there is a selective disruption of vascular PI-3-kinase/Akt-mediated signaling; interestingly, insulin-mediated MAP kinase signaling continues unabated [73,74] and can even further blunt PI-3-kinase signaling by serine-phosphorylation of IRS-1 [75]. Thus, the development of insulin resistance and compensatory hyperinsulinemia can progressively shift the balance of insulin signaling toward a mitogenic state that may contribute to atherosclerosis (see Fig. 2).

Are the direct effects of insulin resistance always pro-atherogenic or can insulin resistance play a paradoxical protective role?

As discussed above, the direct effects of insulin on the vasculature implicate insulin resistance in vascular/endothelial dysfunction. However, it should be noted that there are limited data extending this connection to atherosclerosis; regardless of the experimental system, most published studies use NO-mediated vascular reactivity/signaling as end points rather than more direct ones such as plaque formation/atherosclerotic burden. When one highlights studies assessing the role of insulin signaling in atherogenesis, several interesting observations arise.

ApoE-null mice with selective inactivation of the insulin receptor (IR) in the myeloid lineage have smaller atherosclerotic lesions [76]. In a different approach, bone marrow transplantation of LDLR-null mice with insulin receptor–deficient cells did not affect the number of lesions but created more complex/necrotic lesions [77]. Although whole-animal IRS-2 null mice on an ApoE-null background have increased plaque burden, repopulation of the hematopoietic system of lethally irradiated ApoE-null mice with IRS-2(−/−) cells mitigates the atherosclerotic phenotype [76]. Deletion of the PI-3-kinase p110γ gene in mice, which in contrast to the PI-3-kinase p110α and p110β genes is predominantly expressed in hematopoietic and muscle cells, leads to diminished atherosclerosis [78]. These observations highlight the complexity of insulin signaling at the level of the vasculature and demonstrate the potential disparity between systemic insulin resistance and its direct effects on the forming atherosclerotic lesion.

Emerging themes: the concept of "protective macrophages" in insulin resistance and atherosclerosis

The discovery of adipose tissue as a secretory organ, capable of producing inflammatory markers especially in states of nutrient excess/obesity, was an important step in understanding the initiation of insulin resistance. In the past few years, this concept has been advanced and refined by implicating specific cellular events in the obesity-insulin resistance link.

Immunohistochemical analysis of obesity-induced pathologic changes reveals a progressive accumulation of bone-marrow derived macrophages in the adipose tissue matrix over time [79,80]. These macrophages are the predominant source of adipose tissue TNFα production and a significant contributor to the production of IL-6 as well several other inflammatory markers [80]. Additionally, this macrophage infiltration is observed before overt manifestations of insulin resistance as determined by compensatory increases in insulin levels [79].

It has been known for some time that macrophages are present in numerous tissues even under normal noninflammatory conditions [81]. These resident macrophages are phenotypically different from the more familiar "classically activated"/M1-macrophages (ie, those elicited during acute inflammatory responses) and thus are termed "alternatively activated" or M2-macrophages. Whereas M1 macrophages are activated under inflammatory settings and express numerous proinflammatory markers, M2 macrophages are activated by different stimuli (eg, IL-4 and IL-13) and actually produce anti-inflammatory mediators (eg, IL-10 and IL-1 receptor antagonists) that are involved in tissue healing/remodeling and seem to oppose the effects of their M1 counterparts [82,83]. Interestingly, these observations were recently highlighted in adipose tissue. On a normal diet, the adipose tissue of lean mice is populated with "alternatively activated" macrophages, whereas diet-induced obesity produces a shift toward the M1 phenotype [84]. Curiously, this shift is abrogated in obese C-C motif chemokine receptor-2 (CCR2)-null mice, suggesting that loss of this monocyte chemoattractant receptor presumably disables the robust recruitment of proinflammatory macrophages [84]. This finding extends previous data showing the protective effect of MCP-1 and CCR-2 knockout mice in diet-induced insulin resistance [85,86].

Recently, Odegaard and colleagues [87] provided mechanistic insight into this phenotypic switch by demonstrating that PPARγ is required for the presence and maturation of alternatively activated macrophages in adipose tissue. Furthermore, their macrophage-specific PPARγ-KO mice were more prone to diet-induced obesity and insulin resistance [87]. Using a similar gene-targeting strategy, Hevener and colleagues [88] provided a different perspective on macrophage-specific PPARγ signaling, showing impaired hepatic and skeletal muscle insulin sensitivity, signaling, and lipid accumulation. Interestingly, the insulin-sensitizing effects of thiazolidinediones (TZDs) were only partially effective in these mice, indicating that macrophage PPARγ signaling is at least partially required to achieve the full effects of TZDs on insulin sensitivity [88].

There is also evidence that alternatively activated macrophages may be involved in atherosclerosis [89]. Both M1 and M2 markers are present in human atherosclerotic plaques and are produced by distinct pools of mononuclear cells in these plaques. Also, PPARγ activators such as TZDs are able to drive the differentiation of monocytes into an M2 phenotype, although they are neither able to increase plaque M2 markers nor able to cause a switch of M1 cells to an M2 phenotype [89]. Given the ability of macrophages to take on diametrically opposite fates, the prospect of harnessing such an ability to mitigate proatherogenic states is exciting. Another direct link between macrophages and adipocytes and inflammation has recently emerged in the form of the adipocyte-binding protein aP2 (also known as FABP4). Chemically inhibiting the function of aP2, a protein expressed in macrophages in addition to adipocytes, can suppress inflammatory pathways, decrease atherosclerosis, and treat type 2 diabetes in mice [90].

Insulin resistance, oxidative/mitochondrial stress, and atherosclerosis

Mitochondria are the major source of ATP production by harboring both the enzymes of the tricyclic acid cycle and oxidative phosphorylation. The continuous flow of electrons from complex I through IV of the electron transport chain and pumping of protons though the inner mitochondrial membrane is contingent on steady-state nutrient delivery. In cases of nutrient excess, the surplus of effluxed protons leads to slowed electron transport chain kinetics and augmentation of alternative electron accepting mechanisms [91]. Enhanced production of reactive oxygen species (ROS) such as superoxide is a direct by-product of this process and a contributing factor to vascular dysfunction in insulin resistance (see Fig. 2) [92].

As the predominant site of ROS production, the mitochondrion is a susceptible target for oxidative damage and several lines of evidence point to mitochondrial dysfunction in promoting atherogenesis. Studies in cell culture and rodent models show that increased free fatty acid oxidation in aortic endothelium induces enhanced mitochondrial superoxide generation and inactivation of anti-atherogenic factors (eg, eNOS and prostacyclin synthase); direct inhibition of carnitine palmitoyl transferase I (the rate-limiting mitochondrial enzyme in fatty acid oxidation) reverses this effect [93]. Atherosclerotic lesions from patients undergoing vascular surgery and those from ApoE-null mice show increased mitochondrial DNA damage; this process is observed even in young mice before the overt development of atherosclerotic plaques [94]. Additionally, superoxide dismutase heterozygous-null mice (SOD2±) in the ApoE(−/−) background have accelerated atherosclerosis [94]. In this regard, the fact that mitochondria lack a robust mismatch repair system might make mitochondrial DNA especially susceptible to ROS damage and mitochondrial dysfunction [95].

Another feature of mitochondrial bioenergetics relevant to atherosclerosis is the observed heterogeneity of metabolism in the vasculature (ie, different areas of an arterial wall have varied ATP-generating efficiency probably due to variable uncoupling of respiration and oxidative phosphorylation) [96]. Differences in adequate oxygen delivery to medium and large-size arteries have been proposed to underlie this heterogeneity [96,97]. Intriguingly, although respiratory uncoupling seems to occur in all blood vessels, it is increased in the aorta of atheroma-prone pigeons [98]. Also, a dearth of essential fatty acids, a marker of atherosclerotic lesions, heightens respiratory uncoupling [99,100].

The uncoupling proteins are a family of transporters found in the inner mitochondrial membrane that dissipate the mitochondrial proton-motive force by allowing protons back into the mitochondrial matrix [101]. In a direct test of the relationship between respiratory uncoupling and vascular dysfunction, Bernal-Mizrachi and colleagues [102] created smooth-muscle transgenic mice overexpressing uncoupling protein 1 (UCP1); the choice of smooth muscle cells as the site of uncoupling was based on smooth muscle being a major site for ROS production [91]. These "uncoupled" mice showed significant signs of vascular dysfunction with overt hypertension and when in an ApoE-null background, increased atherosclerosis [102]. Furthermore, superoxide production was elevated and NO availability was decreased.

Taken together, adiposity and insulin resistance create a state of nutrient excess, skewing normally functioning mitochondrial bioenergetics into excess ROS production and by respiratory uncoupling mechanisms, inefficient generation of ATP; the result is vascular dysfunction and a proatherogenic state. In this regard, it is interesting to note that caloric restriction can induce mitochondrial biogenesis, decrease ROS, and lead to more efficient ATP production [103,104].

Insulin resistance, genomic stress, and atherosclerosis

Damage to mitochondrial DNA is not the only consequence of excessive production of ROS; the nuclear genome is also susceptible to damage and alterations of relevant genes involved in DNA repair and stress response contribute to insulin resistance, vascular dysfunction, and atherosclerosis (reviewed in Ref. [105]). Patients with established CAD and diabetes have increased markers of genomic instability and oxidative DNA damage in peripheral blood mononuclear cells [106,107]. FISH analysis of human carotid endarterectomy (CEA) plaques shows chromosomal instability with polyploidy and deletions [108,109]. Markers of oxidative DNA damage such as 8-oxo-deoxyguanosine (8-oxo-dG) are elevated in CEA specimens and this is accompanied by overexpression of several DNA repair proteins [110]. Similarly, diet-induced atherosclerotic plaques in rabbits show increased 8-oxo-dG, DNA strand breaks, and DNA repair enzymes; these markers of DNA damage are significantly but not entirely reversed with normalization of the diet [111].

These data suggesting a causal link between DNA damage and atherosclerosis are corroborated by the phenotypes of several accelerated aging and/or DNA damage disorders [112]. Werner syndrome occurs because of mutations in the WRN gene, encoding a DNA helicase with several functions in DNA replication and repair [113]. In addition to premature aging, Werner patients develop insulin resistance, atherosclerosis, and valvular heart disease [112,114], a phenotype that is partially recapitulated in a mouse model of the disease [115]. Patients with Hutchinson-Gilford Progeria syndrome (HGPS), the prototypical accelerated aging syndrome, also develop insulin resistance and premature atherosclerosis but at even earlier time points than Werner patients and often succumb to MI or strokes by their early teenage years [116,117]. HGPS is caused by mutations in the Lamin A gene, encoding proteins essential for the integrity of the nuclear lamina/ nuclear membrane [117]. The disruption of nuclear lamina is not solely structural and is now known to affect transcriptional regulation, genomic stability, and DNA repair. Recent data show that HGPS patients accumulate a farnesylated precursor of Lamin A that likely imparts genomic instability by impairing formation of DNA repair foci [118,119]. A farnesyltransferase inhibitor can reverse many of the structural and phenotypic abnormalities of a mouse model of HGPS [120]. As statins are also inhibitors of the pathway important for farnesylation, this raises the intriguing possibility that part of the non–lipid-mediated effects of statins are directed at enhancing genomic stability. Another relevant human disease is Ataxia-Telangiectasia (AT), caused by mutations in ATM, a protein kinase with central roles in the response to DNA damage [121]. In addition to progressive ataxia and significant predisposition to cancers, many AT patients also develop insulin resistance [122,123]. Although AT patients die early from a variety of cancers (median age of death 20) [124], carriers of ATM mutations (estimated to comprise 1.4% to 2.0% of the population) have higher CV mortality [125]. In support of a direct pathogenic role for ATM in metabolic and vascular regulation, ATM-null mice in an ApoE-null background indeed develop insulin resistance and accelerated atherosclerosis [126]. Chloroquine, used to treat malaria but also a known activator of ATM, was able to protect against atherosclerosis and many of the metabolic effects of diet-induced insulin resistance in mouse models [126].

Summary

The metabolic syndrome and diabetes are in large part varied manifestations of an underlying process known as insulin resistance. Normally insulin sensitive metabolic organs develop a progressive inability to respond to this signal with resultant metabolic derangements. Cardiovascular disease is associated with insulin-resistant states, although the presence of a myriad of insulin-signaling pathways potentially affecting vascular function precludes a simple explanation for this association. Treatment of insulin-resistant patients with drugs such as statins, ACEi, and ARBs can yield profound improvements in CV mortality. The development of insulin sensitizers such as the thiazolidinediones has been conceptually exciting, but recent data showing lack of/modest benefit or possibly even an increase in CV events combined with a propensity to exacerbate heart failure have dampened enthusiasm for this class of drugs.

Insulin-resistant people tend to have increased adiposity, so novel strategies that exploit the relationship between adipocytes and the inflammatory process in the vasculature to treat atherosclerosis are attractive. Interfering with cellular stress pathways, including those that involve damage to mitochondria and the nuclear genome, may also prove to be useful in the quest for developing new approaches to treat atherosclerosis in people with insulin resistance.

References

[1] Falta WA. Uber Einen Insulinrefraktaren fall von diabetes mellitus. Klinische Wochenschrift 1924;3:1315–7.
[2] Levinson PD. Eighty years of insulin therapy: 1922–2002. Med Health R I 2003;86(4): 101–6.
[3] Executive Summary of the Third Report of the National Cholesterol Education Program (NCEP) Expert Panel on Detection, Evaluation, and Treatment of High Blood Cholesterol in Adults (Adult Treatment Panel III). JAMA 2001;285(19):2486–97.
[4] Alberti KG, Zimmet P, Shaw J. Metabolic syndrome—a new world-wide definition. A consensus statement from the International Diabetes Federation. Diabet Med 2006;23(5): 469–80.
[5] Grundy SM, Cleeman JI, Daniels SR, et al. Diagnosis and management of the metabolic syndrome: an American Heart Association/National Heart, Lung, and Blood Institute Scientific Statement. Circulation 2005;112(17):2735–52.
[6] Haffner SM, Lehto S, Ronnemaa T, et al. Mortality from coronary heart disease in subjects with type 2 diabetes and in nondiabetic subjects with and without prior myocardial infarction. N Engl J Med 1998;339(4):229–34.
[7] Stamler J, Vaccaro O, Neaton JD, et al. Diabetes, other risk factors, and 12-yr cardiovascular mortality for men screened in the Multiple Risk Factor Intervention Trial. Diabetes Care 1993;16(2):434–44.
[8] Kannel WB, McGee DL. Diabetes and cardiovascular risk factors: the Framingham study. Circulation 1979;59(1):8–13.
[9] Vaccaro O, Eberly LE, Neaton JD, et al. Impact of diabetes and previous myocardial infarction on long-term survival: 25-year mortality follow-up of primary screenees of the Multiple Risk Factor Intervention Trial. Arch Intern Med 2004;164(13):1438–43.
[10] Alexander CM, Landsman PB, Teutsch SM, et al. NCEP-defined metabolic syndrome, diabetes, and prevalence of coronary heart disease among NHANES III participants age 50 years and older. Diabetes 2003;52(5):1210–4.
[11] Hunt KJ, Resendez RG, Williams K, et al. National Cholesterol Education Program versus World Health Organization metabolic syndrome in relation to all-cause and cardiovascular mortality in the San Antonio Heart Study. Circulation 2004;110(10):1251–7.
[12] Sattar N, Gaw A, Scherbakova O, et al. Metabolic syndrome with and without C-reactive protein as a predictor of coronary heart disease and diabetes in the West of Scotland Coronary Prevention Study. Circulation 2003;108(4):414–9.
[13] Randomised trial of cholesterol lowering in 4444 patients with coronary heart disease: the Scandinavian Simvastatin Survival Study (4S). Lancet 1994;344(8934):1383–9.
[14] Shepherd J, Cobbe SM, Ford I, et al. Prevention of coronary heart disease with pravastatin in men with hypercholesterolemia. West of Scotland Coronary Prevention Study Group. N Engl J Med 1995;333(20):1301–7.
[15] Collins R, Armitage J, Parish S, et al. Effects of cholesterol lowering with simvastatin on stroke and other major vascular events in 20,536 people with cerebrovascular disease or other high-risk conditions. Lancet 2004;363(9411):757–67.

[16] Ray KK, Cannon CP. The potential relevance of the multiple lipid-independent (pleiotropic) effects of statins in the management of acute coronary syndromes. J Am Coll Cardiol 2005; 46(8):1425–33.

[17] Yusuf S, Pepine CJ, Garces C, et al. Effect of enalapril on myocardial infarction and unstable angina in patients with low ejection fractions. Lancet 1992;340(8829):1173–8.

[18] Pfeffer MA, Braunwald E, Moye LA, et al. Effect of captopril on mortality and morbidity in patients with left ventricular dysfunction after myocardial infarction. Results of the survival and ventricular enlargement trial. The SAVE Investigators. N Engl J Med 1992; 327(10):669–77.

[19] Yusuf S, Sleight P, Pogue J, et al. Effects of an angiotensin-converting-enzyme inhibitor, ramipril, on cardiovascular events in high-risk patients. The Heart Outcomes Prevention Evaluation Study Investigators. N Engl J Med 2000;342(3):145–53.

[20] Lindholm LH, Ibsen H, Dahlof B, et al. Cardiovascular morbidity and mortality in patients with diabetes in the losartan intervention for endpoint reduction in hypertension study (LIFE): a randomised trial against atenolol. Lancet 2002;359(9311):1004–10.

[21] Lehmann JM, Moore LB, Smith-Oliver TA, et al. An antidiabetic thiazolidinedione is a high affinity ligand for peroxisome proliferator-activated receptor gamma (PPAR gamma). J Biol Chem 1995;270(22):12953–6.

[22] Yki-Jarvinen H. Thiazolidinediones. N Engl J Med 2004;351(11):1106–18.

[23] Nissen SE, Wolski K. Effect of rosiglitazone on the risk of myocardial infarction and death from cardiovascular causes. N Engl J Med 2007;356(24):2457–71.

[24] Dormandy JA, Charbonnel B, Eckland DJ, et al. Secondary prevention of macrovascular events in patients with type 2 diabetes in the PROactive Study (PROspective pioglitAzone Clinical Trial In macroVascular Events): a randomised controlled trial. Lancet 2005; 366(9493):1279–89.

[25] Lincoff AM, Wolski K, Nicholls SJ, et al. Pioglitazone and risk of cardiovascular events in patients with type 2 diabetes mellitus: a meta-analysis of randomized trials. JAMA 2007; 298(10):1180–8.

[26] Lago RM, Singh PP, Nesto RW. Congestive heart failure and cardiovascular death in patients with prediabetes and type 2 diabetes given thiazolidinediones: a meta-analysis of randomised clinical trials. Lancet 2007;370(9593):1129–36.

[27] Szapary PO, Rader DJ. The triglyceride-high-density lipoprotein axis: an important target of therapy? Am Heart J 2004;148(2):211–21.

[28] McGarry JD. What if Minkowski had been ageusic? An alternative angle on diabetes. Science 1992;258(5083):766–70.

[29] Ginsberg HN. REVIEW: efficacy and mechanisms of action of statins in the treatment of diabetic dyslipidemia. J Clin Endocrinol Metab 2006;91(2):383–92.

[30] Adiels M, Boren J, Caslake MJ, et al. Overproduction of VLDL1 driven by hyperglycemia is a dominant feature of diabetic dyslipidemia. Arterioscler Thromb Vasc Biol 2005;25(8): 1697–703.

[31] Sparks JD, Sparks CE. Insulin regulation of triacylglycerol-rich lipoprotein synthesis and secretion. Biochim Biophys Acta 1994;1215(1–2):9–32.

[32] Ninomiya JK, L'Italien G, Criqui MH, et al. Association of the metabolic syndrome with history of myocardial infarction and stroke in the Third National Health and Nutrition Examination Survey. Circulation 2004;109(1):42–6.

[33] Bansal S, Buring JE, Rifai N, et al. Fasting compared with nonfasting triglycerides and risk of cardiovascular events in women. JAMA 2007;298(3):309–16.

[34] Nordestgaard BG, Benn M, Schnohr P, et al. Nonfasting triglycerides and risk of myocardial infarction, ischemic heart disease, and death in men and women. JAMA 2007;298(3):299–308.

[35] Sattar N, Williams K, Sniderman AD, et al. Comparison of the associations of apolipoprotein B and non-high-density lipoprotein cholesterol with other cardiovascular risk factors in patients with the metabolic syndrome in the Insulin Resistance Atherosclerosis Study. Circulation 2004;110(17):2687–93.

[36] Austin MA, King MC, Vranizan KM, et al. Atherogenic lipoprotein phenotype. A pro-posed genetic marker for coronary heart disease risk. Circulation 1990;82(2):495–506.

[37] Rashid S, Watanabe T, Sakaue T, et al. Mechanisms of HDL lowering in insulin resistant, hypertriglyceridemic states: the combined effect of HDL triglyceride enrichment and elevated hepatic lipase activity. Clin Biochem 2003;36(6):421–9.

[38] Golay A, Zech L, Shi MZ, et al. High density lipoprotein (HDL) metabolism in noninsulin-dependent diabetes mellitus: measurement of HDL turnover using tritiated HDL. J Clin Endocrinol Metab 1987;65(3):512–8.

[39] Festa A, D'Agostino R Jr, Howard G, et al. Chronic subclinical inflammation as part of the insulin resistance syndrome: the Insulin Resistance Atherosclerosis Study (IRAS). Circula-tion 2000;102(1):42–7.

[40] Shoelson SE, Lee J, Goldfine AB. Inflammation and insulin resistance. J Clin Invest 2006; 116(7):1793–801.

[41] Ross R. Atherosclerosis—an inflammatory disease. N Engl J Med 1999;340(2):115–26.

[42] Hotamisligil GS, Shargill NS, Spiegelman BM. Adipose expression of tumor necrosis factor-alpha: direct role in obesity-linked insulin resistance. Science 1993;259(5091):87–91.

[43] Lau DC, Dhillon B, Yan H, et al. Adipokines: molecular links between obesity and athe-roslcerosis. Am J Physiol Heart Circ Physiol 2005;288(5):H2031–41.

[44] Roytblat L, Rachinsky M, Fisher A, et al. Raised interleukin-6 levels in obese patients. Obes Res 2000;8(9):673–5.

[45] Hotamisligil GS, Arner P, Caro JF, et al. Increased adipose tissue expression of tumor necrosis factor-alpha in human obesity and insulin resistance. J Clin Invest 1995;95(5): 2409–15.

[46] Esposito K, Pontillo A, Di Palo C, et al. Effect of weight loss and lifestyle changes on vascular inflammatory markers in obese women: a randomized trial. JAMA 2003; 289(14):1799–804.

[47] Festa A, D'Agostino R Jr, Tracy RP, et al. Elevated levels of acute-phase proteins and plasminogen activator inhibitor-1 predict the development of type 2 diabetes: the Insulin Resistance Atherosclerosis Study. Diabetes 2002;51(4):1131–7.

[48] Christiansen T, Richelsen B, Bruun JM. Monocyte chemoattractant protein-1 is produced in isolated adipocytes, associated with adiposity and reduced after weight loss in morbid obese subjects. Int J Obes (Lond) 2005;29(1):146–50.

[49] Schwartz EA, Reaven PD. Molecular and signaling mechanisms of atherosclerosis in insulin resistance. Endocrinol Metab Clin North Am. 2006;35(3):525–49, viii.

[50] Baldwin AS Jr. The NF-kappa B and I kappa B proteins: new discoveries and insights. Annu Rev Immunol 1996;14:649–83.

[51] Karin M. The beginning of the end: IkappaB kinase (IKK) and NF-kappaB activation. J Biol Chem 1999;274(39):27339–42.

[52] Thurberg BL, Collins T. The nuclear factor-kappa B/inhibitor of kappa B autoregulatory system and atherosclerosis. Curr Opin Lipidol 1998;9(5):387–96.

[53] Kempe S, Kestler H, Lasar A, et al. NF-kappaB controls the global pro-inflammatory response in endothelial cells: evidence for the regulation of a pro-atherogenic program. Nucleic Acids Res 2005;33(16):5308–19.

[54] Schreyer SA, Peschon JJ, LeBoeuf RC. Accelerated atherosclerosis in mice lacking tumor necrosis factor receptor p55. J Biol Chem 1996;271(42):26174–8.

[55] Kanters E, Pasparakis M, Gijbels MJ, et al. Inhibition of NF-kappaB activation in macro-phages increases atherosclerosis in LDL receptor-deficient mice. J Clin Invest 2003;112(8): 1176–85.

[56] Kanters E, Gijbels MJ, van der Made I, et al. Hematopoietic NF-kappaB1 deficiency results in small atherosclerotic lesions with an inflammatory phenotype. Blood 2004;103(3): 934–40.

[57] Kyriakis JM, Avruch J. Mammalian mitogen-activated protein kinase signal transduction pathways activated by stress and inflammation. Physiol Rev 2001;81(2):807–69.

[58] Sumara G, Belwal M, Ricci R. "Jnking" atherosclerosis. Cell Mol Life Sci 2005;62(21): 2487–94.

[59] Ventura JJ, Kennedy NJ, Lamb JA, et al. c-Jun NH(2)-terminal kinase is essential for the regulation of AP-1 by tumor necrosis factor. Mol Cell Biol 2003;23(8):2871–82.

[60] Manning AM, Davis RJ. Targeting JNK for therapeutic benefit: from junk to gold? Nat Rev Drug Discov 2003;2(7):554–65.

[61] Nishio H, Matsui K, Tsuji H, et al. Immunohistochemical study of the phosphorylated and activated form of c-Jun NH2-terminal kinase in human aorta. Histochem J 2001;33(3): 167–71.

[62] Metzler B, Hu Y, Dietrich H, et al. Increased expression and activation of stress-activated protein kinases/c-Jun NH(2)-terminal protein kinases in atherosclerotic lesions coincide with p53. Am J Pathol 2000;156(6):1875–86.

[63] Ricci R, Sumara G, Sumara I, et al. Requirement of JNK2 for scavenger receptor A-mediated foam cell formation in atherogenesis. Science 2004;306(5701):1558–61.

[64] Hartge MM, Kintscher U, Unger T. Endothelial dysfunction and its role in diabetic vascular disease. Endocrinol Metab Clin North Am 2006;35(3):551–60, viii-ix.

[65] Hsueh WA, Quinones MJ. Role of endothelial dysfunction in insulin resistance. Am J Cardiol 2003;92(4A):10J–7J.

[66] Williams SB, Cusco JA, Roddy MA, et al. Impaired nitric oxide-mediated vasodilation in patients with non-insulin-dependent diabetes mellitus. J Am Coll Cardiol 1996;27(3): 567–74.

[67] Steinberg HO, Tarshoby M, Monestel R, et al. Elevated circulating free fatty acid levels impair endothelium-dependent vasodilation. J Clin Invest 1997;100(5):1230–9.

[68] Perticone F, Ceravolo R, Candigliota M, et al. Obesity and body fat distribution induce endothelial dysfunction by oxidative stress: protective effect of vitamin C. Diabetes 2001; 50(1):159–65.

[69] Scherrer U, Randin D, Vollenweider P, et al. Nitric oxide release accounts for insulin's vascular effects in humans. J Clin Invest 1994;94(6):2511–5.

[70] Montagnani M, Ravichandran LV, Chen H, et al. Insulin receptor substrate-1 and phosphoinositide-dependent kinase-1 are required for insulin-stimulated production of nitric oxide in endothelial cells. Mol Endocrinol 2002;16(8):1931–42.

[71] Zeng G, Nystrom FH, Ravichandran LV, et al. Roles for insulin receptor, PI3-kinase, and Akt in insulin-signaling pathways related to production of nitric oxide in human vascular endothelial cells. Circulation 2000;101(13):1539–45.

[72] Takeda K, Ichiki T, Tokunou T, et al. Critical role of Rho-kinase and MEK/ERK pathways for angiotensin II-induced plasminogen activator inhibitor type-1 gene expression. Arterioscler Thromb Vasc Biol 2001;21(5):868–73.

[73] Jiang ZY, Lin YW, Clemont A, et al. Characterization of selective resistance to insulin signaling in the vasculature of obese Zucker (fa/fa) rats. J Clin Invest 1999;104(4):447–57.

[74] Montagnani M, Golovchenko I, Kim I, et al. Inhibition of phosphatidylinositol 3-kinase enhances mitogenic actions of insulin in endothelial cells. J Biol Chem 2002;277(3):1794–9.

[75] Gual P, Gremeaux T, Gonzalez T, et al. MAP kinases and mTOR mediate insulin-induced phosphorylation of insulin receptor substrate-1 on serine residues 307, 612 and 632. Diabetologia 2003;46(11):1532–42.

[76] Baumgartl J, Baudler S, Scherner M, et al. Myeloid lineage cell-restricted insulin resistance protects apolipoproteinE-deficient mice against atherosclerosis. Cell Metab 2006;3(4): 247–56.

[77] Han S, Liang CP, DeVries-Seimon T, et al. Macrophage insulin receptor deficiency increases ER stress-induced apoptosis and necrotic core formation in advanced atherosclerotic lesions. Cell Metab 2006;3(4):257–66.

[78] Chang JD, Sukhova GK, Libby P, et al. Deletion of the phosphoinositide 3-kinase p110gamma gene attenuates murine atherosclerosis. Proc Natl Acad Sci U S A 2007; 104(19):8077–82.

[79] Xu H, Barnes GT, Yang Q, et al. Chronic inflammation in fat plays a crucial role in the development of obesity-related insulin resistance. J Clin Invest 2003;112(12):1821–30.

[80] Weisberg SP, McCann D, Desai M, et al. Obesity is associated with macrophage accumulation in adipose tissue. J Clin Invest 2003;112(12):1796–808.

[81] Geissmann F, Jung S, Littman DR. Blood monocytes consist of two principal subsets with distinct migratory properties. Immunity 2003;19(1):71–82.

[82] Gordon S. Alternative activation of macrophages. Nat Rev Immunol 2003;3(1):23–35.

[83] Gordon S, Taylor PR. Monocyte and macrophage heterogeneity. Nat Rev Immunol 2005; 5(12):953–64.

[84] Lumeng CN, Bodzin JL, Saltiel AR. Obesity induces a phenotypic switch in adipose tissue macrophage polarization. J Clin Invest 2007;117(1):175–84.

[85] Kanda H, Tateya S, Tamori Y, et al. MCP-1 contributes to macrophage infiltration into adipose tissue, insulin resistance, and hepatic steatosis in obesity. J Clin Invest 2006; 116(6):1494–505.

[86] Weisberg SP, Hunter D, Huber R, et al. CCR2 modulates inflammatory and metabolic effects of high-fat feeding. J Clin Invest 2006;116(1):115–24.

[87] Odegaard JI, Ricardo-Gonzalez RR, Goforth MH, et al. Macrophage-specific PPAR-gamma controls alternative activation and improves insulin resistance. Nature 2007; 447(7148):1116–20.

[88] Hevener AL, Olefsky JM, Reichart D, et al. Macrophage PPAR gamma is required for normal skeletal muscle and hepatic insulin sensitivity and full antidiabetic effects of thiazolidinediones. J Clin Invest 2007;117(6):1658–69.

[89] Bouhlel MA, Derudas B, Rigamonti E, et al. PPARgamma activation primes human monocytes into alternative M2 macrophages with anti-inflammatory properties. Cell Metab 2007;6(2):137–43.

[90] Furuhashi M, Tuncman G, Gorgun CZ, et al. Treatment of diabetes and atherosclerosis by inhibiting fatty-acid-binding protein aP2. Nature 2007;447(7147):959–65.

[91] Droge W. Free radicals in the physiological control of cell function. Physiol Rev 2002;82(1): 47–95.

[92] Brownlee M. The pathobiology of diabetic complications: a unifying mechanism. Diabetes 2005;54(6):1615–25.

[93] Du X, Edelstein D, Obici S, et al. Insulin resistance reduces arterial prostacyclin synthase and eNOS activities by increasing endothelial fatty acid oxidation. J Clin Invest 2006; 116(4):1071–80.

[94] Ballinger SW, Patterson C, Knight-Lozano CA, et al. Mitochondrial integrity and function in atherogenesis. Circulation 2002;106(5):544–9.

[95] Mason PA, Matheson EC, Hall AG, et al. Mismatch repair activity in mammalian mitochondria. Nucleic Acids Res 2003;31(3):1052–8.

[96] Levin M, Leppanen O, Evaldsson M, et al. Mapping of ATP, glucose, glycogen, and lactate concentrations within the arterial wall. Arterioscler Thromb Vasc Biol 2003;23(10): 1801–7.

[97] Bjornheden T, Levin M, Evaldsson M, et al. Evidence of hypoxic areas within the arterial wall in vivo. Arterioscler Thromb Vasc Biol 1999;19(4):870–6.

[98] Santerre RF, Nicolosi RJ, Smith SC. Respiratory control in preatherosclerotic susceptible and resistant pigeon aortas. Exp Mol Pathol 1974;20(3):397–406.

[99] Klein PD, Johnson RM. Phosphorus metabolism in unsaturated fatty acid-deficient rats. J Biol Chem 1954;211(1):103–10.

[100] Cornwell DG, Panganamala RV. Atherosclerosis: an intracellular deficiency in essential fatty acids. Prog Lipid Res 1981;20:365–76.

[101] Echtay KS. Mitochondrial uncoupling proteins—What is their physiological role? Free Radic Biol Med 2007;43(10):1351–71.

[102] Bernal-Mizrachi C, Gates AC, Weng S, et al. Vascular respiratory uncoupling increases blood pressure and atherosclerosis. Nature 2005;435(7041):502–6.

[103] Lopez-Lluch G, Hunt N, Jones B, et al. Calorie restriction induces mitochondrial biogenesis and bioenergetic efficiency. Proc Natl Acad Sci U S A 2006;103(6):1768–73.

[104] Nisoli E, Tonello C, Cardile A, et al. Calorie restriction promotes mitochondrial biogenesis by inducing the expression of eNOS. Science 2005;310(5746):314–7.

[105] Mahmoudi M, Mercer J, Bennett M. DNA damage and repair in atherosclerosis. Cardiovasc Res 2006;71(2):259–68.

[106] Botto N, Rizza A, Colombo MG, et al. Evidence for DNA damage in patients with coronary artery disease. Mutat Res 2001;493(1-2):23–30.

[107] Botto N, Masetti S, Petrozzi L, et al. Elevated levels of oxidative DNA damage in patients with coronary artery disease. Coron Artery Dis 2002;13(5):269–74.

[108] Matturri L, Cazzullo A, Turconi P, et al. Chromosomal alterations in atherosclerotic plaques. Atherosclerosis 2001;154(3):755–61.

[109] Casalone R, Granata P, Minelli E, et al. Cytogenetic analysis reveals clonal proliferation of smooth muscle cells in atherosclerotic plaques. Hum Genet 1991;87(2):139–43.

[110] Martinet W, Knaapen MW, De Meyer GR, et al. Elevated levels of oxidative DNA damage and DNA repair enzymes in human atherosclerotic plaques. Circulation 2002;106(8): 927–32.

[111] Martinet W, Knaapen MW, De Meyer GR, et al. Oxidative DNA damage and repair in experimental atherosclerosis are reversed by dietary lipid lowering. Circ Res 2001;88(7): 733–9.

[112] Capell BC, Collins FS, Nabel EG. Mechanisms of cardiovascular disease in accelerated aging syndromes. Circ Res 2007;101(1):13–26.

[113] Gray MD, Shen JC, Kamath-Loeb AS, et al. The Werner syndrome protein is a DNA helicase. Nat Genet 1997;17(1):100–3.

[114] Yamada K, Ikegami H, Yoneda H, et al. All patients with Werner's syndrome are insulin resistant, but only those who also have impaired insulin secretion develop overt diabetes. Diabetes Care 1999;22(12):2094–5.

[115] Massip L, Garand C, Turaga RV, et al. Increased insulin, triglycerides, reactive oxygen species, and cardiac fibrosis in mice with a mutation in the helicase domain of the Werner syndrome gene homologue. Exp Gerontol 2006;41(2):157–68.

[116] DeBusk FL. The Hutchinson-Gilford progeria syndrome. Report of 4 cases and review of the literature. J Pediatr 1972;80(4):697–724.

[117] Eriksson M, Brown WT, Gordon LB, et al. Recurrent de novo point mutations in lamin A cause Hutchinson-Gilford progeria syndrome. Nature 2003;423(6937):293–8.

[118] Liu Y, Rusinol A, Sinensky M, et al. DNA damage responses in progeroid syndromes arise from defective maturation of prelamin A. J Cell Sci 2006;119(Pt 22):4644–9.

[119] Manju K, Muralikrishna B, Parnaik VK. Expression of disease-causing lamin A mutants impairs the formation of DNA repair foci. J Cell Sci 2006;119(Pt 13):2704–14.

[120] Fong LG, Frost D, Meta M, et al. A protein farnesyltransferase inhibitor ameliorates disease in a mouse model of progeria. Science 2006;311(5767):1621–3.

[121] Savitsky K, Bar-Shira A, Gilad S, et al. A single ataxia telangiectasia gene with a product similar to PI-3 kinase. Science 1995;268(5218):1749–53.

[122] Schalch DS, McFarlin DE, Barlow MH. An unusual form of diabetes mellitus in ataxia telangiectasia. N Engl J Med 1970;282(25):1396–402.

[123] Bar RS, Levis WR, Rechler MM, et al. Extreme insulin resistance in ataxia telangiectasia: defect in affinity of insulin receptors. N Engl J Med 1978;298(21):1164–71.

[124] Morrell D, Cromartie E, Swift M. Mortality and cancer incidence in 263 patients with ataxia-telangiectasia. J Natl Cancer Inst 1986;77(1):89–92.

[125] Su Y, Swift M. Mortality rates among carriers of ataxia-telangiectasia mutant alleles. Ann Intern Med 2000;133(10):770–8.

[126] Schneider JG, Finck BN, Ren J, et al. ATM-dependent suppression of stress signaling reduces vascular disease in metabolic syndrome. Cell Metab 2006;4(5):377–89.

ELSEVIER
SAUNDERS

Endocrinol Metab Clin N Am
37 (2008) 623–633

ENDOCRINOLOGY
AND METABOLISM
CLINICS
OF NORTH AMERICA

Obesity and Dyslipidemia

Remco Franssen, MD, Houshang Monajemi, MD,
Erik S.G. Stroes, MD, PhD,
John J.P. Kastelein, MD, PhD*

*Department of Vascular Medicine, Academic Medical Center, Meibergdreef 9,
Room F4-159.2, 1105 AZ, Amsterdam, The Netherlands*

Cardiovascular (CV) disease is a major cause of mortality worldwide. Traditional risk factors for cardiovascular disease are smoking, hypertension, dyslipidemia, hyperinsulinemia, and obesity. Because these risk factors tend to cluster and most patients have multiple risk factors, the term "metabolic syndrome" has been introduced. Although the precise cause, definition, and additional CV risk of the metabolic syndrome are still under debate, in 2001 the National Cholesterol Education Program Adult Treatment Panel III defined the metabolic syndrome as an independent risk factor for atherosclerosis [1]. Currently, three different definitions are being used to classify the metabolic syndrome. Recently, the International Diabetes Foundation has added yet another classification to the available options, in which waist circumference can be corrected for ethnicity [2,3]. During the last 2 decades, there has been an unprecedented increase in the prevalence of obesity, as well as the metabolic syndrome, closely associated with an increased CV risk. The prevalence of obesity (body mass index or BMI $\geq$ 30 kg/m^2) in the United States now exceeds 30%, which makes obesity a leading public health problem [4]. The United States has the highest rates of obesity worldwide. From 1980 to 2002, obesity prevalence has doubled in adults and, even more compelling, overweight prevalence has tripled in children and adolescents [5]. The prevalence of overweight adolescence in 2000 was 16.7% in boys and 15.4% in girls; based on these data it is predicted that by 2020 30% to 37% of adolescent boys and 34% to 44% of adolescent girls will be overweight. Based on the current child obesity numbers in the United States, it

---

* Corresponding author.
E-mail address: j.j.kastelein@amc.uva.nl (J.J.P. Kastelein).

0889-8529/08/$ - see front matter © 2008 Elsevier Inc. All rights reserved.
doi:10.1016/j.ecl.2008.06.003

is speculated that by 2035 the prevalence of chronic heart disease (CHD) will increase by a range of 5% to 16% [6]. Not only in the United States but also in socioeconomic upcoming countries, such as India and Poland, childhood obesity is already progressing rapidly [7].

The dyslipidemia associated with obesity predicts the majority of the increased CV risk seen in obese subjects. The dyslipidemic phenotype, commonly associated with obesity, is characterized by increased triglyceride (TG) levels, decreased high-density lipoproteins (HDL) levels, and a shift in low-density lipoproteins (LDL) to a more pro-atherogenic composition (small dense LDL). Whereas all components of the obesity-associated dyslipidemia have been linked with increased CV risk, low HDL has emerged as one of the most potent risk factors. The strong inverse relationship between HDL-cholesteral (HDL-c) levels and the incidence of CV disease has been substantiated in numerous large observational studies. Even if LDL-c levels are lowered to levels below 70 mg-dl, low HDL-c is still associated with a clearly increased CV disease risk [8]. This potent atheroprotective effect of HDL is traditionally attributed to the role of HDL-c in the reverse cholesterol transport (RCT) pathway, resulting in cholesterol transport from peripheral tissues to the liver followed by excretion in the feces. In the last decade, a wide variety of additional protective effects have been attributed to HDL, comprising inhibition of thrombosis, oxidation, and inflammation [9]. However, low HDL-c is not the only important lipid disorder associated with obesity. High-fasting TGs have also been shown to have independent predictive value for CV risk [10–12]. Although it has proven difficult to dissect the effects mediated by high TGs per se from those conveyed by the concomitant low HDL-c, TGs are shown to convey increased CV risk even after adjusting for HDL-c levels. In a meta-analysis of 21 population-based prospective studies involving a total of 65,863 men and 11,089 women [13], investigators found that each 1-mmol/L (89-mg/dL) TG increase was associated with a 32% increase in CHD risk in men (relative risk or RR = 1.30; 95% confidence interval or CI, 1.25–1.35) and a 76% increase in women (RR = 1.69; 95% CI, 1.45–1.97). After adjustment for total cholesterol, LDL-c, HDL-c, BMI, blood pressure, and diabetes, the increase in CHD risk associated with each 1-mmol/L increase in TG remained statistically significant: 12% in men (RR = 1.12; 95% CI, 1.06–1.19) and 37% in women (RR = 1.37; 95% CI, 1.13–1.66). Of note, subjects with high TG are invariably characterized by a shift toward small dense LDL. Numerous studies have pointed toward a particular proatherogenic impact of these small dense LDLs. These particles are more likely to be glycosylated and oxidized and, therefore, important in the initiating process of atherosclerosis [14].

This article focuses on the mechanisms involved in the development of the pro-atherogenic lipid changes associated with obesity. Therefore, it is necessary to first briefly describe normal lipid metabolism before focusing on the obesity associated abnormalities.

Normal lipid metabolism

Cholesterol and TGs are both essential for membrane integrity and structure, but also serve as an energy source as well as signaling molecules. Because they are water-insoluble, cholesterol and TGs have to be transported in special water-soluble particles, such as lipoproteins. Triglyceride-rich lipoproteins are secreted in the circulation either by the gut (as chylomicrons) or by the liver (as very low-density lipoprotein [VLDL]) (Fig. 1). After a meal, dietary TGs are first digested by pancreatic lipase before they can be absorbed by the intestine and transported into the circulation as chylomicrons. These particles transport the TGs to target tissues, adipose tissue and muscle, where they can be hydrolyzed by the enzyme lipoprotein lipase (LPL) located on the endothelial surface. Upon hydrolysis of TGs, nonesterified fatty acids (NEFA) are formed, which can be taken up by adipose tissue for storage or by skeletal muscle for use as an energy source. The LPL involved in this process is mainly produced by adipose tissue and muscle itself, and its synthesis and function are under strict control of insulin. This control mechanism through insulin results in activation of LPL in adipose tissue, with a concomitant decrease in LPL activity in muscle during the fed state [15,16]. During the fasted state, when the body relies on fatty acids as an energy source, the hormone glucagon signals the breakdown of TGs by hormone-sensitive lipase (HSL) to release NEFA.

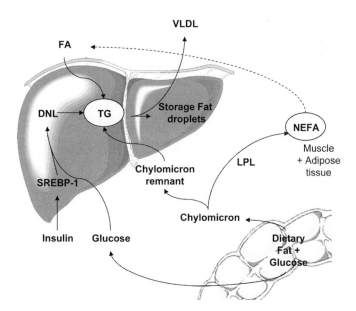

Fig. 1. Schematic representation of normal triglyceride metabolism. DNL, de novo lipogenesis; FA, fatty acids; LPL, lipoprotein lipase; NEFA, nonesterified fatty acids; SREBP1, sterol regulatory element binding protein.

The liver itself is also able to produce TGs from fatty acids and glycerol, also under the influence of insulin. These TGs are then secreted into the blood as VLDL. The fatty acids used by the liver for TG formation are either derived from the plasma or newly formed within the liver by a process called de novo lipogenesis (DNL). In DNL, glucose serves as a substrate for fatty acid synthesis. The uptake of fatty acids in the liver from the plasma is uncontrolled and driven by free fatty acid (FFA) plasma levels. If the liver is taking up more fatty acids than it can use in the VLDL formation and excretion, these surplus fatty acids will be stored in the liver in the form of fat droplets. Through the study of these processes, part of the problem with surplus dietary intake becomes immediately clear: more dietary TGs (chylomicrons), fatty acids, and glucose (source for VLDL) intake can promote liver fat accumulation. Besides up-regulating LPL and stimulation of gene expression of multiple intracellular lipogenic enzymes, insulin controls the uptake and processing of NEFA in adipose tissue and muscle during the fed state. Insulin also acts in the liver on the sterol regulatory element binding protein (SREBP) 1-c, a protein located on hepatocyte cell membranes which transcriptionally activates most genes involved in DNL [17].

Obesity-associated dyslipidemia

The unraveling of the metabolic mechanisms underlying these proatherogenic lipid changes has made large strides in the last decade. In fact, the lipid changes associated with obesity are similar to those seen in patients with type-2 diabetes or insulin resistance (IR) [18]. Insulin resistance itself is a hallmark of the metabolic syndrome, and has a profound impact on the lipid profiles seen in patients suffering from the syndrome [19]. The presence of IR has also been shown to precede the onset of dyslipidemia in most obese individuals.

In the IR state, a reduced efficiency of insulin to inhibit hepatic glucose production and stimulate glucose use in skeletal muscle and adipose tissue leads to hyperglycemia and a subsequent compensatory hyperinsulinemia [19]. In IR, insulin is also no longer capable of inhibiting TG-lipolysis by HSL in fat stores [20,21]. As a consequence, the flux of FFAs to the liver increases profoundly, and this will contribute to increased fat accumulation within the liver. Unfortunately, the IR also results in impaired activation of LPL within the vasculature, contributing to a further increase in circulating TG levels. Thus, in the IR state the responses of both LPL and HSL are blunted and the resulting inefficient trapping of dietary energy will produce a postprandial lipemia and an increase in NEFA, as is seen in both obesity and hyperinsulinemia. This increase in NEFA will result in an increased NEFA flux to tissues, like the liver and muscle, during the fed state. The liver will be the major recipient of this increased flux because of the uncontrolled plasma level-driven uptake. To maintain TG homeostasis, VLDL production is increased in the liver, particularly large VLDL1 particles [22], as is also observed in obese- and IR patients [23]. When plasma NEFA are raised in normal individuals, VLDL secretion will increase [24]. The formation and excretion of VLDL is then the consequential rate-limiting step and the newly synthesized, but not excreted surplus TGs, will therefore be stored as lipid droplets in the liver that ultimately might lead to nonalcoholic fatty liver disease (NAFLD) [25]. NAFLD has numerous causes, but is often encountered in patients with obesity or other components of the metabolic syndrome. The prevalence of NAFLD increases to 74% in obese and up to 90% in morbidly obese individuals [26,27].

Even when these changes in peripheral energy metabolism caused by IR are not sufficient to disturb lipid profiles and increase liver fat content, hyperinsulinemia per se is also capable of stimulating DNL in the liver through activation of the previously described SREBP-1 pathway. And the hyperglycemia resulting from the IR can also stimulate lipogenesis directly by activation of the carbohydrate response element-binding protein, which in its turn activates the transcription of numerous genes also involved in DNL [28].

Lipid composition in obesity

These changes will also have a dramatic impact on the lipid composition and levels of, for instance, HDL-c particles, that are (besides hypertriglyceridemia) commonly low in both obesity and hyperinsulinemia. The increased assembly, secretion, and decreased clearance of VLDL, and the resulting hypertriglyceridemia, all contribute to lower HDL-c levels. This results partly from the decreased flux of apolipoproteins and phospholipids from chylomicrons and VLDL particles, which are normally used in HDL-c maturation [15]. The enzyme cholesteryl ester transfer protein (CETP), the mass of which and activity are found to be increased in obese patients, also contributes to the decreased HDL-c levels through facilitating transfer of cholesteryl esters from HDL to TG-rich lipoproteins (chylomicrons, VLDL) [29]. CETP is also secreted by adipose tissue, which is thought of as an important source of plasma CETP in human beings [30,31]. This cholesteryl ester transfer decreases HDL-c levels but also creates a TG-rich HDL that serves as a better substrate for clearance by hepatic lipase [32–34]. Increased CETP mass and activity also cause the shift that is observed in the LDL composition in obesity. Because of the increased VLDL pool size and delayed particle clearance, an induction of cholesteryl ester exchange in LDL takes place for TGs in VLDL. These LDL particles enriched with TGs are similarly like HDL-c, a better substrate for lipolysis by hepatic lipase.

Besides the decrease of HDL-c levels, there is also evidence that the changes in HDL composition result in a less antiatherogenic function of HDL [35]. HDL isolated from patients with metabolic syndrome was shown to be less capable of attenuating anti-apoptotic activities, indicating defective protection of endothelial cells from oxLDL-induced apoptosis. This antiapopototic function was inversely correlated with abdominal obesity, atherogenic dyslipidemia, and systemic oxidative stress.

Adipocyte dysfunction and obesity

During the last decade, it has become widely accepted that adipose tissue is not only a storage organ, but also an active endocrine organ with key regulatory functions in both inflammation and metabolism, capable of excreting a wide array of cytokines called adipokines [36,37]. These molecules have been shown to exert significant effects on total body glucose metabolism, insulin sensitivity, and satiety. During obesity an expansion of adipose tissue is associated with an increased influx of mononuclear white blood cells [38], resulting in the generation of "dysfunctional" fat, characterized by disturbances in the excretion of these adipokines. Defective insulin signaling is also thought to play a role in this expansion of adipose tissue. When the insulin receptor is selectively knocked out in adipose tissue in mice, these mice become resistant to obesity, suggesting that a defect in insulin signaling in adipocytes is important for developing obesity [39].

Some of the more extensively researched adipokines, such as leptin, adiponectin, resistin, and interleukin (IL)-6 exhibit interactions with lipid metabolism and IR. Leptin was one of the first adipokines discovered, and underlined the impact of adipokines on human energy and fat metabolism [40]. Leptin is the protein, encoded by the ob gene which, when deficient, is responsible for the obesity in the ob/ob mouse and plays a major role in the food intake and energy homeostasis. Absence of leptin drives hunger and suppresses energy expenditure. Notably, leptin has both central as well as peripheral actions. Central administration of leptin increases resting metabolic rates, resulting in reduced TG content in tissues with a concomitant decrease in plasma TG levels [37,41]. In contrast, peripheral leptin stimulates lipolysis of TGs. The complete absence of leptin in both animal models and human patients is associated with a lipotoxicity that can be reversed by administration of leptin itself [42,43]. Patients with lipoatrophy, who have no fat tissue at all or who experienced a loss of fat tissue, suffer from IR, diabetes, and leptin deficiency. When these patients are treated with recombinant leptin the IR can be reversed [44]. Although leptin administration can reverse metabolic disturbances in these patients, this is not a potential cure for obesity because many obese individuals already have high plasma leptin levels and are somewhat leptin resistant [45].

Whereas attention has now shifted from leptin to novel adipokines, the metabolic consequences of these adipokines are less clear. Adiponectin is a unique adipokine in the sense that as far as we know, it is the only adipokine with antiatherothrombotic effects. In line, plasma levels are reduced in obese, insulin resistant, diabetic, and dyslipidemic patients. Adiponectin-deficient mice develop IR on a high fat diet. When recombinant adiponectin is administrated in obese mouse models, this results in multiple beneficial effects, including a reduction of glucose and lipid levels, increased lipid oxidation, and reduced vascular thickening [46,47]. Adiponectin levels are inversely related to plasma TG and positively correlated with HDL-c levels in human beings [48]. The correlation between HDL-c levels and adiponectin is independent of BMI and IR; however, whether adiponectin directly influences HDL-c metabolism has as of yet to be proven [49,50].

The gene encoding for another adipokine involved in obesity, resistin, was found to be suppressed by treatment with antidiabetic thiazoladinediones, and therefore also thought to play a role in IR and obesity. However, the precise mechanism of action of this molecule remains unclear. Resistin levels are elevated in diet-induced or genetic mouse models of obesity; however, in human beings data are conflicting [51]. IL-6 is an immune modulating cytokine and its expression in adipose tissue is increased in obesity. IL-6 deficient mice develop late onset obesity that can be prevented by low-dose IL-6 infusion into the brain. Obviously, IL-6 is not really an adipokine. Whereas fat cells have the capacity to produce IL-6, the majority of this cytokine is likely to derive from macrophages located within the fat tissue, actively recruited by local expression of monocyte chemotactic protein 1 (MCP-1) [38].

Central regulation of lipid metabolism and obesity

Certain parts of the brain are devoted to the control of energy homeostasis and food intake. Foremost, the hypothalamus is known to play a major role in the regulation of satiety and energy expenditure [45]. There are now numerous hormonal mechanisms shown to participate in the regulation of appetite and food intake, relative size of lean and fat mass, and the development of IR. For instance leptin and ghrelin, which are both produced peripherally, are able to exert their effect on appetite through the central nervous system via the hypothalamus. Ghrelin is produced by the stomach and was first found to stimulate growth hormone release from the pituary gland, but is now seen as a short-term appetite controller that is released in response to stretch of the stomach with a function complementary to leptin [52]. The arcuate nucleus has several circuits linking it to different parts of the hypothalamus: the lateral hypothalamus, which is important in feeding, and the ventromedial hypothalamus, which is important in satiety [53]. The arcuate nucleus contains two distinct groups of neurons to exert its effects. The first group coexpresses neuropeptide Y (NPY) and agouti-related peptide (AgRP) and has stimulatory inputs to the lateral hypothalamus and inhibitory inputs to the ventromedial hypothalamus [54,55]. The second group coexpresses pro-opiomelanocortin (POMC) and cocaine- and amphetamine-regulated transcript (CART), and has stimulatory inputs to the ventromedial hypothalamus and inhibitory inputs to the lateral hypothalamus. Consequently, the NPY/AgRP neurons will stimulate feeding and inhibit satiety, while the POMC/CART neurons stimulate satiety and inhibit feeding. Leptin exerts its action to both groups of these arcuate nucleus neurons by inhibiting the NPY/AgRP group while stimulating the POMC/CART group [56]. Besides neuropetides and neurocytokines coming from the adipose tissue, metabolic substrates can influence these hypothalamic regions as well. Glucose and fatty acids also have a central influence on satiety feeling and the metabolic pathways. When an inhibitor of fatty acid synthesis is given centrally, both food intake and body weight are decreased [57]. More recently, central glucose levels were also shown to play a pivotal role in the obesity-associated dyslipidemia. A selective increase in hypothalamic glucose is able to inhibit VLDL secretion by the liver and, therefore, to decrease TG levels in rats. These effects are lost during diet-induced obesity, indicating a role for defective brain glucose signaling in the etiology of the dyslipidemia associated with the metabolic syndrome [58].

Summary

Dyslipidemia associated with obesity and the metabolic syndrome is one of the central features contributing to the increased CV risk in these patients. In view of the pandemic of the metabolic syndrome, it is imperative to fully understand the mechanisms leading to the metabolic lipid phenotype before embarking upon optimal treatment strategies. The traditional concept that insulin resistance causes increased FFA flux via increased TG hydrolysis in adipose tissue is still of a central theme in the general hypothesis. The combination of increased hepatic VLDL secretion with impaired LPL-mediated TG clearance explains the hypertriglyceridemia phenotype of the metabolic syndrome. Hence, central IR may be an important factor contributing to peripheral hypertriglyceridemia. Recently recognized regulatory systems include the profound impact of the hypothalamus on TG secretion and glucose control. In addition, dysfunctional (or inflamed) intra abdominal adipose tissue has emerged as a potent regulator of dyslipidemia and IR. It will be a challenge to design novel treatment modalities that target "dysfunctional" fat or central IR to attempt to prevent the epidemic of CV disease secondary to the metabolic syndrome.

References

[1] Third report of the National Cholesterol Education Program (NCEP) Expert Panel on detection, evaluation, and treatment of high blood cholesterol in adults (Adult Treatment Panel III) final report. Circulation 2002;106:3143–421.
[2] Alberti KG, Zimmet P, Shaw J. The metabolic syndrome—a new worldwide definition. Lancet 2005;366:1059–62.
[3] Alberti KG, Zimmet PZ. Definition, diagnosis and classification of diabetes mellitus and its complications. Part 1: diagnosis and classification of diabetes mellitus provisional report of a WHO consultation. Diabet Med 1998;15:539–53.

[4] Mokdad AH, Ford ES, Bowman BA, et al. Prevalence of obesity, diabetes, and obesity-related health risk factors, 2001. JAMA 2003;289:76–9.

[5] Ford ES. Prevalence of the metabolic syndrome defined by the International Diabetes Federation among adults in the U.S. Diabetes Care 2005;28:2745–9.

[6] Bibbins-Domingo K, Coxson P, Pletcher MJ, et al. Adolescent overweight and future adult coronary heart disease. N Engl J Med 2007;357:2371–9.

[7] Kelishadi R. Childhood overweight, obesity, and the metabolic syndrome in developing countries. Epidemiol Rev 2007;29:62–76.

[8] Castelli W. Lipoproteins and cardiovascular disease: biological basis and epidemiological studies. Value Health 1998;1:105–9.

[9] Ansell BJ, Watson KE, Fogelman AM, et al. High-density lipoprotein function: recent advances. J Am Coll Cardiol 2005;46:1792–8.

[10] Onat A, Sari I, Yazici M, et al. Plasma triglycerides, an independent predictor of cardiovascular disease in men: a prospective study based on a population with prevalent metabolic syndrome. Int J Cardiol 2006;108:89–95.

[11] Bansal S, Buring JE, Rifai N, et al. Fasting compared with nonfasting triglycerides and risk of cardiovascular events in women. JAMA 2007;298:309–16.

[12] Jacobson TA, Miller M, Schaefer EJ. Hypertriglyceridemia and cardiovascular risk reduction. Clin Ther 2007;29:763–77.

[13] Abdel-Maksoud MF, Hokanson JE. The complex role of triglycerides in cardiovascular disease. Semin Vasc Med 2002;2:325–33.

[14] Sobenin IA, Tertov VV, Orekhov AN. Atherogenic modified LDL in diabetes. Diabetes 1996;45(Suppl 3):S35–9.

[15] Goldberg IJ. Lipoprotein lipase and lipolysis: central roles in lipoprotein metabolism and atherogenesis. J Lipid Res 1996;37:693–707.

[16] Merkel M, Eckel RH, Goldberg IJ. Lipoprotein lipase: genetics, lipid uptake, and regulation. J Lipid Res 2002;43:1997–2006.

[17] Horton JD, Goldstein JL, Brown MS. SREBPs: activators of the complete program of cholesterol and fatty acid synthesis in the liver. J Clin Invest 2002;109:1125–31.

[18] Taskinen MR. Diabetic dyslipidaemia: from basic research to clinical practice. Diabetologia 2003;46:733–49.

[19] Ginsberg HN. Insulin resistance and cardiovascular disease. J Clin Invest 2000;106:453–8.

[20] Arner P. Human fat cell lipolysis: biochemistry, regulation and clinical role. Best Pract Res Clin Endocrinol Metab 2005;19:471–82.

[21] Kraemer FB, Shen WJ. Hormone-sensitive lipase: control of intracellular tri-(di-)acylglycerol and cholesteryl ester hydrolysis. J Lipid Res 2002;43:1585–94.

[22] Adiels M, Boren J, Caslake MJ, et al. Overproduction of VLDL1 driven by hyperglycemia is a dominant feature of diabetic dyslipidemia. Arterioscler Thromb Vasc Biol 2005;25:1697–703.

[23] Ginsberg HN, Zhang YL, Hernandez-Ono A. Metabolic syndrome: focus on dyslipidemia. Obes Res 2006;14:S41–9.

[24] Lewis GF. Fatty acid regulation of very low density lipoprotein production. Curr Opin Lipidol 1997;8:146–53.

[25] Qureshi K, Abrams GA. Metabolic liver disease of obesity and role of adipose tissue in the pathogenesis of nonalcoholic fatty liver disease. World J Gastroenterol 2007;13:3540–53.

[26] Angulo P, Lindor KD. Treatment of nonalcoholic fatty liver: present and emerging therapies. Semin Liver Dis 2001;21:81–8.

[27] Abrams GA, Kunde SS, Lazenby AJ, et al. Portal fibrosis and hepatic steatosis in morbidly obese subjects: a spectrum of nonalcoholic fatty liver disease. Hepatology 2004;40:475–83.

[28] Yamashita H, Takenoshita M, Sakurai M, et al. A glucose-responsive transcription factor that regulates carbohydrate metabolism in the liver. Proc Natl Acad Sci U S A 2001;98:9116–21.

[29] Arai T, Yamashita S, Hirano K, et al. Increased plasma cholesteryl ester transfer protein in obese subjects. A possible mechanism for the reduction of serum HDL cholesterol levels in obesity. Arterioscler Thromb 1994;14:1129–36.

[30] Radeau T, Lau P, Robb M, et al. Cholesteryl ester transfer protein (CETP) mRNA abundance in human adipose tissue: relationship to cell size and membrane cholesterol content. J Lipid Res 1995;36:2552–61.

[31] Dullaart RP, Sluiter WJ, Dikkeschei LD, et al. Effect of adiposity on plasma lipid transfer protein activities: a possible link between insulin resistance and high density lipoprotein metabolism. Eur J Clin Invest 1994;24:188–94.

[32] Lewis GF, Lamarche B, Uffelman KD, et al. Clearance of postprandial and lipolytically modified human HDL in rabbits and rats. J Lipid Res 1997;38:1771–8.

[33] Rashid S, Uffelman KD, Lewis GF. The mechanism of HDL lowering in hypertriglyceridemic, insulin-resistant states. J Diabet Complications 2002;16:24–8.

[34] Horowitz BS, Goldberg IJ, Merab J, et al. Increased plasma and renal clearance of an exchangeable pool of apolipoprotein A-I in subjects with low levels of high density lipoprotein cholesterol. J Clin Invest 1993;91:1743–52.

[35] de Souza JA, Vindis C, Hansel B, et al. Metabolic syndrome features small, apolipoprotein A-I-poor, triglyceride-rich HDL3 particles with defective anti-apoptotic activity. Atherosclerosis 2008;197(1):84–94.

[36] Yu YH, Ginsberg HN. Adipocyte signaling and lipid homeostasis: sequelae of insulin-resistant adipose tissue. Circ Res 2005;96:1042–52.

[37] Ahima RS. Adipose tissue as an endocrine organ. Obes Res 2006;14:242S–9S.

[38] Wellen KE, Hotamisligil GS. Obesity-induced inflammatory changes in adipose tissue. J Clin Invest 2003;112:1785–8.

[39] Bluher M, Michael MD, Peroni OD, et al. Adipose tissue selective insulin receptor knockout protects against obesity and obesity-related glucose intolerance. Dev Cell 2002;3:25–38.

[40] Zhang F, Basinski MB, Beals JM, et al. Crystal structure of the obese protein Ieptin-E100. Nature 1997;387:206–9.

[41] Ahima RS, Saper CB, Flier JS, et al. Leptin regulation of neuroendocrine systems. Front Neuroendocrinol 2000;21:263–307.

[42] Farooqi IS, Jebb SA, Langmack G, et al. Effects of recombinant leptin therapy in a child with congenital leptin deficiency. N Engl J Med 1999;341:879–84.

[43] Halaas JL, Gajiwala KS, Maffei M, et al. Weight-reducing effects of the plasma protein encoded by the obese gene. Science 1995;269:543–6.

[44] Oral EA, Ruiz E, Andewelt A, et al. Effect of leptin replacement on pituitary hormone regulation in patients with severe lipodystrophy. J Clin Endocrinol Metab 2002;87:3110–7.

[45] Flier JS. Obesity wars: molecular progress confronts an expanding epidemic. Cell 2004;116: 337–50.

[46] Pajvani UB, Scherer PE. Adiponectin: systemic contributor to insulin sensitivity. Curr Diab Rep 2003;3:207–13.

[47] Berg AH, Combs TP, Scherer PE. ACRP30/adiponectin: an adipokine regulating glucose and lipid metabolism. Trends Endocrinol Metab 2002;13:84–9.

[48] Yamamoto Y, Hirose H, Saito I, et al. Correlation of the adipocyte-derived protein adiponectin with insulin resistance index and serum high-density lipoprotein-cholesterol, independent of body mass index, in the Japanese population. Clin Sci 2002;103:137–42.

[49] Cote M, Mauriege P, Bergeron J, et al. Adiponectinemia in visceral obesity: impact on glucose tolerance and plasma lipoprotein and lipid levels in men. J Clin Endocrinol Metab 2005; 90:1434–9.

[50] Martin LJ, Woo JG, Daniels SR, et al. The relationships of adiponectin with insulin and lipids are strengthened with increasing adiposity. J Clin Endocrinol Metab 2005;90:4255–9.

[51] Steppan CM, Bailey ST, Bhat S, et al. The hormone resistin links obesity to diabetes. Nature 2001;409:307–12.

[52] Kojima M, Hosoda H, Date Y, et al. Ghrelin is a growth-hormone-releasing acylated peptide from stomach. Nature 1999;402:656–60.

[53] Fan W, Boston BA, Kesterson RA, et al. Role of melanocortinergic neurons in feeding and the agouti obesity syndrome. Nature 1997;385:165–8.

[54] Batterham RL, Cowley MA, Small CJ, et al. Physiology: does gut hormone PYY3-36 decrease food intake in rodents? [reply]. Nature 2004;430:3–4.

[55] Ollmann MM, Wilson BD, Yang YK, et al. Antagonism of central melanocortin receptors in vitro and in vivo by agouti-related protein. Science 1997;278:135–8.

[56] Cowley MA, Smith RG, Diano S, et al. The distribution and mechanism of action of ghrelin in the CNS demonstrates a novel hypothalamic circuit regulating energy homeostasis. Neuron 2003;37:649–61.

[57] Loftus TM, Jaworsky DE, Frehywot GL, et al. Reduced food intake and body weight in mice treated with fatty acid synthase inhibitors. Science 2000;288:2379–81.

[58] Lam TK, Gutierrez-Juarez R, Pocai A, et al. Brain glucose metabolism controls the hepatic secretion of triglyceride-rich lipoproteins. Nat Med 2007;13:171–80.

ELSEVIER
SAUNDERS

Endocrinol Metab Clin N Am
37 (2008) 635–646

ENDOCRINOLOGY
AND METABOLISM
CLINICS
OF NORTH AMERICA

Obesity and Free Fatty Acids

Guenther Boden, MD

Department of Medicine, Division of Endocrinology/Diabetes/Metabolism,
Temple University School of Medicine, Temple University Hospital,
3401 North Broad Street, Philadelphia, PA 19140, USA

Obesity is closely associated with insulin resistance (peripheral and hepatic) [1] and with a low-grade state of inflammation characterized by the elevation of proinflammatory cytokines in blood and tissues [2]. Insulin and inflammation contribute to the development of type 2 diabetes mellitus (T2DM), hypertension, atherogenic dyslipidemias, and disorders of blood coagulation and fibrinolysis. All of these disorders are independent risk factors for atherosclerotic vascular disease (ASVD) such as heart attacks, strokes, and peripheral arterial disease [3].

The reason why obesity is associated with insulin resistance is not well understood. This article reviews the evidence demonstrating that free fatty acids (FFAs) cause insulin resistance and inflammation in the major insulin target tissues (skeletal muscle, liver, and endothelial cells) and thus are an important link between obesity, insulin resistance, inflammation, and the development of T2DM, hypertension, dyslipidemia, disorders of coagulation, and ASVD (Fig. 1).

The central nervous system effects of FFAs, including the demonstration that infusion of oleic acid into the third ventricle of rats reduced food intake and hepatic glucose production (HGP), are reviewed separately elsewhere in this issue.

Free fatty acids and insulin resistance

The recognition that adipose tissue not only stores and releases fatty acids but also synthesizes and releases a large number of other active compounds [4] has provided a conceptual framework that helps to understand

This work was supported by National Institutes of Health grants RO1-DK-68895, RO1-HL-733267, and RO1-DK-066003.

E-mail address: bodengh@tuhs.temple.edu

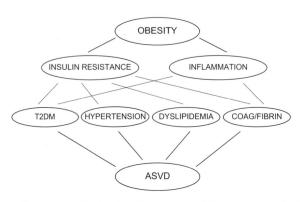

Fig. 1. Relationship between obesity, insulin resistance, inflammation, and ASVD. Obesity causes insulin resistance and a state of low-grade inflammation. Both conditions contribute to the development of several disorders, including T2DM, hypertension, dyslipidemia, and disorders of coagulation and fibrinolysis, which are independent risk factors for the development of ASVD.

how obesity can result in the development of insulin resistance. According to this concept, an expanding fat mass releases increasing amounts of compounds such as FFAs, angiotensin 2, resistin, tumor necrosis factor α (TNF-α), interleukin (IL)-6, IL-1β, and others. Some of these compounds, when infused in large amounts, can produce insulin resistance; however, any substance, to qualify as a physiologic link between obesity and insulin resistance, should meet at least the following three criteria: (1) the substance should be elevated in the blood of obese people; (2) raising its blood level (within physiologic limits) should increase insulin resistance; and (3) lowering its blood level should decrease insulin resistance. So far, only FFAs meet these three criteria in human subjects. Plasma FFA levels are elevated in most obese individuals [5]; raising plasma FFA levels increases insulin resistance [6] and lowering FFA levels improves insulin resistance [7].

Free fatty acid levels are elevated in obesity

Plasma FFA levels are usually elevated in obesity because (1) the enlarged adipose tissue mass releases more FFAs and (2) FFA clearance may be reduced [8]. Moreover, after plasma FFA levels are elevated, they will inhibit insulin's antilipolytic action, which will further increase the rate of FFA release into the circulation [9].

Raising free fatty acid levels increases insulin resistance

In skeletal muscle, acutely raising plasma FFA levels—for instance, by infusing heparinized lipid emulsions—reduces insulin-stimulated glucose uptake (more than 80% of which occurs in skeletal muscle) dose dependently in all individuals irrespective of sex and age [6,10]. Under these conditions, insulin resistance develops within 2 to 4 hours after plasma FFA levels increase, and disappears within 4 hours after normalization of FFA levels [11].

In the liver, FFA-induced hepatic insulin resistance is more difficult to demonstrate because the liver is more insulin sensitive than skeletal muscle [12]. Nevertheless, there is convincing evidence that physiologic elevations of FFAs (such as seen after a fat-rich meal) inhibit insulin suppression of HGP, resulting in an increase in HGP [1]. Acutely (1–4 hours), this rise in HGP is due to FFA-mediated inhibition of insulin suppression of glycogenolysis [13]. Longer-lasting elevations of FFAs, however, are likely to also increase gluconeogenesis.

In endothelial cells, intravenous infusion of insulin has been shown to increase nitric oxide (NO) production, resulting in increased peripheral vascular blood flow [14,15]. Physiologic elevations of plasma FFAs produce insulin resistance in endothelial cells by inhibiting the insulin-induced increase in NO and blood flow [16].

Lowering free fatty acid levels reduces insulin resistance

Chronically elevated plasma FFA levels, as commonly seen in obese diabetic and nondiabetic individuals, also cause insulin resistance. This relationship was demonstrated by normalizing elevated plasma FFA levels for 12 hours, which resulted in the normalization of insulin-stimulated glucose uptake in obese nondiabetic individuals but improved insulin sensitivity from approximately one fourth to one half of normal in obese patients who had T2DM [7]. These results suggest that high plasma FFA levels may have been the sole cause for insulin resistance in obese nondiabetic subjects but were responsible for only approximately one half of the insulin resistance in obese patients who had T2DM [7]. Similar results have been reported in nondiabetic subjects genetically predisposed to T2DM [17].

Mechanisms of free fatty acid–mediated insulin resistance

FFAs have been shown to produce a defect in insulin-stimulated glucose transport and/or phosphorylation that is caused by a defect in insulin signaling [10,18]. Plasma FFAs can easily enter cells, where they are oxidized to generate energy in the form of ATP or are re-esterified for storage as triglycerides. Not surprisingly, therefore, raising blood FFA levels results in intracellular (intramyocellular or intrahepatocellular) accumulation of triglycerides [19]. For reasons that are not well understood, raising plasma FFA levels also results in accumulation of several metabolites involved in FFA re-esterification, including long-chain acyl coenzyme A and diacylglycerol (DAG) [20]. DAG is a potent activator of conventional and novel protein kinase C (PKC) isoforms [21]. In addition to PKC, several other serine/threonine kinases, including IKβ kinase (IKK-β) and c-Jun NH$_2$

terminal kinase (JNK), can also be activated by acutely raising plasma FFA levels [22,23]. Exactly how these kinases are activated by FFAs is not clear but may include FFA-mediated generation of reactive oxygen species (ROS) [24], activation of the Toll-like receptor 4 (TLR-4) pathway [25], or endoplasmic reticulum stress [23]. After being activated, one or several of these serine/threonine kinases can interrupt insulin signaling by decreasing tyrosine phosphorylation of the insulin receptor substrate 1 or 2 (IRS 1/2) [26]. This interruption inhibits the activity of the IRS/phosphatidylinositol 3-kinase/Akt pathway, which controls most of the metabolic actions of insulin, including glucose uptake, glycogen synthesis, glycogenolysis, and lipolysis [27]. The IRS/phosphatidylinositol 3-kinase/Akt pathway is also important for the activation of endothelial NO synthase and the production of NO. In addition, FFAs can reduce NO production through a second mechanism, namely, by stimulation of NAD(P)H oxidase. This stimulation has been shown to occur in a PKC-dependent manner, and leads to increased production of ROS and a decrease in NO (Fig. 2) [24].

FFAs may also interfere with insulin stimulation of glucose transport by modulating glucose transporter gene transcription and mRNA stability [28,29].

Free fatty acids and inflammation

Obesity is associated with elevated levels of proinflammatory cytokines and chemokines in the circulation and in tissues [2]. As mentioned earlier, adipose tissue produces and releases a large number of cytokines and chemokines (collectively called adipokines) [4], some of which are proinflammatory. Recent studies have shed some light on the reasons for the increased release of proinflammatory cytokines in obesity. In one study, mice fed a high-fat diet for 3 months developed low-grade hepatic inflammation that was associated with increased production and secretion of several proinflammatory cytokines [30]. These results suggest that the inflammatory state was caused by a component of the diet or by a substance released from the enlarged adipose tissue. FFAs are good candidates for both possibilities because they are elevated in most obese individuals during a fat meal [31] and under basal and postprandial conditions [5].

The recent demonstration that acute elevation of plasma FFAs (in addition to producing peripheral and hepatic insulin resistance) activated the proinflammatory nuclear factor (NF)κB pathway [20] and resulted in increased hepatic expression of several proinflammatory cytokines including TNF-α, IL-1β, and IL-6 and an increase in circulating monocyte chemoattracting protein (MCP)-1 [22] supported the notion that FFAs are a primary link between obesity or high-fat feeding and the development of inflammatory changes (see Fig. 2). In this context, the increase in circulating MCP-1 in response to an acute rise in plasma FFAs is particularly interesting because MCP-1 is well established to regulate macrophage recruitment

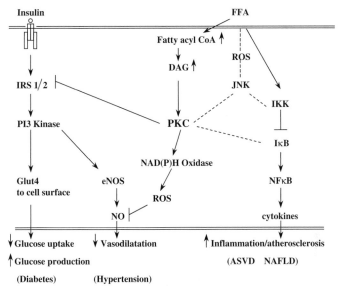

Fig. 2. Potential mechanisms of FFA-induced insulin resistance and inflammation. The key event is an increase in plasma FFA concentration, which leads to the accumulation of fatty acyl coenzyme A (CoA) and DAG and to the activation of PKC in skeletal muscle, liver, and vascular endothelial cells. It is assumed that activation of PKC interrupts insulin signaling by serine phosphorylation of IRS 1/2, resulting in a decrease in tyrosine phosphorylation of IRS 1/2. In endothelial cells, PKC has been shown to activate NAD(P)H oxidase, which produces ROS and destroys NO. Elevation of plasma FFA levels also leads to the production of inflammatory and proatherogenic proteins through activation of the IKK/IκB–α/NFκB and JNK pathways. The broken lines indicate that activation of PKC by the IKK/IκB–α/NFκB pathway and by ROS is a possibility that has not yet been demonstrated in human muscle or liver. Increased FFA-induced insulin resistance reduces glucose uptake in muscle and increases glucose production in the liver, which together results in hyperglycemia. In endothelial cells, FFA-mediated insulin resistance results in decreased NO and decreased vasodilatation, which may contribute to the development of hypertension. In muscle and liver, FFA activation of the IKK/IκB–α/NFκB and JNK pathways results in low-grade inflammation, which may promote ASVD and nonalcoholic fatty liver disease (NAFLD). NFκB, nuclear factor κB; PI, phosphatidylinositol.

to sites of inflammation [32]. The rise in plasma MCP-1 levels, therefore, may explain the recent observation of macrophage infiltration into the adipose tissue of obese animals [33].

The early events leading from a rise in circulating FFAs to activation of the NFκB pathway are not clear but include several possibilities. First, as discussed previously, an increase in plasma FFAs results in intramyocellular accumulation of DAG and activation of several PKC isoforms [20,22]. Gao and colleagues [34] recently showed that the FFA-mediated activation of IKK (a kinase involved in the activation of NFκB) in fat cells was PKC dependent. Thus, DAG-mediated PKC activation may be an upstream effector of NFκB activation. Second, some recent evidence suggests that

FFA-mediated activation of IKK and NFκB may be, at least partially, mediated by the TLR-4 [25]. The TLR-4 pathway, which is essential for the development of innate immunity to pathogens, triggers production of inflammatory cytokines [35]. Thus, it appears that sensing of excess nutrients such as FFAs and sensing of infectious pathogens may use the same signaling pathway and result in the same downstream effects, that is, inflammation. Third, obesity and FFAs have been shown to induce endoplasmic reticulum stress that can result in activation of IKK, JNK, and inflammatory responses [36], and lastly, several G protein–coupled receptors, including GRP-40 and GRP-120, have been shown to bind FFAs [37,38]. There is as yet, however, no evidence that these receptors are involved in any of the FFA activities discussed here.

Free fatty acids and the metabolic syndrome

The increase in the metabolic syndrome (also called the insulin-resistance syndrome) is mainly driven by the worldwide increase in obesity. Not surprisingly, therefore, obesity-associated and fatty acid–mediated insulin resistance is intimately connected with all major components of this syndrome; that is, T2DM, hypertension, atherogenic dyslipidemia, and other components that have not yet been formally included in the metabolic syndrome complex such as disorders of blood coagulation and fibrinolysis.

Type 2 diabetes mellitus

FFA-mediated insulin resistance results in the development of T2DM unless the insulin resistance is compensated by oversecretion of insulin. There is increasing evidence that FFAs stimulate insulin secretion, acutely and chronically, and that FFA-induced insulin resistance is compensated by FFA-mediated oversecretion of insulin in obese but otherwise healthy individuals [39]. In prediabetic individuals (subjects who have inherited predisposition to develop T2DM, including first-degree relatives of those who have T2DM), however, this compensation fails and the consequence of FFA-induced insulin resistance is T2DM [17,39]. This explains why only approximately 50% of all obese insulin-resistant individuals, namely those who are unable to compensate, develop T2DM during their lifetime [40].

Hypertension

FFA-induced insulin resistance also reduces endothelial production of NO through PKC-dependent activation of NAD(P)H oxidase, resulting in increased production of ROS (see the section "Mechanisms of free fatty acid–mediated insulin resistance" and Ref. [24]). NO deficiency decreases vasodilatation and promotes the development of hypertension.

Atherogenic dyslipidemia

Obesity and insulin resistance are associated with increased production of very low-density lipoproteins and triglycerides. A major factor for this is believed to be the increased flux of FFAs to the liver in combination with insulin resistance–associated hyperinsulinemia. The precise mechanism of this insulin resistance–driven hepatic very low-density lipoprotein overproduction, however, remains uncertain [41].

Disorders of coagulation and fibrinolysis

Hyperinsulinemia, the hallmark of insulin resistance, is now recognized to create a procoagulant state in diabetic and nondiabetic individuals by increasing circulatory levels of tissue factor procoagulant activity, increased generation of thrombin, elevated plasma levels of coagulation factors VII and VIII, and activation of platelets [42,43].

Obesity, insulin resistance, and T2DM are also associated with impaired fibrinolysis [44]. Plasma concentrations of plasminogen activator inhibitor 1 (PAI-1), which is the primary inhibitor of fibrinolysis, are increased in obese insulin-resistant individuals and in patients who have T2DM [45,46]. PAI-1 down-regulates fibrinolysis by inhibiting the production of plasmin, thus promoting thrombosis. PAI-1 is synthesized in endothelial cells and hepatocytes and is present in platelets and in plasma (reviewed in Ref. [47]). In vitro, PAI-1 secretion is stimulated by insulin in human adipocytes and by FFAs in hepatocytes. Hence, elevated plasma FFA levels, by way of producing insulin resistance and hyperinsulinemia (with or without hyperglycemia), promote a state of increased tendency for thrombosis (see previous discussion) and the decreased ability to lyse blood clots, which together, increase the risk for acute vascular events.

Free fatty acids and matrix metalloproteinases

Smoking, together with the established insulin resistance–related risk factors for ASVD such as T2DM, hypertension, atherogenic dyslipidemia, and disorders of blood coagulation and fibrinolysis, probably cannot completely explain the obesity/insulin resistance–related ASVD risk [48]. This suggests that there may be other ways by which insulin resistance can increase this risk. Indeed, one such risk factor may be increased activity of several matrix metalloproteinases (MMPs). MMPs are enzymes with proteolytic activities against connective tissue proteins such as collagen, proteoglycans, and elastin. They control degradation and remodeling of extracellular matrix. There is accumulating evidence that MMP-2, MMP-9, and MT-MMP play important roles in the development and progression of heart attacks, strokes, peripheral arterial disease, and aortic aneurysms [49–52]. The author and colleagues [53] recently found that acutely increasing plasma levels of FFAs, particularly when combined with hyper-insulinemia, strongly increased the activities of MMP-2, MMP-9, and MT-MMP in rat aorta. As mentioned previously, FFAs also promote the release of proinflammatory cytokines, which are known to be potent stimulators of MMP synthesis and release [49]. Thus, the combination of increased MMP activity and inflammatory cytokines may lead to progression of atherosclerotic lesions and contribute to the increased risk for cardiovascular disease in obese insulin-resistant individuals.

Free fatty acids as target for therapy

Because insulin resistance is at the core of several serious health problems associated with obesity, insulin resistance should be a major focus of therapy. Whereas weight loss through diet and exercise is clearly the most desirable way to reduce insulin resistance in obese people, diet and exercise programs and presently available pharmacologic approaches have not been very successful. As noted earlier, elevated plasma FFA levels are responsible for much of the insulin resistance in obese individuals. Therefore, normalizing plasma FFA levels can be expected to improve insulin sensitivity. The author and colleagues [7] showed that normalization of plasma FFA levels overnight with Acipimox, a nicotinic analog, normalized insulin resistance in obese nondiabetic subjects and improved insulin resistance in obese patients who had T2DM. Nicotinic acid or long-acting nicotinic acid analogs effectively lower plasma FFA levels. It is unfortunate that their use is associated with a rebound of plasma FFAs to very high levels [54], which makes this class of drugs unsuitable for the long-term control of plasma FFAs. Thiazolidinediones (TZD) lower plasma FFA levels long-term and without rebound. They do this primarily by stimulating fat oxidation through a coordinated induction of genes in adipose tissue related to FFA uptake, binding, β-oxidation, and oxidative phosphorylation [55]. TZD-mediated lowering of plasma FFA levels is modest, however, ranging from less than 10% to approximately 20% in most studies [56,57]. Moreover, this class of drug has several unwanted effects that limit their use [58]. Fibrates, another class of lipid-lowering drugs, also lower plasma FFA levels modestly and without rebound, primarily by stimulating fat oxidation in the liver [59]. Because both classes of drugs work in different organs (TZDs in fat; fibrates in the liver) and through different mechanisms (TZDs through activation of peroxisomal proliferator-activated receptor [PPAR]-γ; fibrates through activation of PPAR-α), their use in combination produces greater decreases in plasma FFA levels and greater improvements in insulin sensitivity than the use of either drug alone [60].

Lowering of plasma FFAs, in addition to improving insulin sensitivity, may prevent activation of the proinflammatory and proatherogenic NFκB pathway and thus may reduce the incidence of atherosclerotic vascular problems. Therefore, the challenges for the future include the prevention or correction of obesity and elevated plasma FFA levels through methods that include decreased caloric intake and increased caloric expenditure, the development of easy, fast, and reliable methods to measure FFAs in small blood samples (comparable to portable blood sugar–monitoring devices), and the development of efficient pharmacologic approaches to normalize increased plasma FFA levels.

Summary

Plasma FFA levels are elevated in obesity. FFAs cause insulin resistance in all major insulin target organs (skeletal muscle, liver, endothelial cells) and have emerged as a major link between obesity, the development of the metabolic syndrome, and ASVD. Mechanisms through which FFAs induce insulin resistance involve intramyocellular and intrahepatic accumulation of DAG and triglycerides, activation of several serine/threonine kinases, reduction of tyrosine phosphorylation of the IRS 1/2, and impairment of the IRS/phosphatidylinositol 3-kinase pathway of insulin signaling. FFAs also produce low-grade inflammation in skeletal muscle, liver, and fat through activation of the NFκB and JNK pathways, resulting in release of

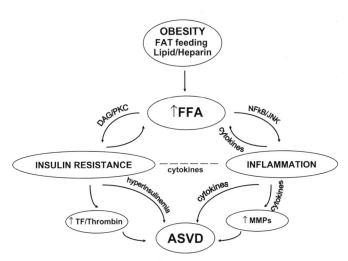

Fig. 3. Summary of the relationship between obesity, FFAs, and ASVD. Obesity, fat feeding, and lipid/heparin infusion all raise plasma FFA levels. Elevated plasma FFAs produce insulin resistance by way of DAG/PKC by decreasing insulin signaling at the IRS 1/2 level. Insulin resistance promotes ASVD by way of chronic hyperinsulinemia, a state of increased tendency to blood coagulation and decreased fibrinolysis and by mechanisms not shown here, including hypertension and atherogenic dyslipidemia. Elevated plasma FFAs also cause inflammation by way of activation of the NFκB and JNK pathways. Inflammation can promote ASVD by increasing the production of inflammatory cytokines and by activation of MMPs. TF, tissue factor.

proinflammatory and proatherogenic cytokines. In addition, FFAs contribute to cardiovascular events by promoting a prothrombotic state by reducing fibrinolysis and by activating platelets and arterial MMPs (Fig. 3).

Acknowledgments

The author thanks Maria Mozzoli, BS, and Karen Kresge, BS, for technical assistance, and Constance Harris Crews for typing the manuscript.

References

[1] Boden G. Role of fatty acids in the pathogenesis of insulin resistance and NIDDM. Diabetes 1997;46:3–10.
[2] Tataranni PA, Ortega EA. Burning question. Does an adipokines-induced activation of the immune system mediate the effect of overnutrition on type 2 diabetes? Diabetes 2005;54: 917–27.
[3] Bray GA. Medical consequences of obesity. J Clin Endocrinol Metab 2004;89:2583–9.
[4] Kershaw EE, Flier JS. Adipose tissue as an endocrine organ. J Clin Endocrinol Metab 2004; 89:2548–56.
[5] Reaven GM, Hollenbeck C, Jeng C-Y, et al. Measurement of plasma glucose, free fatty acid, lactate and insulin for 24 h in patients with NIDDM. Diabetes 1988;37:1020–4.
[6] Boden G, Chen X, Ruiz J, et al. Mechanisms of fatty acid-induced inhibition of glucose uptake. J Clin Invest 1994;93:2438–46.
[7] Santomauro ATMG, Boden G, Silva M, et al. Overnight lowering of free fatty acids with acipimox improves insulin resistance and glucose tolerance in obese diabetic and nondiabetic subjects. Diabetes 1999;48:1836–41.
[8] Bjorntorp P, Bergman H, Varnauskas E. Plasma free fatty acid turnover in obesity. Acta Med Scand 1969;185:351–6.
[9] Jensen MD, Haymond MW, Rizza RA, et al. Influence of body fat distribution on free fatty acid metabolism in obesity. J Clin Invest 1989;83:1168–73.
[10] Boden G, Chen X. Effects of fat on glucose uptake and utilization in patients with non-insulin-dependent diabetes. J Clin Invest 1995;96:1261–8.
[11] Boden G, Jadali F, White J, et al. Effects of fat on insulin stimulated carbohydrate metabolism in normal men. J Clin Invest 1991;88:960–6.
[12] Rizza RA, Mandarino LJ, Gerich JE. Dose-response characteristics for effects of insulin on production and utilization of glucose in man. Am J Phys 1981;240:E630–9.
[13] Boden G, Cheung P, Stein TP, et al. FFA cause hepatic insulin resistance by inhibiting insulin suppression of glycogenolysis. Am J Phys 2002;283:E12–9.
[14] Baron AD. Insulin resistance and vascular function. J Diabet Complications 2002;16: 92–102.
[15] Zeng G, Nystrom FH, Ravichandran LV, et al. Roles for insulin receptor, PI3-kinase and Akt in insulin-signaling pathways related to production of nitric oxide in human vascular endothelial cells. Circulation 2000;101:L1539–45.
[16] Steinberg HO, Tarshoby M, Monestel R, et al. Elevated circulating free fatty acid levels impair endothelium-dependent vasodilation. J Clin Invest 1997;100:1230–9.
[17] Cusi K, Kashyap S, Gastaldelli A, et al. Effect on insulin secretion and insulin action of a 48-h reduction of plasma free fatty acids with acipimox in nondiabetic subjects genetically predisposed to type 2 diabetes. Am J Physiol Endocrinol Metab 2007;292:E1775–81.
[18] Dresner A, Laurent D, Marcucci M, et al. Effects of free fatty acids on glucose transport and IRS-1 associated phosphatidylinositol 3-kinase activity. J Clin Invest 1999;103:253–9.

[19] Boden G, Lebed B, Schatz M, et al. Effects of acute changes of plasma free fatty acids on intramyocellular fat content and insulin resistance in healthy subjects. Diabetes 2001;50: 1612–7.

[20] Itani SI, Ruderman NB, Schmieder F, et al. Lipid-induced insulin resistance in human muscle is associated with changes in diacylglycerol, protein kinase C, and IκB-α. Diabetes 2002; 51:2005–11.

[21] Farese R. Diabetes mellitus: a fundamental and clinical text. In: LeRoith D, Taylor SI, Olefsky JM, editors. Philadelphia: Lippincott; 2000. p. 239–51.

[22] Boden G, She P, Mozzoli M, et al. Free fatty acids produce insulin resistance and activate the proinflammatory nuclear factor-κB pathway in rat liver. Diabetes 2005;54:3458–65.

[23] Hotamisligil GS. Role of endoplasmic reticulum stress and c-Jun NH2-terminal kinase pathways in inflammation and origin of obesity and diabetes. Diabetes 2005;54:S73–8.

[24] Inoguchi T, Li P, Umeda F, et al. High glucose level and free fatty acid stimulate reactive oxygen species production through protein kinase C-dependent activation of NAD(P)H oxidase in cultured vascular cells. Diabetes 2000;49:1939–45.

[25] Shi A, Kokoeva V, Inouye K, et al. TLR4 links innate immunity and fatty acid-induced insulin resistance. J Clin Invest 2006;116:3015–25.

[26] Yu C, Chen Y, Cline GW, et al. Mechanism by which fatty acids inhibit activation of insulin receptor substrate-1 (IRS-1)-associated phosphatidylinositol 3-kinase activity in muscle. J Biol Chem 2002;277:50230–6.

[27] Saltiel AR, Kahn CR. Insulin signaling and the regulation of glucose and lipid metabolism. Nature 2001;414:799–806.

[28] Long SD, Pekala PH. Regulation of Glut4 gene expression by arachidonic acid. Evidence for multiple pathways, one of which requires oxidation to prostaglandin. European Journal of Biological Chemistry 1996;271:1138–44.

[29] Armoni M, Harel C, Bar-Yoseph F, et al. Free fatty acids repress the Glut4 gene expression in cardiac muscle via novel response elements. J Biol Chem 2005;280:34786–95.

[30] Xu H, Barnes GT, Yang Q, et al. Chronic inflammation in fat plays a crucial role in the development of obesity-related insulin resistance. J Clin Invest 2003;112:1821–30.

[31] van Oostrom AJ, van Dijk H, Verseyden C, et al. Addition of glucose to an oral fat load reduces postprandial free fatty acids and prevents the postprandial increase in complement component 31-3. Am J Clin Nutr 2004;79:5–10.

[32] Rollins BJ, Walz A, Baggiolini M. Recombinant human MCP-1/JE induces chemotaxis, calcium flux, and the respiratory burst in human monocytes. Blood 1991;78:1112–6.

[33] Weisberg SP, McCann D, Desai M, et al. Obesity is associated with macrophage accumulation in adipose tissue. J Clin Invest 2003;112:1796–808.

[34] Gao Z, Zhang X, Zuberi A, et al. Inhibition of insulin sensitivity by free fatty acids requires activation of multiple serine kinases in 3T3-L1 adipocytes. Mol Endocrinol 2004;18: 2024–34.

[35] Medzhitov R. Toll-like receptors and innate immunity. Nat Rev Immunol 2001;1:135–45.

[36] Ozcan U, Cao Q, Yilmaz E, et al. Endoplasmic reticulum stress links obesity, insulin action, and type 2 diabetes. Science 2004;306:457–61.

[37] Hirasawa A, Tsumaya K, Awali T, et al. Free fatty acids regulate gut incretin glucagon-like peptide-1 secretion through GPR 120. Nat Med 2005;1:90–4.

[38] Itoh Y, Kawamata Y, Harada M, et al. Free fatty acids regulate insulin secretion from pancreatic beta cells through GPR40. Nature 2003;422:173–6.

[39] Boden G. Free fatty acids and insulin secretion in humans. Curr Diab Rep 2005;5:167–70.

[40] Benjamin SM, Valdez R, Geiss LS, et al. Estimated number of adults with prediabetes in the US in 2000: opportunities for prevention. Diabetes Care 2003;26:645–9.

[41] Bamba V, Rader DJ. Obesity and atherogenic dyslipidemia. Gastroenterology 2007;132: 2181–90.

[42] Boden G, Rao AK. Effects of hyperglycemia and hyperinsulinemia on the tissue factor pathway of blood coagulation. Curr Diab Rep 2007;7:223–7.

[43] Boden G, Vaidyula VR, Homko C, et al. Circulating tissue factor procoagulant activity and thrombin generation in patients with type 2 diabetes: Effects of insulin and glucose. J Clin Endocrinol Metab 2007;92:4352–8.

[44] Vague P, Juhan-Vague I, Aillaud MF, et al. Correlation between blood fibrinolytic activity, plasminogen activator inhibitor level, plasma insulin level and relative body weight in normal and obese subjects. Metabolism 1986;35:250–3.

[45] Pannacciulli N, De Mitrio R, Giorgino R, et al. Effect of glucose tolerance status on PAI-1 plasma levels in overweight and obese subjects. Obes Res 2002;10:717–25.

[46] Festa A, D'Agostino R Jr, Tracy RP, et al. Elevated levels of acute-phase proteins and plasminogen activator inhibitor-1 predict the development of type 2 diabetes: the insulin resistance atherosclerosis study. Diabetes 2002;51:1131–7.

[47] Sobel BE, Schneider DJ. Platelet function, coagulopathy, and impaired fibrinolysis in diabetes. Cardiol Clin 2004;22:511–26.

[48] Hennekens CH. Increasing burden of cardiovascular disease: current knowledge and future directions for research on risk factors. Circulation 1998;97:1095–102.

[49] Newby AC. Dual role of matrix metalloproteinases (Matrixins) in intimal thickening of atherosclerotic plaque rupture. Physiol Rev 2005;85:1–31.

[50] Galis ZS, Sukhova GK, Lark MW, et al. Increased expression of matrix metallo-proteinases and matrix degrading activity in vulnerable regions of human atherosclerotic plaques. J Clin Invest 1994;94:2493–503.

[51] Pasterkamp G, Schoneveld AH, Hijnen DJ, et al. Atherosclerotic arterial remodeling and the localization of macrophages and matrix metalloproteinases 1, 2 and 9 in the human coronary artery. Atherosclerosis 2000;150:245–53.

[52] Longo GM, Xiong W, Greiner TC, et al. Matrix metalloproteinases 2 and 9 work in concert to produce aortic aneurysms. J Clin Invest 2002;110:625–32.

[53] Boden G, Song W, Pashko L, et al. In vivo effects of insulin and free fatty acids on matrix metalloproteinases in rat aorta. Diabetes 2008;57:476–83.

[54] Chen X, Iqbal N, Boden G. The effects of free fatty acids on gluconeogenesis and glycogenolysis in normal subjects. J Clin Invest 1999;103:365–72.

[55] Boden G, Homko C, Mozzoli M, et al. Thiazolidinediones upregulate fatty acid uptake and oxidation in adipose tissue of diabetic patients. Diabetes 2005;54:880–5.

[56] Ghazzi MN, Perez JE, Antonucci TK, et al. Cardiac and glycemic benefits of troglitazone treatment in NIDDM: the Troglitazone Study Group. Diabetes 1997;46:433–9.

[57] Maggs DG, Buchanan TA, Burant CF, et al. Metabolic effects of troglitazone monotherapy in type 2 diabetes mellitus. A randomized, double-blind, placebo-controlled trial. Ann Intern Med 1998;128:176–85.

[58] Boden G, Zhang M. Recent findings concerning thiazolidinediones in the treatment of diabetes. Expert Opin Investig Drugs 2006;15:243–50.

[59] Staels B, Fruchart J-C. Therapeutic roles of peroxisome proliferator-activated receptor agonists. Diabetes 2005;54:2460–70.

[60] Boden G, Homko C, Mozzoli M, et al. Combined use of rosiglitazone and fenofibrate in patients with type 2 diabetes. Prevention of fluid retention. Diabetes 2007;56:248–55.

ELSEVIER
SAUNDERS

Endocrinol Metab Clin N Am
37 (2008) 647–662

ENDOCRINOLOGY
AND METABOLISM
CLINICS
OF NORTH AMERICA

Hypertension in Obesity

L. Romayne Kurukulasuriya, MD[a,b,*],
Sameer Stas, MD[a,b], Guido Lastra, MD[a,b],
Camila Manrique, MD[a,b],
James R. Sowers, MD[a,c,d,e]

[a]Department of Internal Medicine, University of Missouri-Columbia School of Medicine,
Columbia, MO 65212, USA
[b]Cosmopolitan International Diabetes and Endocrinology Center, University
of Missouri-Columbia, Columbia, MO 65212, USA
[c]Department of Medical Pharmacology and Physiology, University of Missouri-Columbia
School of Medicine, Columbia, MO 65212, USA
[d]Thomas W. Burns Center of Diabetes and Cardiovascular Research,
University of Missouri-Columbia
School of Medicine, Colmbia, MO 65212, USA
[e]Harry S. Truman VA Medical Center, University of Missouri-Columbia
School of Medicine, Columbia, Columbia, MO 65212, USA

There have been significant increases in hypertension (HTN), obesity, and diabetes in the last several years. The increase in these comorbid conditions will contribute to an increased incidence of cardiovascular disease (CVD) and chronic kidney disease (CKD). Central or visceral obesity is much more closely related to metabolic risk factors, CVD, and CKD, than peripheral or lower-body obesity. Furthermore, the European Prospective Investigation into Cancer Norfolk (EPIC) study of 22,090 men and women showed that systolic blood pressure (SBP) and diastolic blood pressure (DBP) increased linearly across the whole range of waist-to-hip ratio in both men and women [1]. As per National Health and Nutrition

Dr. Sowers's research is supported by grants from the National Institutes of Health (R01 HL73101-01A1 NIH/NHLBI) and from the Veterans Affairs Research Service (VA Merit Review). Dr. Sowers is a member of the Speakers' Bureau and has received grant funding from Novaritis Pharmaceutical Company. Dr. Sowers is also a member of the Speakers' Bureau for Merck Pharmaceutical Company and has received grant funding from Forest Research Institute and is on their Advisory Board.

* Corresponding author. Division of Internal Medicine, University of Missouri-Columbia, Columbia, MO 65212.

E-mail address: romaynel@health.missouri.edu (L.R. Kurukulasuriya).

Examination Survey (NHANES) data, in 1999 to 2000 only 68.9% of people with HTN were aware of their high blood pressure (BP), only 58.4% were treated, and HTN was controlled in only 31%. Women, Mexican Americans, and those aged 60 years or older had significantly lower rates of control when compared with men, younger individuals, and non-Hispanic whites [2]. In the United States population with HTN, inadequate BP control was estimated to result in 39,702 cardiovascular events, 8,374 CVD deaths, and $964 million in direct medical expenditures. In the medicated population with CVD, the incremental costs of failure to attain BP goals reached approximately $467 million. These results reflect the importance of adequate BP control (in particular, SBP control) in reducing CVD morbidity, mortality, and overall health care expenditures among patients with HTN [3]. Based on the NHANES III sample, approximately 63% of men and 55% of women aged 25 years or older in the United States population, were overweight or obese [4]. Obesity is becoming recognized as one of the most important risk factors for the development of HTN in both males and females [5]. Several genetic and environmental factors play a role in the pathogenesis of obesity, HTN, and CVD (Fig. 1). This article discusses the underlying mechanisms of obesity-related HTN and their clinical implications.

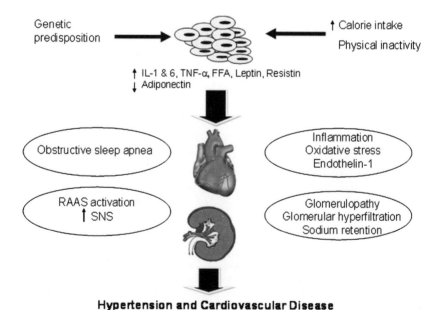

Fig. 1. Pathophysiologic events implicated in the relationship between obesity and development of hypertension and cardiovascular disease. FFA, free fatty acids; IL, interleukin; RAAS, renin-angiotensin-aldosterone syste; SNS, sympathetic nervous system; TNFα, tumor necrosis factor alpha.

Mechanisms of hypertension in obesity

The mechanisms involved in obesity-related HTN are complex and involve derangements in multiple systems. They include increased activation of the renin-angiotensin-aldosterone system (RAAS), increased sympathetic nervous system (SNS) activity, and insulin resistance. In addition, obesity is associated with increased renal sodium reabsorption, impaired pressure natriuresis, and volume expansion. Furthermore, obesity may also cause marked structural changes in the kidneys that will eventually lead to CKD and further increases in BP [6]. In addition, alterations in adipokines, free fatty acids (FFA), endothelial dysfunction, systemic inflammation, and sleep apnea promote hypertension and CVD (Box 1).

Renin angiotensin aldosterone system

There is evidence to suggest that the activation of the RAAS plays an important role in obesity-related HTN. This system has a crucial role in regulating fluid volume and vascular tone. In a study of 449 individuals from Jamaica, serum angiotensin converting enzyme (ACE) and circulating angiotensinogen levels were significantly higher in individuals with a body mass index (BMI) over 31 [6]. A study of postmenopausal women showed

---

Box 1. Factors involved in obesity-related hypertension

Insulin resistance
RAAS activation
SNS activation
Endothelial dysfunction and oxidative stress
Endothelin-1
Adiposity
   Leptin resistance
   Resistin
   Low adiponectin
   FFAs
   Hydroxysteroid dehydrogenase type 1 enzyme
   Increased abdominal pressure
   Local RAAS and SNS activiation
Renal derangement
   Sodium retention
   Obesity-related glomerulopathy
   Perirenal fat accumulation
   Renal RAAS and SNS activation
Obstructive sleep apnea

that obese women had higher circulating angiotensinogen, renin, aldosterone, and ACE levels than lean women. Weight reduction by 5% reduced plasma angiotensinogen by 27%, renin by 43%, aldosterone by 31%, ACE activity by 12%, and angiotensinogen expression by 20% in adipose tissue (all $P < .05$). The decrease in plasma angiotensinogen levels was highly correlated with the waist circumference decline ($r = 0.74$; $P < .001$) [7]. Studies on animal models have demonstrated that angiotensinogen produced by adipose tissue plays a role in local adipose tissue differentiation. In addition, angiotensinogen produced in the adipose tissue can be released into the blood stream (an endocrine effect). This suggests that high blood angiotensinogen levels and associated HTN seen in obese patients may be because of the increased fat mass [8]. Furthermore, activation of systemic and tissue RAAS can cause increased renal sodium reabsorption and a hypertensive shift of pressure natriuresis [9].

Plasma aldosterone levels are higher in obese subjects. This cannot be explained by the impact of increased plasma renin activity or other factors promoting aldosterone production. Some predictors of plasma aldosterone include abdominal obesity, measured as waist/hip ratio or by CT scan, and insulin resistance measured by glucose tolerance tests or euglycemic clamp techniques. These studies suggest that aldosterone participates in HTN associated with insulin resistance, both components of the cardiometabolic syndrome (CMS) [10]. Aldosterone increases BP in obesity by its action on both mineralocorticoid and glucocorticoid receptors located in different tissues, including brain, heart, kidney, and vasculature [11].

In a study of 223 obese patients, lisinopril was shown to be as effective as hydrochlorothiazide in treating obese subjects with HTN. This study also showed that ACE inhibitors may show greater efficacy as monotherapy at lower doses (compared with thiazide diuretics), may have a more rapid rate of response, and may offer advantages in patients at high risk of metabolic disorders [12].

Aldosterone antagonist eplerenone markedly attenuated glomerular hyperfiltration, sodium retention, and HTN associated with chronic dietary-induced obesity in dogs fed a high fat diet. Collectively, these data indicate that aldosterone plays an important role in the pathogenesis of obesity HTN [13].

Sympathetic nervous system

The SNS plays an important role in the regulation of cardiovascular homeostasis. There are several proposed mechanisms linking obesity with SNS activation. These include baroreflex dysfunction, hypothalamic-pituitary axis dysfunction, hyperinsulinemia/insulin resistance, hyperleptinemia, and elevated circulating angiotensin II concentrations [14,15]. Muscle sympathetic nervous system activity (MSNA) in men is more closely associated with the level of abdominal visceral fat than total fat mass or abdominal subcutaneous fat. MSNA does not differ in subcutaneous obese and nonobese men with similar levels of abdominal visceral fat [16]. Furthermore, these findings may have important implications in understanding the increased risk of developing CVD in individuals with visceral obesity. Men with higher visceral adiposity seem to be at higher risk for CVD than their total body fat-matched peers [15]. The increase in renal sympathetic activity in obesity may possibly be necessary for the development of HTN in obese individuals, but not a sufficient cause, being present in both normotensive and hypertensive obese individuals. The discriminating feature of obesity-related HTN has been shown to be an absence of the suppression of the cardiac sympathetic outflow seen in normotensive obese individuals [17]. Interestingly, the lack of increase in SNS activity with increasing adiposity and insulinemia in Pima Indians may contribute to the low prevalence of HTN in this population [18]. Nevertheless, increased renal sodium absorption associated with increased renal SNS activity appears to contribute to obesity-related HTN in many individuals. A study of both lean and obese hypertensives has shown that BP is more sensitive to alpha and beta adrenergic blockade in obese than in lean hypertensive patients, and suggests that increased sympathetic activity may be an important factor in the development and maintenance of HTN in obesity [19].

Insulin resistance

Diabetes mellitus is commonly associated with HTN. One link between diabetes and essential HTN may be hyperinsulinemia. When hypertensive patients, whether obese or of normal body weight, are compared with age- and weight-matched normotensive control subjects, a heightened plasma insulin response to a glucose challenge is consistently found. Insulin resistance predisposes an individual to hyperinsulinism [20]. Most glucose uptake under control of insulin occurs in skeletal muscle tissue. Interestingly, the insulin resistance in skeletal muscle accompanying essential HTN is limited to nonoxidative pathways of glucose disposal (glycogen synthesis). This resistance correlates directly with the severity of HTN. Mechanisms involved in the association of insulin resistance and essential HTN include renal sodium retention, SNS overactivity, disturbed membrane cation transport, and proliferation of vascular smooth muscle cells [20]. The conclusion of a study of 2,475 subjects was that insulin resistance or hyperinsulinemia is present in the majority of hypertensives, and constitutes a common pathophysiologic feature linking obesity, glucose intolerance, and HTN. Insulin resistance is associated with decreased metabolic signaling, which normally modulates intracellular calcium levels. With insulin resistance there is increased intracellular calcium and calcium sensitization, resulting in increased peripheral vascular resistance [21].

Despite this evidence, the direct role of insulin resistance or hyperinsulinemia in the pathophysiology of HTN is not well understood. In a study of obese dogs, chronic hyperinsulinemia did not raise BP, even though they were resistant to the metabolic and vasodilator effects of insulin [22].

A study of 14 normotensive subjects infused with high and low doses of insulin showed that the acute increases in plasma insulin within the physiologic range elevate sympathetic neural outflow but do not elevate arterial pressure in normal human beings [23]. Insulinoma patients have inappropriately high plasma concentrations of insulin and proinsulin, but their BP levels do not typically differ from those of normal control subjects, and surgical removal of the insulinomas does not reduce their BP. These findings argue against the hypothesis that hyperinsulinemia is an independent causal factor in the development of essential hypertension in humans [24]. Studies with spontaneously hypertensive rats support the view that HTN does not lead to insulin resistance, hyperinsulinemia, and hypertriglyceridemia [25]. Interestingly, the relationship between plasma insulin levels and HTN seen in essential HTN does not occur with secondary forms of HTN [26]. Therefore, insulin resistance and hyperinsulinemia are not consequences of HTN; instead, a genetic predisposition may exist that contributes to both disorders [27]. This concept is supported by the occurrence of hyperinsulinemia and insulin resistance in normotensive offspring of hypertensive adults [28,29]. Even though hyperinsulinemia may not be a major cause of obesity-related HTN, insulin resistance may contribute to HTN by other mechanisms involving inflammation and oxidative stress superimposed on abnormalities in glucose and lipid metabolism. Mechanisms for the development of HTN in insulin resistance/hyperinsulinemia include activation of the SNS, renal sodium retention, altered membrane cation transport, vascular smooth muscle growth and remodeling, and vasoconstriction [27].

Renal structural and functional changes

There is substantial evidence that abnormal kidney function plays a key role in obesity-related HTN. Obesity increases tubular sodium reabsorption and shifts pressure natriuresis toward higher BP. Increased tubular sodium reabsorption is closely linked to activation of the SNS and RAAS, and possible changes in intrarenal physical forces. For example, medullary compression because of accumulation of adipose tissue around the kidney and increased extracellular matrix within the kidney can result in enhanced tubular reabsorption and altered pressure natriuresis. Obesity is also associated with marked afferent renal artery vasodilatation and increased glomerular filtration rate, which are compensatory responses that help overcome the increased tubular sodium reabsorption and maintain sodium balance. However, chronic renal vasodilation causes increased hydrostatic pressure and wall stress in the glomeruli that, along with increased lipids and glucose, may cause glomerulosclerosis and loss of nephron function in obese patients. Obesity is increasingly a primary cause of essential HTN as well as type 2 diabetes, and consequently is an increasingly frequent cause of end-stage renal disease [30]. Kambham and colleagues [31] have defined obesity related glomerulopathy (ORG) as a focal segmental glomerulosclerosis (FSG) and glomerulomegaly in patients with a BMI of over $30 \, \text{kg/m}^2$. They showed that ORG is distinct from idiopathic FSGS, with a lower incidence of nephrotic syndrome, a more indolent course, consistent presence of glomerulomegaly, and milder foot process fusion. The 10-fold increase in incidence over the past 15 years suggests a newly emerging epidemic. Increased intra abdominal pressure (IAP) produced by progressively inflating an intra-abdominal balloon in dogs caused significant increases in SBP and DBP that resolved with balloon deflation. This has lead to the concept that increased IAP and accompanying changes in renal dynamics may be a cause for systemic HTN in those with central obesity [32].

In summary, persistent obesity causes renal injury and functional nephron loss, contributing to an elevated BP. This in turn leads to further renal injury, thereby setting off a vicious cycle of events leading to further BP elevation and renal injury. It is difficult to dissociate the cause from the effect in this nexus, as the overall burden of obesity on renal injury and BP may be strongly time dependent [33].

Role of adipocytes

Excess energy-intake leads to an expansion of adipose tissue, which is a hallmark of obesity, but the location and adipocyte morphology of the expanded adipose tissue differs among individuals. The presence of large adipocytes is associated with functional and structural abnormalities of adipose tissue. These include: (1) the increased production of bioactive molecules, such as leptin, resistin, angiotensinogen, proinflammatory cytokines, and reactive oxygen species (ROS); (2) an insufficient capacity to accommodate excess energy-intake related increases in serum lipids, leading to ectopic fat storage in tissues such as skeletal muscle and liver, which, in turn, enhances insulin resistance and hyperinsulinemia; (3) augmented macrophage infiltration of the adipose tissue enhancing the production of proinflammatory cytokines and ROS. This "dysfunctional" adipose tissue may, in turn, induce activation of the SNS and RAAS, and enhance systemic oxidative stress, all of which promote the development of obesity-associated HTN [34]. It has been shown that weight reduction is associated with a marked decrease in fat cell volume, leptin secretion, and serum leptin concentration. Fat cell volume, but not percent body fat or BMI, was directly proportional to leptin secretion and serum leptin concentrations [35].

It has been shown that secretory products from human adipocytes stimulated steroidogenesis in human adrenocortical cells with a predominant effect on mineralocorticoid secretion, suggesting a direct link between obesity, RAAS activation, and HTN [36].

Resistin

Resistin (named for resistance to insulin) is a recently discovered polypeptide that antagonizes insulin action and may play a part in the pathogenesis of insulin resistance. Resistin is increased in diet-induced and genetic forms of obesity [37]. A Chinese study with 1,102 subjects has shown resistin gene polymorphism to be an independent factor associated with elevated SBP and DBP in patients with type 2 diabetes. These findings suggest that resistin may play a part in the pathogenesis of type 2 diabetes and insulin resistance-related HTN [38]. Another study from China, with 71 subjects, showed that resistin was not related to systolic or diastolic HTN [39].

Endothelin

Some hypertensive patients have increased endothelin-1 (ET-1) dependent vasoconstrictor tone. It has been shown in subjects with a BMI of over 25 kg/m^2, that DBP is significantly associated with G/T polymorphism of ET-1 [40]. In human HTN, increased BMI may be associated with enhanced ET_A receptor-dependent vasoconstrictor activity, suggesting that this abnormality may play a role in the pathophysiology of obesity-related HTN. Therefore, targeting the ET-1 system may be useful in the treatment of these patients [41]. In addition, BP increases in relation to BMI in carriers of the T allele of ET-1/C198 polymorphism when compared with GG homozygotes. As a consequence of this interaction, the T allele was associated with a significant increase of SBP and DBP levels in overweight subjects with a BMI over 26 kg/m^2, whereas no significant effect was observed in lean subjects (BMI <26 kg/m^2) [42]. Endothelin antagonism unmasks or augments nitric oxide synthesis capacity in obese patients. Thus, in addition to direct vasoconstrictor effects of endothelin, impaired nitric oxide bioavailability as a result of elevated endogenous endothelin may also contribute to endothelial dysfunction in obesity [43].

Free fatty acids

It has been shown that increases in portal venous delivery of FFA (ie, oleic acid- a cis unsaturated nonesterified fatty acid or NEFA) to the liver, stimulates a neurally mediated reflex that results in an increase in vascular sympathetic tone and an increase in BP [44]. In vivo data from both animal and human studies support the notion that acute plasma NEFA elevation leads to an increase in BP levels. Epidemiologic evidence suggests a link between increased NEFA levels and HTN. Accumulating evidence indicates the existence of several pathways through which NEFA could promote BP elevation. These include alpha (1)-adrenergic stimulation, endothelial dysfunction, increases in oxidant stress, and stimulation of vascular smooth muscle cell growth and remodeling. Collectively, these data support a possibly important role of NEFA in the development of HTN in patients with obesity and CMS [45].

Glucocorticoid excess

Glucocorticoids play an essential role in adaptation to stress, regulation of metabolism, and inflammatory responses. Patients with Cushing's Syndrome develop insulin resistance, dyslipidemia, and HTN. Adipose stromal cells from omental fat, but not subcutaneous fat, can generate active cortisol from inactive cortisone mediated via 11 beta- hydroxysteroid dehydrogenase type 1 (11beta-HSD1) enzyme activity. In vivo, such a mechanism would ensure a constant exposure of glucocorticoid specifically to omental adipose tissue, suggesting that central obesity may reflect "Cushing's disease of the omentum" [46]. Type 1 enzyme (11beta-HSD1) in vitro is an NADP(H)-dependent bidirectional enzyme; it promotes conversion of cortisone to active cortisol. In contrast, 11beta HSD type 2 enzyme, residing in the distal tubule and collecting duct of the kidney, converts cortisol to cortisone, thus protecting the mineralocorticoid receptor from occupation by cortisol. HSD1 amplifies glucocorticoid receptor activation and promotes preadipocyte differentiation and adipocyte hypertrophy. Although initial studies in transgenic mice and human beings support this concept, more data is required to conclusively demonstrate that the adipose-tissue specific overexpression of HSD1 and increases in adipose tissue cortisol lead to obesity, insulin resistance, high BP, and CMS [47]. Patients with essential HTN usually do not have overt signs of mineralocorticoid excess, but nevertheless can show a positive correlation between BP and increased serum sodium levels, or a negative correlation with potassium concentrations, suggesting a mineralocorticoid influence. Recent studies revealed a prolonged half-life of cortisol and an increased ratio of urinary cortisol to cortisone metabolites in some patients with essential HTN. These abnormalities may be genetically determined [48]. For example, the P2-HSD1 mouse with over expression of HSD1 is hypertensive with apparent activation of the circulating RAAS and features of the CMS [49]. These mice highlight the potential role of adipose glucocorticoid activation in the pathophysiology of HTN seen in the CMS. They develop visceral obesity, salt-sensitive HTN, insulin resistance, dyslipidemia, and increased plasma levels of angiotensinogen, angiotensin II, and aldosterone [49].

Leptin

Leptin is important in regulating appetite, body weight, and energy balance. It plays a vital role in the cross-talk between the brain and adipose tissue. Moreover, leptin has a wide range of biologic actions, including effects on the SNS, glucose and insulin metabolism, lipolysis, vascular tone, the hypothalamic-pituitary-adrenal axis, and reproduction [50]. Normally, leptin alters energy intake by decreasing appetite and increasing energy expenditure via SNS stimulation [50]. Leptin deficiency, or disruption of leptin signaling in the hypothalamus, can lead to obesity [51]. Plasma leptin levels are typically elevated in obese people and are positively correlated with the amount of adipose tissue. In fact, hyperleptinemia is an independent risk factor for coronary artery disease [52]. The failure of high levels of leptin in most obese individuals to promote weight loss is thought to be because of hypothalamic insensitivity to leptin action. It was proposed that hypothalamic leptin resistance in obesity is selective; the appetite-controlling and weight-reducing effects of leptin are disrupted while the excitatory effects on SNS are maintained [53].

The cardiovascular effects of leptin have recently been reviewed [54,55]. The mechanisms of leptin's vascular effects are complex. Despite the experimental reports of beneficial vascular effects, including improved nitric oxide production and endothelium-dependent vasodilatation [56], the predominant vascular effect of chronic hyperleptinemia is a pressor effect mediated by increased SNS activity. Leptin infusion in animal models causes increases in arterial BP, heart rate, and sympathetic nerve signals in several tissues [50,57,58]. Finally, leptin has been found to increase ROS and ET-1, which might contribute to HTN [59,60].

Adiponectin

Adiponectin has insulin-sensitizing, antiatherogenic, and anti-inflammatory effects [61]. Plasma levels of adiponectin are inversely related to obesity. Cross-sectional studies have shown that hypoadiponectinemia is an independent risk factor for HTN [62–64]. Recently, in a prospective 5-year nested study in a nondiabetic Chinese cohort, hypoadiponectinemia predicted the development of HTN in normotensive subjects, independent of sex, age, C-reactive protein, waist circumference, or BMI [65].

Several mechanisms might be involved in the association between hypoadiponectinemia and HTN [61,65,66]. Reduced adiponectin levels can be caused by interactions of genetic factors and environmental factors, such as lifestyle changes that cause obesity. Hypoadeponectinemia, in turn, appears to play an important causal role in the development of insulin resistance and HTN [67]. Studies of overexpression or knock-down of adiponectin receptors suggest that adiponectin increases adenosine monophosphate kinase and peroxisome proliferaltor-activator receptor (PPAR) ligand activity [61]. Adiponectin replenishment reduces BP in the hypertensive obese KKAy mice (a model of obesity-related HTN). Independent of obesity and insulin resistance, salt-fed adiponectin knockout mice develop HTN and adiponectin delivery improves HTN [68]. Furthermore, adiponectin induces nitric oxide production and increases nitric oxide bioavailability by up-regulating eNOS expression and reducing ROS production in endothelial cells [69,70]. It was shown both in human beings and in adiponectin-deficient mice that hypoadiponectinemia is associated with endothelial dysfunction and impaired endothelium-dependent vasodilatation [71]. It is likely that angiotensin receptor blocker induced adiponectin production is mediated by way of PPARγ activation [72].

Obstructive sleep apnea

Obesity, especially upper body obesity, is a major risk factor for obstructive sleep apnea (OSA). OSA frequently coexists with HTN. Approximately 5% to 10% of the general population and 50% to 60% of hypertensive patients have OSA [73]. The association between sleep-disordered breathing and the risk of developing HTN were studied prospectively in the Wisconsin Sleep Cohort Study. After adjustment for base-line HTN status, BMI, neck and waist circumference, age, sex, and weekly use of alcohol and cigarettes, there was a dose-response association between sleep-disordered breathing at base line and the presence of HTN 4 years later [74]. Despite its common prevalence, OSA is largely undetected and undertreated.

OSA results from a partial or complete collapse of the upper respiratory airways because of physiologic or anatomic causes. There is a wide spectrum of the manifestations of OSA, ranging from intermittent simple snoring to frequent episodes of apneas (absence of airflow), hypoxia, and hypercapnia with frequent arousals. The arousals from sleep, which are usually unrecognized by the patient, are associated with acute spikes in SBP [75]. People with OSA lose the physiologic nocturnal drop in arterial BP and have an average mean pressure that is higher during OSA episodes than it is during wakefulness. Symptoms of OSA include frequent snoring, nocturnal apnea and choking, diurnal hypersomnolence despite getting 8 hours of sleep, dyspnea, and nocturia.

Mechanisms of hypertension in obstructive sleep apnea

Patients with untreated OSA have increased SNS activity. Plasma and urine norepinephrine levels and baseline MSNA are also elevated in individuals with OSA [76–78]. Intermittent hypoxia in an animal model of sleep apnea results in prolonged high BP. Surgical denervation of peripheral chemoreceptors, adrenal demedullation, and chemical denervation of the peripheral SNS prevented such increases in arterial BP [79]. Moreover, in OSA hypoxia-induced autonomic and ventilatory responses in the peripheral chemoreceptor activation are exaggerated, with a blunted response to hypotensive stimulation [77]. There is evidence that patients with OSA have attenuated baroreflex control [80]. Finally, continuous positive airway pressure (CPAP) administered during the night, the most widely used treatment for OSA, decreases sympathetic activity and improves baroreflex control of heart rate, thus improving HTN [73].

There is accumulating evidence of endothelial dysfunction in OSA. For instance, endothelium-dependent vasodilatation of resistance vessels is impaired in patients with OSA [81]. This effect is subsequently reversed with CPAP treatment [82]. ET-1 seems to be a pathogenic factor in provoking HTN in OSA. A recent study, in patients with OSA, showed that they had higher plasma levels of ET-1 than did healthy controls. In this study, the mean nocturnal level of ET-1 was related significantly to the severity of OSA. This correlation remained statistically significant after correction for confounders [83]. In a study of 22 patients who had OSA, CPAP treatment reduced plasma ET-1 and the changes in ET-1 levels were correlated with changes in mean arterial blood pressure and oxygen saturation [84].

Plasma Ang II and aldosterone are both elevated in OSA patients compared with control subjects. In addition, long-term CPAP therapy resulted in correlated decreases in BP, plasma renin activity, and plasma Ang II concentrations [85]. Activation of the SNS seems to play a role in RAAS activation in OSA. In an animal model of episodic hypoxia, both renal-artery denervated and angiotensin receptor blocker-treated animals did not develop high BP in response to hypoxia, while control rats had progressive and sustained elevation in arterial BP [86]. This finding implicates the role of an activated RAAS and the kidney in OSA-related HTN.

Recent work suggests that hypoadiponectemia is independently associated with OSA [87–89]. Moreover, 14 days of CPAP treatment in overweight people with moderate to severe OSA decreased mean arterial pressure and increased adiponectin levels [90]. In summary, the etiology of HTN in OSA is complex. SNS hyperactivity plays a major role, while other factors include abnormalities in baroreflex control, the RAAS system, adipokines, and renal function.

Summary

Obesity and HTN are on the rise in the world. HTN seems to be the most common obesity-related health problem and visceral obesity seems to be the major culprit. Unfortunately, only 31% of hypertensives are treated to goal. This translates into an increased incidence of CVD and related morbidity and mortality. Several mechanisms have been postulated as the causes of obesity-related HTN. Activation of the RAAS, SNS, insulin resistance, leptin, adiponectin, dysfunctional fat, FFA, resistin, 11 Beta dehydrogenase, renal structural and hemodynamic changes, and OSA are some of the abnormalities in obesity-related HTN. Many of these factors are interrelated. Treatment of obesity should begin with weight loss via lifestyle modifications, medications, or bariatric surgery. According to the mechanisms of obesity-related HTN, it seems that drugs that blockade the RAAS and target the SNS should be ideal for treatment. There is not much evidence in the literature that one drug is better than another in controlling obesity-related HTN. There have only been a few studies specifically targeting the obese hypertensive patient, but recent trials that emphasize the importance of BP control have enrolled both overweight and obese subjects.

Until we have further studies with more in-depth information about the mechanisms of obesity-related HTN and what the targeted treatment should be, the most important factor necessary to control the obesity-related HTN pandemic and its CVD and CKD consequences is to prevent and treat obesity and to treat HTN to goal.

References

[1] Canoy D, Luben R, Welch A, et al. Fat distribution, body mass index and blood pressure in 22,090 men and women in the Norfolk cohort of the European Prospective Investigation into Cancer and Nutrition (EPIC-Norfolk) study. J Hypertens 2004;22(11):2067–74.

[2] Hajjar I, Kotchen TA. Trends in prevalence, awareness, treatment, and control of hypertension in the United States, 1988–2000. JAMA 2003;290(2):199–206.

[3] Flack JM, Casciano R, Casciano J, et al. Cardiovascular disease costs associated with uncontrolled hypertension. Manag Care Interface 2002;15(11):28–36.

[4] Must A, Spadano J, Coakley EH, et al. The disease burden associated with overweight and obesity. JAMA 1999;282(16):1523–9.

[5] Narkiewicz K. Diagnosis and management of hypertension in obesity. Obes Rev 2006;7(2): 155–62.

[6] Cooper R, McFarlane-Anderson N, Bennett FI, et al. ACE, angiotensinogen and obesity: a potential pathway leading to hypertension. J Hum Hypertens 1997;11(2):107–11.

[7] Engeli S, Böhnke J, Gorzelniak K, et al. Weight loss and the renin-angiotensin-aldosterone system. Hypertension 2005;45(3):356–62.

[8] Massiera F, Bloch-Faure M, Ceiler D, et al. Adipose angiotensinogen is involved in adipose tissue growth and blood pressure regulation. FASEB J 2001;15(14):2727–9.

[9] Hall JE, Brands MW, Henegar JR. Mechanisms of hypertension and kidney disease in obesity. Ann N Y Acad Sci 1999;892:91–107.

[10] Goodfriend TL, Egan BM, Kelley DE. Aldosterone in obesity. Endocr Res 1998;24(3–4): 789–96.

[11] Rahmouni K, Correia ML, Haynes WG, et al. Obesity induced hypertension: new insights into mechanism. Hypertension 2005;45(1):9–14.

[12] Reisin E, Weir MR, Falkner B, et al. Lisinopril versus hydrochlorothiazide in obese hypertensive patients: a multicenter placebo-controlled trial. Treatment in obese patients with hypertension (TROPHY) study group. Hypertension 1997;30(1 Pt 1):140–5.

[13] De Paula RB, Da Silva AA, Hall JE. Aldosterone antagonism attenuates obesity-induced hypertension and glomerular hyperfiltration. Hypertension 2004;43(1):41–7.

[14] Davy KP, Hall JE. Obesity and hypertension: two epidemics or one? Am J Physiol Regul Integr Comp Physiol 2004;286(5):R803–13.

[15] Alvarez GE, Beske SD, Ballard TP, et al. Sympathetic neural activation in visceral obesity. Circulation 2002;106(20):2533–6.

[16] Alvarez G, Ballard T, Beske S, et al. Subcutaneous obesity is not associated with sympathetic neural activation. Am J Physiol Heart Circ Physiol 2004;287(1):H14–8.

[17] Rumantir MS, Vaz M, Jennings GL, et al. Neural mechanisms in human obesity-related hypertension. J Hypertens 1999;17(8):1125–33.

[18] Weyer C, Pratley RE, Snitker S, et al. Ethnic differences in insulinemia and sympathetic tone as links between obesity and hypertension. Hypertension 2000;36(4):531–7.

[19] Wofford MR, Anderson DC Jr, Brown CA, et al. Antihypertensive effect of alpha- and beta-adrenergic blockade in obese and lean hypertensive subjects. Am J Hypertens 2001; 14(7 Pt 1):694–8.

[20] DeFronzo RA, Ferrannini E. Insulin resistance. A multifaceted syndrome responsible for NIDDM, obesity, hypertension, dyslipidemia, and atherosclerotic cardiovascular disease. Diabetes Care 1991;14(3):173–94.

[21] Modan M, Halkin H, Almog S, et al. Hyperinsulinemia. A link between hypertension obesity and glucose intolerance. J Clin Invest 1985;75(3):809–17.

[22] Hall JE, Brands MW, Zappe DH, et al. Hemodynamic and renal responses to chronic hyper-
    insulinemia in obese, insulin resistant dogs. Hypertension 1995;25(5):994–1002.
[23] Anderson EA, Hoffman RP, Balon TW, et al. Hyperinsulinemia produces both sympathetic
    neural activation and vasodilation in normal humans. J Clin Invest 1991;87(6):2246–52.
[24] Sawicki PT, Baba T, Berger M, et al. Normal blood pressure in patients with insulinoma
    despite hyperinsulinemia and insulin resistance. J Am Soc Nephrol 1992;3(Suppl 4):S64–8.
[25] Reaven GM, Chang H. Relationship between blood pressure, plasma insulin and triglyceride
    concentration, and insulin action in spontaneous hypertensive and Wistar-Kyoto rats. Am
    J Hypertens 1991;4(1 Pt 1):34–8.
[26] Sechi LA, Melis A, Tedde R. Insulin hypersecretion: a distinctive feature between essential
    and secondary hypertension. Metabolism 1992;41(11):1261–6.
[27] McFarlane SI, Banerji M, Sowers JR. Insulin resistance and cardiovascular disease. J Clin
    Endocrinol Metab 2001;86(2):713–8.
[28] Grunfeld B, Balzareti H, Romo H, et al. Hyperinsulinemia in normotensive offspring of
    hypertensive parents. Hypertension 1994;23(Suppl 1):I12–5.
[29] Beatty OL, Harper R, Sheridan B, et al. Insulin resistance in offspring of hypertensive
    parents. BMJ 1993;307(6896):92–6.
[30] Hall JE, Brands MW, Henegar JR, et al. Abnormal kidney function as a cause and a conse-
    quence of obesity hypertension. Clin Exp Pharmacol Physiol 1998;25(1):58–64.
[31] Kambham N, Markowitz GS, Valeri AM, et al. Obesity related glomerulopathy: an emerg-
    ing epidemic. Kidney Int 2001;59(4):1498–509.
[32] Bloomfield GL, Sugerman HJ, Blocher CR, et al. Chronically increased intra-abdominal pres-
    sure produces systemic hypertension in dogs. Int J Obes Relat Metab Disord 2000;24(7):819–24.
[33] Aneja A, El-Atat F, McFarlane S, et al. Hypertension and obesity. Recent Prog Horm Res
    2004;59:169–205.
[34] Pausova Z. From big fat cells to high blood pressure: a pathway to obesity-associated hyper-
    tension. Curr Opin Nephrol Hypertens 2006;15(2):173–8.
[35] Lofgren P, Andersson I, Adolfsson B, et al. Long-term prospective and controlled studies
    demonstrate adipose tissue hypercellularity and relative leptin deficiency in the postobese
    state. J Clin Endocrinol Metab 2005;90(11):6207–13.
[36] Ehrhart-Bornstein M, Lamounier-Zepter V, Schraven A, et al. Human adipocytes secrete
    mineralocorticoid-releasing factors. Proc Natl Acad Sci U S A 2003;100(24):14211–6.
[37] Steppan CM, Bailey ST, Bhat S, et al. The hormone resistin links obesity to diabetes. Nature
    2001;409(6818):307–12.
[38] Tan MS, Chang SY, Chang DM, et al. Association of resistin gene 3'-untranslated region
    +62G→A polymorphism with type 2 diabetes and hypertension in a Chinese population.
    J Clin Endocrinol Metab 2003;88(3):1258–63.
[39] Zhang J, Qin Y, Zheng X, et al. [The relationship between human serum resistin level and
    body fat content, plasma glucose as well as blood pressure]. Chung-Hua i Hsueh Tsa
    Chih. [Chinese Medical Journal] 2002;82(23):1609–12 [in Chinese].
[40] Asai T, Ohkubo T, Katsuya T, et al. Endothelin-1 gene variant associates with blood pres-
    sure in obese Japanese subjects. Hypertension 2001;38(6):1321–4.
[41] Cardillo C, Campia U, Iantorno M, et al. Enhanced vascular activity of endogenous endo-
    thelin-1 in obese hypertensive patients. Hypertension 2004;43(1):36–40.
[42] Tiret L, Poirier O, Hallet V, et al. The Lys198Asn polymorphism in the endothelin-1 gene is
    associated with blood pressure in overweight people. Hypertension 1999;33(5):1169–74.
[43] Mather KJ, Lteif A, Steinberg H, et al. Interactions between endothelin and nitric oxide in
    the regulation of vascular tone in obesity and diabetes. Diabetes 2004;53(8):2060–6.
[44] Grekin RJ, Vollmer AP, Sider RS. Pressor effects of portal venous oleate infusion.
    A proposed mechanism for obesity hypertension. Hypertension 1995;26(1):193–8.
[45] Sarafidis PA, Bakris GL. Non-esterified fatty acids and blood pressure elevation: a mecha-
    nism for hypertension in subjects with obesity/insulin resistance? J Hum Hypertens 2007;
    21(1):12–9.

[46] Bujalska IJ, Kumar S, Stewart PM. Does central obesity reflect "Cushing's disease of the omentum"? Lancet 1997;349(9060):1210–3.

[47] Sukhija R, Kakar P, Mehta V, et al. Enhanced 11beta-hydroxysteroid dehydrogenase activity, the metabolic syndrome, and systemic hypertension. Am J Cardiol 2006;98(4):544–8.

[48] Ferrari P, Lovati E, Frey FJ. The role of the 11beta-hydroxysteroid dehydrogenase type 2 in human hypertension. J Hypertens 2000;18(3):241–8.

[49] Masuzaki H, Yamamoto H, Kenyon CJ, et al. Transgenic amplification of glucocorticoid action in adipose tissue causes high blood pressure in mice. J Clin Invest 2003;112(1):83–90.

[50] Haynes WG, Morgan DA, Walsh SA, et al. Receptor mediated regional sympathetic nerve activation by leptin. J Clin Invest 1997;100(2):270–8.

[51] Münzberg H, Björnholm M, Bates SH, et al. Leptin receptor action and mechanisms of leptin resistance. Cell Mol Life Sci 2005;62(6):642–52.

[52] Wallace AM, McMahon AD, Packard CJ, et al. Plasma leptin and the risk of cardiovascular disease in the West of Scotland Cornary Prevention Study (WOSCOPS). Circulation 2001; 104(25):3052–6.

[53] Mark AL, Correia ML, Rahmouni K, et al. Selective leptin resistance: a new concept in leptin physiology with cardiovascular implications. J Hypertens 2002;20(7):1245–50.

[54] Yang R, Barouch LA. Leptin signaling and obesity: cardiovascular consequences. Circ Res 2007;101(6):545–59.

[55] Katagiri H, Yamada T, Oka Y. Adiposity and cardiovascular disorders: disturbance of the regulatory system consisting of humoral and neuronal signals. Circ Res 2007;101(1):27–39.

[56] Vecchione C, Aretini A, Maffei A, et al. Cooperation between insulin and leptin in the modulation of vascular tone. Hypertension 2003;42(2):166–70.

[57] Dunbar JC, Hu Y, Lu H. Intracerebroventricular leptin increases lumbar and renal sympathetic nerve activity and blood pressure in normal rats. Diabetes 1997;46(12):2040–3.

[58] Shek EW, Brands MW, Hall JE. Chronic leptin infusion increases arterial pressure. Hypertension 1998;31(1 Pt 2):409–14.

[59] Quehenberger P, Exner M, Sunder-Plassmann R, et al. Leptin induces endothelin-1 in endothelial cells in vitro. Circ Res 2002;90(6):711–8.

[60] Bouloumie A, Marumo T, Lafontan M, et al. Leptin induces oxidative stress in human endothelial cells. FASEB J 1999;13(10):1231–8.

[61] Kadowaki T, Yamauchi T. Adiponectin and adiponectin receptors. Endocr Rev 2005;26(3): 439–51.

[62] Adamczak M, Wiecek A, Funahashi T, et al. Decreased plasma adiponectin concentration in patients with essential hypertension. Am J Hypertens 2003;16(1):72–5.

[63] Francischetti EA, Celoria BM, Duarte SF, et al. Hypoadiponectinemia is associated with blood pressure increase in obese insulin-resistant individuals. Metabolism 2007;56(11): 1464–9.

[64] Iwashima Y, Katsuya T, Ishikawa K, et al. Hypoadiponectinemia is an independent risk factor for hypertension. Hypertension 2004;43(6):1318–23.

[65] Chow WS, Cheung BM, Tso AW, et al. Hypoadiponectinemia as a predictor for the development of hypertension: a 5-year prospective study. Hypertension 2007;49(6):1455–61.

[66] Schillaci G, Pirro M. Hypoadiponectinemia: a novel link between obesity and hypertension? Hypertension 2007;49(6):1217–9.

[67] Kadowaki T, Yamauchi T, Kubota N, et al. Adiponectin and adiponectin receptors in insulin resistance, diabetes, and the metabolic syndrome. J Clin Invest 2006;116(7):1784–92.

[68] Ohashi K, Kihara S, Ouchi N, et al. Adiponectin replenishment ameliorates obesity-related hypertension. Hypertension 2006;47(6):1108–16.

[69] Chen H, Montagnani M, Funahashi T, et al. Adiponectin stimulates production of nitric oxide in vascular endothelial cells. J Biol Chem 2003;278(45):45021–6.

[70] Motoshima H, Wu X, Mahadev K, et al. Adiponectin suppresses proliferation and superoxide generation and enhances eNOS activity in endothelial cells treated with oxidized LDL. Biochem Biophys Res Commun 2004;315(2):264–71.

[71] Ouchi N, Ohishi M, Kihara S, et al. Association of hypoadiponectinemia with impaired vasoreactivity. Hypertension 2003;42(3):231–4.

[72] Clasen R, Schupp M, Foryst-Ludwig A, et al. PPARgamma-activating angiotensin type-1 receptor blockers induce adiponectin. Hypertension 2005;46(1):137–43.

[73] Baguet JP, Narkiewicz K, Mallion JM. Update on hypertension management: obstructive sleep apnea and hypertension. J Hypertens 2006;24(1):205–8.

[74] Peppard PE, Young T, Palta M, et al. Prospective study of the association between sleep-disordered breathing and hypertension. N Engl J Med 2000;342(19):1378–84.

[75] Davies RJ, Crosby J, Vardi-Visy K, et al. Non-invasive beat to beat arterial blood pressure during non-REM sleep in obstructive sleep apnoea and snoring. Thorax 1994;49(4):335–9.

[76] Dimsdale JE, Coy T, Ziegler MG, et al. The effect of sleep apnea on plasma and urinary catecholamines. Sleep 1995;18(5):377–81.

[77] Narkiewicz K, Pesek CA, Kato M, et al. Baroreflex control of sympathetic activity and heart rate in obstructive sleep apnea. Hypertension 1998;32(6):1039–43.

[78] Robinson GV, Stradling JR, Davies RJ. Sleep 6: obstructive sleep apnea/hypopnea syndrome and hypertension. Thorax 2004;59(12):1089–94.

[79] Lesske J, Fletcher EC, Bao G, et al. Hypertension caused by chronic intermittent hypoxia–influence of chemoreceptors and sympathetic nervous system. J Hypertens 1997;15(12 Pt 2): 1593–603.

[80] Carlson JT, Hedner JA, Sellgren J, et al. Depressed baroreflex sensitivity in patients with obstructive sleep apnea. Am J Respir Crit Care Med 1996;154(5):1490–6.

[81] Kato M, Roberts-Thomson P, Phillips BG, et al. Impairment of endothelium-dependent vasodilation of resistance vessels in patients with obstructive sleep apnea. Circulation 2000;102(21):2607–10.

[82] Duchna HW, Stoohs R, Guilleminault C, et al. Vascular endothelial dysfunction in patients with mild obstructive sleep apnea syndrome. Wien Med Wochenschr 2006;156(21–22): 596–604.

[83] Gjorup PH, Sadauskiene L, Wessels J, et al. Abnormally increased endothelin-1 in plasma during the night in obstructive sleep apnea: relation to blood pressure and severity of disease. Am J Hypertens 2007;20(1):44–52.

[84] Phillipps BG, Narkiewicz K, Pesek CA, et al. Effects of obstructive sleep apnea on endothelin-1 and blood pressure. J Hypertens 1999;17(1):61–6.

[85] Moller DS, Lind P, Strunge B, et al. Abnormal vasoactive hormones and 24-hour blood pressure in obstructive sleep apnea. Am J Hypertens 2003;16(4):274–80.

[86] Fletcher EC, Bao G, Li R. Renin activity and blood pressure in response to chronic episodic hypoxia. Hypertension 1999;34(2):309–14.

[87] Zhang XL, Yin KS, Wang H, et al. Serum adiponectin levels in adult male patients with obstructive sleep apnea hypopnea syndrome. Respiration 2006;73(1):73–7.

[88] Makino S, Handa H, Suzukawa K, et al. Obstructive sleep apnoea syndrome, plasma adiponectin levels, and insulin resistance. Clin Endocrinol (Oxf) 2006;64(1):12–9.

[89] Masserini B, Morpurgo PS, Donadio F, et al. Reduced levels of adiponectin in sleep apnea syndrome. J Endocrinol Invest 2006;29(8):700–5.

[90] Zhang XL, Yin KS, Li C, et al. Effect of continuous positive airway pressure treatment on serum adiponectin level and mean arterial pressure in male patients with obstructive sleep apnea syndrome. Chin Med J (Engl) 2007;120(17):1477–81.

ELSEVIER
SAUNDERS

Endocrinol Metab Clin N Am
37 (2008) 663–684

ENDOCRINOLOGY
AND METABOLISM
CLINICS
OF NORTH AMERICA

Impact of Obesity
on Cardiovascular Disease

Kerstyn C. Zalesin, MD[a],*, Barry A. Franklin, PhD[b],
Wendy M. Miller, MD[c],
Eric D. Peterson, MD, MPH[d],
Peter A. McCullough, MD, MPH[a]

[a]*Department of Medicine, Division of Nutrition and Preventative Medicine, William Beaumont
Hospital, 4949 Coolidge Highway, Royal Oak, MI 48073, USA*
[b]*Cardiac Rehabilitation and Exercise Laboratories, William Beaumont Hospital,
4949 Coolidge Highway, Royal Oak, MI 48073, USA*
[c]*Weight Control Center, Division of Nutrition and Preventative Medicine, William Beaumont
Hospital, 4949 Coolidge Highway, Royal Oak, MI 48073, USA*
[d]*Duke Clinical Research Institute, Duke University School of Medicine, 2400 Pratt Street,
Durham, NC 22705, USA*

The growing prevalence of obesity has created a global public health threat. Two thirds of the American population is overweight or obese [1]; moreover, the prevalence of obesity is rising in developing countries and now is reaching many impoverished nations [2]. Overweight and obesity portends metabolic and cardiovascular consequences, placing individuals at higher risk for premature coronary heart disease (CHD) morbidity and mortality (Fig. 1). The cascade of obesity-related conditions accrues at the upper end of normal body mass index (BMI), highlighting the curious relationship that overweight and obesity share with CHD and metabolic risks [3]. In the United States, it is estimated that obesity causes an excess of 300,000 deaths annually [4], and potentially reduces lifespan by as much as 5 to 20 years in the morbidly obese [5]. The spread of the obesity epidemic will likely inversely impact life expectancy trends. Accordingly, today's generation of youth may be the first in the United States to not outlive their parents [6].

In past years, the role of obesity as an independent modulator of coronary risk has been controversial. Recent evidence, however, directly links

---

* Corresponding author.
E-mail address: kzalesin@beaumont.edu (K.C. Zalesin).

0889-8529/08/$ - see front matter © 2008 Elsevier Inc. All rights reserved.
doi:10.1016/j.ecl.2008.06.004
endo.theclinics.com

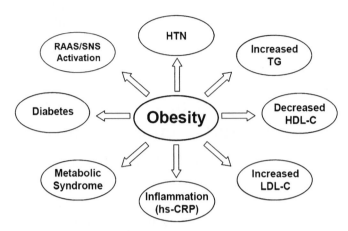

Fig. 1. Obesity is positioned as the only central and reversible cardiovascular risk factor that favorably influences all the other associated factors. HDL-C, high-density lipoprotein cholesterol; hs-CRP, high-sensitivity C-reactive protein; HTN, hypertension; LDL-C, low-density lipoprotein cholesterol; RAAS/SNS, renin-angiotensin-aldosterone system/sympathetic nervous system; TG, triglycerides.

obesity to intrinsic cardiac conditions including coronary artery disease (CAD), heart failure (HF), cardiomyopathy, and atrial fibrillation (AF), which collectively carry important health implications. In addition, excess adiposity appears to amplify Framingham CHD risk in patients who are followed over time for actual CHD events (Fig. 2). Potentially, many of the obesity-associated risks are partially remediable or preventable with treatment, education, and lifestyle modification. This article explores the impact of obesity on cardiovascular disease.

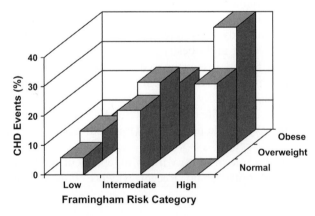

Fig. 2. Amplification of Framingham CHD risk by excess adiposity in 827 apparently healthy siblings (mean age, 46 years) over a mean follow-up of 8.7 years. (*From* Mora S, Yanek LR, Moy TF, et al. Interaction of body mass index and Framingham risk score in predicting incident coronary disease in families. Circulation 2005;111(15):1871–6; with permission.)

Obesity and coronary heart disease risk factors in the pediatric population

For youth, the prevalence of obesity—defined as a BMI (weight in kilograms divided by height in meters squared) at or above the 95th percentile for age and sex—is 10% for children aged 2 to 5 years and 15% for 6- to 19-year-olds [7]. This prevalence represents a doubling in children and a near tripling among adolescents over the last 2 decades [8]. Childhood obesity significantly increases morbidity and mortality from cardiovascular disease and has great prognostic significance [9]. The presence of cardiovascular risk factors among the pediatric population has become a modern phenomenon. Using the Bogalusa Heart Study database, Freedman and colleagues [10] studied 5- to 10-year-old obese children and reported significant odds ratios (ORs) for systolic blood pressure (OR 4.5, defined as >95th percentile), diastolic blood pressure (OR 2.4, defined as >95th percentile), low-density lipoprotein cholesterol (LDL-C; OR 3.0, defined as >130 mg/dL), triglycerides (OR 7.1, defined as >130 mg/dL), insulin concentration (OR 12.1, defined as >95th percentile), and low levels of high-density lipoprotein cholesterol (HDL-C; OR 3.4, defined as <35 mg/dL). The investigators noted that 58% of the study population had at least one of these cardiovascular risk factors and that 25% had two or more. Similar to the adult population, the presence of atherosclerotic lesions can be predicted by the number of coronary risk factors [11]. Childhood obesity substantially raises the risk of obesity in adulthood, which augments CHD morbidity and mortality risks for future generations.

Definition of obesity and abdominal obesity

The conventional measurements that define overweight and obesity (ie, BMI, weight, waist circumference, and waist-to-hip ratio) are not sensitive to body composition and merely represent surrogate markers for adiposity. Waist circumference, which is measured halfway between the last rib and the iliac crest, has independently been correlated with visceral obesity and abdominal fat [12]. Abdominal obesity, which is defined as a waist circumference of 103 cm (40 in) or more in men or 88 cm (35 in) or more in women, is associated with several metabolic risks including insulin resistance, type 2 diabetes mellitus (DM), the metabolic syndrome, and CHD. These metabolic alterations are excessively inflammatory in nature and are likely involved in the development of atherosclerosis. Waist circumference measurements among the American population have increased in the last several decades, perhaps even more so than BMI levels, which may be a surrogate marker of greater CHD risks, even among the nonobese.

Leading risks for cardiovascular disease: the obesity link

Cardiovascular disease continues to be a leading cause of morbidity and mortality throughout the world. In 2008 alone, 770,000 Americans will experience an acute myocardial infarction (AMI) and an additional 430,000 will have a recurrent event [13]. There are strong associations between cardiovascular disease risks and obesity. In a prospective study of over a million people followed for 14 years, obesity was strongly associated with an increased risk of all-cause and cardiovascular mortality. This study directly correlated CHD mortality risk with increasing BMI, reporting a twofold to threefold greater risk in individuals who had a BMI of 35 kg/m^2 or higher compared with leaner persons (BMI 18.5–24.9 kg/m^2). An increased risk of cardiovascular mortality was apparent at BMIs greater than 26.5 kg/m^2 and 25.0 kg/m^2 for men and women, respectively (Fig. 3) [14].

Data from the INTERHEART study, which evaluated a large controlled population and represented many diverse ethnic groups, confirmed that higher waist-to-hip ratios are associated with greater risks of cardiovascular disease and identified this measurement as a more discriminating risk factor than BMI in men and women of all ages [15]. A recent meta-analysis involving more than 258,000 subjects reported a progressive increase in cardiovascular risk with increasing waist circumference and waist-to-hip ratios [16]. In this study, every 1-cm increase in waist circumference was associated with a 2% increased relative risk of a cardiovascular event (95% confidence interval [CI]: 1%–3%) for men and women. These findings emphasize the importance of using this simple screening measure as a potential tool in assessing and predicting cardiometabolic risk.

Whether obesity is an independent mediator of CHD risk, apart from its comorbid associations, remains unclear. The Munster Heart Study [17], which followed more than 23,000 patients over a 7-year span, noted an association of increasing BMI with CHD mortality. After multivariate analysis, however, the increase in death was attributed to confounding medical conditions including hypertension and hypercholesterolemia, negating obesity as an independent mediator of risk. Others studies suggest that

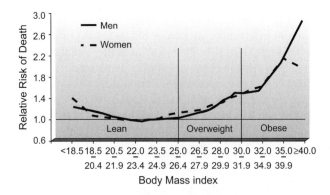

Fig. 3. Mortality risks across the BMI spectrum (*Data from* Calle EE, Thun MJ, Petrelli JM, et al. Body-mass index and mortality in a prospective cohort of US adults. N Eng J Med 1999;341:1097–105.)

obesity augments CHD risk through a codependent mechanism. A recent meta-analysis of more than 300,000 healthy patients identified a 45% increased risk of CHD with overweight and obesity, partially owing to the association with hypertension and hypercholesterolemia. Obesity and over-weight, however, were confirmed as significant risk factors warranting treatment [18]. The Framingham Heart Study 26-year follow-up identified obesity as an independent risk factor associated with CHD, stroke, HF, and death from cardiovascular disease [19]. These studies highlight the controversies in the literature with regard to the influence of obesity on cardiovascular risk.

Obesity appears to accelerate established CAD. Obese patients who have acute coronary syndromes tend to be younger at the time of their first cardiovascular event than their normal-weight counterparts and tend to suffer worse outcomes [20]. Based on strong current supportive evidence, the American Heart Association has identified obesity as a major modifiable risk factor for CHD [21]. Despite contemporary guidelines and improved technology for diagnosis, cardiovascular disease remains the leading cause of morbidity and mortality in America [13]. Moreover, the disease often presents without warning, that is, the first clinical manifestation is often an AMI [22]. Heart disease rates are escalating, making primary prevention of cardiovascular disease a major public health objective. Screening for those at elevated risk in the general population is crucial. Arguably, for much of the obese population, excess adiposity serves as a metabolic barometer, which can be highly indicative of excess risk.

Obesity and heart failure

Obesity is gaining support as an independent risk factor for HF, as verified in small population-based studies [23,24]. This hypothesis was strengthened in a prospective population study of approximately 6000 subjects followed for over 14 years that reported a twofold increase in the risk of developing HF among those individuals who had a BMI greater than 30 kg/m^2, even after adjusting for CAD, hypertension, and left ventricular hypertrophy. This study detailed increased HF rates of 5% and 7% for men and women, respectively, with each incremental unit increase in BMI [25]. Furthermore, the risk increased with escalating BMI categories for men and for women and was associated with both diastolic and systolic HF [25].

Although the mechanisms by which obesity causes HF remains unclear, the relationship may be attributed, at least in part, to the stress of an enlarged body habitus in conjunction with obesity-specific comorbid processes. Obesity is associated with several compensatory structural cardio-vascular alterations that result from the increased demands of an excessive body mass and a hyperdynamic circulation. These pathologic changes may stem from the associated increases in blood volume, cardiac output, stroke volume, and filling pressures, culminating in left ventricular hypertrophy and dilation that may induce diastolic dysfunction through impairment in diastolic relaxation [26].

The established metabolic consequences of obesity also impact HF. There is frequent overlap of obstructive sleep apnea (OSA) with increased vascular tone through activation of the renin-angiotensin and sympathetic systems, resulting in hypertension that can exacerbate left ventricular hypertrophy and diastolic dysfunction and contribute to HF [27–29]. The atherogenic, prothrombotic, and proinflammatory states noted in overweight and obesity enhance atherogenesis and CAD as precursors to HF [24]. It has been suggested that the likelihood of left ventricular dysfunction may be increased by the metabolic syndrome because the components of this medical condition have now been correlated to the degree of myocardial dysfunction [30].

An emerging hypothesis describes a direct influence of obesity on the myocardium through an accumulation of lipids in the muscle and vasculature, which increases with the extent of adiposity [31]. This association was first described in 1933 from autopsy findings that suggested fatty degeneration of the myocardial tissues as a direct consequence of obesity [32]. The theory suggests that when excessive body fat accumulates, visceral storage sites fill to capacity, promoting a release of triglycerides and free fatty acids into the circulation that then accumulate within the myocardium itself. There is also an abnormal aggregation of epicardial and paracardial adipose tissue, which are forms of visceral fatty accumulation [33]. These pathologic fatty depots secrete hormones, inflammatory cytokines, and proteins that apply a direct and continued exposure of the myocardium to an inflammatory milieu through a paracrine influence. This proximal association may intensify the progression of atherosclerosis and serve as a unique marker for cardiovascular disease risk [33]. The accumulation of lipid metabolism by-products within the myocardium promotes lipotoxicity through a pathologic activation of adverse signaling cascades, which can culminate in cellular death [34]. Animal research has also established the relationship of steatosis and interstitial dysfunction in other organ systems [35]. Collectively, these consequences induce left ventricular remodeling and diastolic dysfunction that in some cases may culminate in an obesity-specific dilated nonischemic cardiomyopathy. The term *obesity-specific lipotoxic cardiomyopathy* has been used to describe the relationship between obesity and HF and includes pathologic changes that may be arrhythmogenic [36].

Obesity and atrial fibrillation

Incidence rates of AF have increased dramatically over the last several decades. Approximately 2.5 million Americans now have AF, and these numbers are expected to soar with the aging of the population and the obesity epidemic [37]. The obese population demonstrates a twofold to fivefold increased risk of stroke and a twofold increase in early mortality as a consequence of its excessive adiposity [38]. Although previous reports regarding the link between obesity and AF have been inconsistent, a recent large community-based observational long-term follow-up (mean 13.7 years) of Framingham subjects delineated a close association between these two syndromes [39]. In this multivariate model adjusted for cardiovascular diseases (including a history of myocardial infarction and HF), a 4% increase in AF risk per 1-unit increase in BMI among men ($P = .02$) and women ($P = .009$) was reported. Adjusted hazard ratios for AF associated with obesity were 1.52 (95% CI: 1.09–2.13; $P = .02$) for men and 1.46 (95% CI: 1.03–2.07; $P = .03$) for women compared with normal-weight participants. In this study, left atrial diameter enlargement emerged as the strongest echocardiographic predictor of AF and has been directly correlated with increasing BMI levels [40]. These associations have been substantiated in another large population-based prospective cohort study, further strengthening the connection between obesity and AF [41]. Using many of the same hypotheses that explain the association of obesity and HF, researchers have now described common modulators that promote left atrial enlargement and AF, including elevated plasma volume, hypertension, left ventricular hypertrophy, diastolic dysfunction, stimulation of sympathetic tone, and OSA [30,42]. A theoretic direct influence of lipotoxicity promoting atrial enlargement has also been offered as a potential mechanism [36].

The obesity outcome paradox: findings after disease manifestation and treatment

Despite the fact that obesity is tightly linked to earlier CHD presentation, there has been a frequently reported "survival paradox" associated with overweight and obesity in patients who experience acute coronary events and in those who undergo emergent or elective coronary revascularization procedures [43,44]. A large population-based cohort study found that although there was a higher prevalence of overweight and obesity and related comorbidities among patients who had previous myocardial infarction, there were no adverse outcomes associated with obesity [45]. Recently, Uretsky and colleagues [46] noted this paradox among hypertensive patients who had known cardiovascular disease. This study evaluated 22,576 obese and overweight patients and found a decreased risk of primary end points (defined as death, nonfatal myocardial infarction, or nonfatal stroke) compared with a normal-weight control group. The results from the Arterial Revascularization Therapy Study trial (ARTS), a multicenter randomized trial comparing normal, overweight, and stage 1 obese patients who underwent coronary artery bypass grafting (CABG) or coronary stenting, reported a significant decrease in repeat revascularizations in the stage 1 obese subgroup ($P = .03$). At the 3-year end point, obese subjects who underwent CABG demonstrated a superior outcome with regard to survival and had a significantly decreased rate of major cardiac and cerebrovascular events ($P = .008$) [47].

The obesity survival benefit has been substantiated in similar multicenter randomized trials, whereby lower mortality rates after coronary angioplasty among hospitalized patients, at 30 days, and at 1-year intervals compared with patients who had normal BMI levels were noted [48]. Similar findings highlighting the existence of an obesity paradox have been noted in HF patients. Curtis and colleagues [49] reported that overweight and obesity provided a relative risk reduction of 12% and 19%, respectively, for all-cause mortality compared with a normal-weight group in patients who had established HF.

A meta-analysis [50] of 40 different studies with over 250,000 subjects who had known coronary disease followed for over a mean of 3.8 years revealed an inverse relationship with increasing BMI and CHD mortality rates that persisted through class II obesity. In this study, a BMI of less than 20 kg/m^2 was associated with an increased relative risk for CHD mortality of 1.45 (1.16–1.81). In the overweight group (BMI 25–29.9 kg/m^2), CHD mortality was lowest, with a relative risk of 0.88 (0.75–1.02), whereas class I obesity (BMI 30–35 kg/m^2) had a relative risk of 0.97 (0.82–1.15). Among patients who had class II obesity and above (BMI ≥ 35 kg/m^2), the cardiac mortality was significantly elevated and corresponded to a relative risk of 1.88 (1.05–3.34). Similarly, Kaplan and colleagues [51] correlated obesity with a higher mortality after AMI, reporting a U-shaped mortality curve by BMI levels, highlighting the complex association of mortality risks at BMI extremes (see Fig. 2).

Although this U-shaped association has been found in most studies, a few have reported decreased survival with increasing BMI levels after coronary revascularization. In the Bypass Angioplasty Revascularization Investigation (BARI) trial [52], there was a strikingly worse long-term prognosis after CABG as BMI increased, described as an 11% higher adjusted 5-year cardiac mortality rate among CABG-treated subjects with each incremental unit of BMI. These cumulative findings describe the controversy that surrounds the obesity paradox.

The mechanism underlying higher survival rates among obese CHD individuals is not fully clear. Some of these observed differences are due to the fact that the disease is manifest in patients at an earlier age [53]. It is also possible that obese cardiac patients tolerate the catabolic stress of myocardial ischemia or HF better than their normal-weight counterparts [53]. Conversely, weight loss due to chronic disease and cachexia may serve as a confounding variable, worsening outcomes in lower-weight individuals.

Obesity and diabetes mellitus

The worldwide prevalence of DM is rapidly increasing and is projected to increase to roughly 300 million by the year 2025. At least 95% of the new cases are a result of type 2 DM [54]. Obesity is strongly associated with the development of type 2 DM, and nearly 90% of individuals who have this metabolic condition are overweight or obese [55]. A recent study reported a reduction of 8 years in life expectancy in an individual who is diagnosed with DM by the age of 40 years compared with an individual who is not diagnosed with DM [56]. Approximately 65% of patients who have type 2 DM die from a cardiovascular event [57], and 7-year outcomes of patients who have CHD are similar to those of patients who have DM without known coronary disease. In a meta-analysis of 27 studies that evaluated mortality from CHD in the presence of diabetes, the risk of a fatal coronary event was three times higher in those affected with type 2 DM [58]. These sobering statistics support diabetes as risk equivalent to known cardiovascular disease [59].

Hyperglycemia with insulin resistance in conjunction with dyslipidemia, chronic inflammation, and procoagulability all contribute to endothelial dysfunction and macrovascular disease, leading to the development of CHD. Aggressive strategies to improve these metabolic markers are useful to prevent initial and recurrent cardiovascular events. The United Kingdom Prospective Diabetes Study found that poor diabetic control (hemoglobin A_{1c} >7.9%) was associated with a greater cardiovascular mortality rate when compared with tight glycemic control (hemoglobin A_{1c} <6%). In patients who have type 1 DM, intensive control of blood glucose involving three or more injections of insulin per day with appropriate adjustments has been shown to reduce the incidence of cardiovascular disease. Among the intensively treated group, there was a 42% reduction in the risk of cardiovascular events and a 57% decrease in the risk for nonfatal myocardial infarction, cerebrovascular accidents, and death from cardiovascular disease [60].

To achieve comprehensive cardiovascular risk reduction in a diabetic patient, optimization of risk factors is required from a multifactorial approach, including sustaining blood glucose levels (hemoglobin A_{1c} around 7%), appropriate blood pressure levels (<130/80 mm Hg), and targeted lipid levels (triglycerides <150 mg/dL, LDL-C <100 mg/dL, and HDL-C >40 mg/dL and >50 mg/dL in men and women, respectively). Gaede and colleagues [61] compared conventional treatment with intensive behavioral modification in patients who had type 2 DM that was aimed at achieving these goals and reported that the latter was superior, with behavioral modification resulting in a 53% cardiovascular risk reduction over 7-year period.

The reduction of cardiovascular risk factors has been repeatedly documented with therapeutic lifestyle intervention. Three separate large randomized controlled studies have concluded that lifestyle modification in an at-risk population is a successful method of diabetes prevention and is superior to pharmacologic intervention alone [62–64]. These strategies, however, employ behavior modification, which is labor-intensive and subject to recidivism.

Obesity and hypertension

Obesity is strongly associated with hypertension, which is a major risk factor for the development of CHD. The Framingham Heart Study reported that 79% of the hypertension in men and 65% in women was a direct result of excess weight [65]. Data from the Third National Health and Nutritional Examination Survey indicate a linear relationship between BMI and systolic and diastolic blood pressure [66]. In age-adjusted regression models, an increase in BMI of 1.25 kg/m^2 and 1.70 kg/m^2 and an increase in waist circumference of 2.5 cm and 4.5 cm among women and men, respectively, was associated with a 1-mm Hg increase in systolic blood pressure [67]. Uncontrolled hypertension increases CHD risks and exacerbates vascular complications including CAD, chronic kidney disease, stroke, peripheral vascular disease, and retinopathy [68]. The risk of developing CHD and of coronary death is increased in a progressive manner, with higher systolic and diastolic blood pressure levels seen among all age categories including the elderly [69,70].

The etiologic mediators of these increased risks are likely multifactorial. The consequence of obesity combined with hypertension promotes hemodynamic cardiac compensations from increased preload, stroke work, and blood volume, producing an eccentric cardiac hypertrophy [71]. These alterations are clinically meaningful because they are mediators of HF, ventricular arrhythmias, and sudden cardiac death. Obesity is associated with sympathetic stimulation and renin-angiotensin-aldosterone activation, exacerbating these hemodynamic alterations and increasing the likelihood of hypertension [72]. Collectively, these changes may heighten the risk of chronic kidney disease, which by way of a viscous feedback mechanism may accelerate the development of CHD.

Blood pressure lowering has been shown to be a successful strategy to reduce cardiovascular events. A meta-analysis of 10 randomized trials revealed that a 12- to 13-mm Hg lowering in systolic blood pressure over a 4-year follow-up was associated with a 21% reduction in CHD, a 37% reduction in stroke, and a 25% decrease in total cardiovascular mortality [73]. To minimize the likelihood of cardiovascular events, lowering blood pressure to normal ranges, especially in patients who have known cardiovascular disease, is of utmost importance. The last Joint National Committee guidelines recommended a blood pressure goal of less than 130/85 mm Hg and acknowledged that higher-risk patients who have known chronic kidney disease and proteinuria (>1 g) may benefit from even lower pressures (125/75 mm Hg) [74]. Concomitant diet/lifestyle intervention and pharmacotherapy are recommended strategies to achieve these goals. Currently, there is no evidence-based approach to direct obesity-related hypertension treatment other than empiric experience. Angiotensin-converting enzyme inhibitors or angiotensin-receptor blockers, however, may produce benefits beyond blood pressure lowering by improving modulators in DM, HF, and microalbuminuria, delaying the onset of DM and potentially reducing the risk of death, MI, and stroke [75,76]. β-blockers are routinely prescribed for patients who have known coronary disease and are an attractive treatment option for inhibition of the adrenergic response [77,78]; however, these agents may promote weight gain and potentially worsen glycemic control, limiting their appeal.

Obesity and dyslipidemia

Cholesterol is one of the greatest mediators for cardiovascular risk in visceral obesity. Indeed, approximately 70% of patients who have premature CHD also have dyslipidemia [79]. Increasing BMI levels mediate a common pattern of dyslipidemia characterized by higher triglycerides, lower HDL-C, and increased small, dense LDL particles, which are all independent risk factors for coronary disease [80,81]. This abnormal pattern of cholesterol is typically compounded in obesity by secondary associations to type 2 DM, the metabolic syndrome, and dietary influences from high fat and high sugar intakes. The small, dense LDL particles are excessively atherogenic due to their tendency for oxidation and their ability to penetrate the endothelial barrier of vessel walls, impairing nitric oxide production, blunting endothelial-mediated vasodilation, and augmenting inflammation, smooth muscle proliferation, and platelet aggregation [82–84].

The National Cholesterol Education Program Expert Panel on Detection, Evaluation, and Treatment of High Blood Cholesterol in Adults (Adult Treatment Panel III) guidelines provide evidence-based recommendations on the management of LDL-C using the Framingham Score, a 10-year prognostic assessment for identifying those at risk of developing cardiovascular disease. This score is derived from a formula using age, sex, tobacco use, HDL-C, LDL-C, blood pressure, and presence of diabetes. Modifying LDL-C is the major treatment goal for risk reduction within this model that incorporates lifestyle modifications and pharmacologic intervention, when appropriate. This validated model has the power to predict greater than 90% of all cardiac events, identifying those individuals at greatest risk [59]. A significant limitation of this common risk assessment tool is the absence of the variables obesity, physical inactivity, and insulin resistance—the metabolic syndrome parameters that are uniquely associated with cardiovascular disease and that are highly modifiable. If these variables were included in traditional risk assessments, then a significantly higher proportion of the population would meet criteria for treatment.

Treatment of these lipid/lipoprotein markers may decrease systemic inflammation, improve endothelial dysfunction, and stabilize and promote regression of atherosclerotic plaques, which all serve to reduce cardiovascular event rates and total mortality [85]. Statin therapy is highly effective for treating elevated LDL-C and triglycerides and reduced HDL-C. Certain patients who have elevated triglycerides and low HDL-C may benefit from the addition of a fibrate, which also has anti-inflammatory and antiatherosclerotic properties [86]. The Veterans Affairs HDL Intervention trial [87] found that the benefits of fibrate therapy depended on insulin resistance and, to a lesser extent, triglyceride or HDL-C abnormalities, supporting their potential use in the patient who has DM or the metabolic syndrome. Fibrate therapy was evaluated in the treatment of diabetic dyslipidemia in the Fenofibrate Interventions and Event-Lowering in Diabetes study [88], which found a significant benefit in secondary treatment outcomes among the intervention group; however, there was no significant benefit with respect to primary prevention. The Action to Control Cardiovascular risk in Diabetes study is currently investigating the use of statins and fibrate therapy in diabetics to determine the value of combined treatments with regard to cardiovascular and all-cause mortality outcomes [89].

Obesity and the metabolic syndrome

The association of visceral obesity and cardiovascular risks stems from the clustering of metabolic conditions (including hypertension, dyslipidemia, and type 2 DM) that are mediated through insulin resistance, leading to the metabolic syndrome. The purpose of this unique designation was to identify those at higher metabolic risk for cardiovascular disease and the development of diabetes and to respond with more aggressive strategies for prevention. The metabolic syndrome, as defined by the guidelines from the National Cholesterol Education Program Adult Treatment Panel III, is characterized by three or more of the criteria listed in Box 1. The metabolic syndrome is present in 24% of all adults in the United States and in more than 40% of men and women over the age of 65 years [90]. Each component of the metabolic syndrome is associated with a heightened risk for developing cardiovascular disease and diabetes [91]. Patients who have the metabolic syndrome have a 1.5- to 3-fold increased risk for developing CHD or stroke [92]. In the primary prevention arm of the San Antonio Heart Study (mean follow-up, 12.7 years), the metabolic syndrome was associated with a twofold higher risk for developing cardiovascular disease [93], which distinguishes the metabolic syndrome as a unique marker for increased cardiovascular risk and highlights the need for aggressive risk-factor reduction in this population.

Box 1. National Cholesterol Education Program Adult Treatment Panel III guidelines for diagnosing the metabolic syndrome

- Abdominal obesity defined as a waist circumference of 102 cm (40 in) in men and 88 cm (35 in) in women
- TG levels of 150 mg/dL or more (1.7 mmol/L)
- HDL-C levels of less than 40 mg/dL (1 mmol/L) in men and less than 50 mg/dL (1.3 mmol/L) in women
- Blood pressure levels of 130/85 mm Hg or higher
- Fasting glucose levels of 100 mg/dL or greater (5.5 mmol/L)

Links with nontraditional risk factors

Recent studies suggest that traditional risk factors do not fully encompass global cardiovascular risks. A new set of nontraditional risk factors are emerging (Box 2) [85,94]. Insulin resistance is the primary mediator in the development of diabetes (along with visceral obesity) and is a significant and independent risk factor for cardiovascular disease [95]. This condition adversely impacts insulin action and glucose disposal. β cells of the pancreas secrete higher levels of insulin to maintain blood glucose concentrations, which leads to hyperinsulinemia. These changes promote an impairment of lipolysis and the release of free fatty acids, leading to hypertriglyceridemia and the accumulation of fatty acids in the muscle and liver, which exacerbates insulin resistance and dyslipidemia [96].

Visceral obesity also promotes an inflammatory environment and increased levels of resistin, free fatty acids, and interleukin-6, which are the primary mediators of insulin resistance that accelerate atherogenic dyslipidemia and the likelihood of the metabolic syndrome and type 2 DM [97]. Obesity and insulin resistance contribute to vascular dysfunction by inhibiting the release of nitric oxide, a natural promoter of endothelial integrity and a mediator of vascular homeostasis. A recent study noted that increasing BMI was paralleled by abnormal vascular reactivity, increased vasoconstriction, and procoagulant influences [98]. Hyperinsulinemia with insulin resistance promotes multiple other metabolic derangements and is proportional to the risk of cardiovascular mortality [99].

Numerous studies have demonstrated beneficial effects of insulin sensitizers in modifying cardiovascular risk factors. Insulin sensitivity can be moderated by up-regulating peroxisome proliferator–activated receptors within adipose tissue, which favorably alters lipid and carbohydrate metabolism. Thiazolidinediones are peroxisome proliferator–activating receptor gamma agonists that are used in the treatment of type 2 DM. These agents

---

Box 2. Emerging risk factors for cardiovascular risk

- Insulin resistance
- Abnormal fibrinolysis
- Endothelial dysfunction
- Microalbuminuria
- Inflammation
- Procoagulation
- Obstructive sleep apnea

Data from Grundy SM, Cleeman JI, Mez CNB, et al. Implications of recent clinical trials for the National Cholesterol Education Program Adult Treatment Panel III Guidelines. Circulation 2004;110:227–39.

improve lipid/lipoprotein profiles and emerging vascular risk factors by enhancing vascular reactivity and inhibiting markers of thrombosis and inflammation, distinguishing this class of medications as an attractive intervention [100]. The carotid intima-media thickness is highly correlated with the risk of developing cardiovascular disease. In the Carotid Intima-Media Thickness in Atherosclerosis Using Pioglitazone trial, diabetic subjects were randomized to pioglitazone or glimepiride. Using carotid intima-media thickness as the criterion measure, investigators reported a significant benefit in the thiazolidinedione group compared with the glimepiride group [101].

Thiazolidinediones, however, are associated with weight gain and a more resistant adipose mass, which represent potential limitations. In contrast, fibrate therapy used in the treatment of dyslipidemia may up-regulate insulin receptors, facilitating glucose disposal in adipose and muscle tissue, thereby improving insulin sensitivity [102].

Microalbuminuria is now recognized as an early independent risk factor for chronic kidney disease, cardiovascular disease, insulin resistance, type 2 DM, and hypertension [103]. The exact mechanisms by which microalbuminuria is associated with cardiovascular disease are not known; however, it has been suggested that proteinuria serves as a generalized marker for endothelial dysfunction and, in this manner, signals a greater risk of generalized vascular disease and atherosclerosis [104].

There is an inverse relationship between microalbuminuria and insulin sensitivity. Conversely, with the reduction of urinary protein concentrations, there are associated metabolic improvements that translate to a markedly diminished cardiovascular risk [105]. DeZeaw and colleagues [106] examined type 2 DM patients who had nephropathy and reported that a decrease in proteinuria of 50% translated to an 18% reduction in cardiovascular risk. Pharmacologic treatment aimed at improving glycemia and hypertension has also proved to be beneficial at lowering microalbuminuria. Adequate blood pressure control is essential in improving the degree of urinary albumin excretion and hence the degree of nephropathy. Angiotensin-converting enzyme inhibitors and angiotensin II–receptor blockers improve albuminuria through their antihypertensive effects and lowering of intraglomerular pressure, reducing the progression of chronic kidney disease risks [107].

Visceral adipose cells were once considered inert but have now been shown to behave similarly to endocrine tissue, releasing cytokines and adhesion molecules including tumor necrosis factor α, which stimulates high-sensitivity C-reactive protein; P-selectin; and interleukin-6, which limits adiponectin release and is known for its antiatherogenic and insulin sensitivity–promoting properties. Excessive visceral adipose tissue secretions have been confirmed in biopsy studies in obese compared with normal-weight subjects [108]. These inflammatory changes further exacerbate hyperinsulinemia, hyperglycemia, and dyslipidemia in the obese patient, promoting oxidative stress, endothelial dysfunction, and cardiovascular alterations that are compatible with atherosclerotic heart disease. Rosito and colleagues [109] studied over 3230 subjects and found that increasing BMI values and hip-to-waist ratios were independently associated with prothrombotic factors, including impaired fibrinolytic activity, as well as abnormalities with fibrinogen, factor VII, plasminogen activating inhibitor 1, and tPA antigen in men and women ($P < .002$). Accordingly, the investigators found greater thrombotic potential in overweight and obese subjects.

Higher levels of plasminogen activator inhibitor 1, increased platelet aggregation, and elevated levels of fibrinogen promote a thrombotic state that exacerbates atherogenesis and cardiovascular risks [110]. These conditions function in concert with the metabolic syndrome and are highly atherogenic in nature. Presumably, the mechanisms involve an up-regulation of adhesion molecules and the inhibition of endothelial synthesis of nitrous oxide, which promote an increased risk for atherogenesis.

Using the notion that inflammation plays a key role in the development of cardiovascular disease, clinicians have increasingly examined the role of inflammatory markers in predicting risks for CAD. C-reactive protein levels of 2 mg/L or higher may be a powerful predictor for future cardiovascular events [111]. The current American Heart Association/Centers for Disease Control and Prevention Scientific Statement on Markers of Intervention and Cardiovascular Disease recommends that in the patient who has an intermediate Framingham 10-year risk (10%–20%) and an LDL-C level below the cut-off for initiation of pharmacotherapy it may be appropriate to measure C-reactive protein to aid in risk stratification and assessment [112]. The Justification for the Use of Statins in Primary Prevention (JUPITER) trial [113], which is currently ongoing, will assist in evaluating the utility of this inflammatory marker to help identify patients who may require more aggressive treatment. More recently, lipoprotein-associated phospholipase A_2 has emerged as a promising inflammatory marker associated with cardiovascular risk that may be able to predict atherosclerosis independent from obesity or other nonspecific inflammatory conditions. This ability would distinguish it as a potentially more sensitive screening tool that may further enhance risk assessments [114].

OSA is characterized by repeated partial or complete cessation of airflow during sleep, causing transient oxygen desaturation. Obesity is also a major determinant in risk for OSA [115]. Approximately 70% of patients diagnosed with OSA are obese, and the risk of OSA increases incrementally with escalating BMI levels [116]. For example, for every 10-kg increase in body weight, the risk of OSA doubles [117]. This condition contributes to the risks of hypertension, fatal and nonfatal cardiovascular events, stroke, HF, and cardiac arrhythmias [42]. Some of the metabolic disruptions associated with OSA stem from the activation of the sympathetic nervous system and the concurrent associations with systemic and pulmonary hypertension, atherosclerotic heart disease, dilated cardiomyopathy with or without HF, and cerebrovascular disease, arrhythmias, and AF [118–121]. Observational studies suggest that OSA is associated with a threefold increased risk for coronary disease apart from these related comorbid conditions [122]. There are also numerous thrombotic parameters that are associated with OSA that may increase cardiovascular events, including the exacerbation of coagulation defects, inflammatory responders, and endothelial dysfunction [123]. Despite these associations, OSA continues to be underdiagnosed and undertreated. In patients who have known coronary disease, OSA bears important prognostic significance, in that those patients who have untreated OSA experience a significantly higher mortality rate (38%) than their counterparts who do not have OSA (9%), which distinguishes OSA as a risk factor in need of diagnosis and of treatment.

Summary

Obesity promotes a cascade of secondary pathologies including diabetes, insulin resistance, dyslipidemia, inflammation, thrombosis, hypertension, the metabolic syndrome, and OSA, which collectively heighten the risk for cardiovascular disease. Obesity may also be an independent moderator of cardiac risk apart from these comorbid conditions. Rates of obesity and cardiac disease continue to rise in a parallel and exponential manner. Because obesity is potentially one of the most modifiable mediators of cardiovascular morbidity and mortality, effective treatment and prevention interventions should have a profound and favorable impact on public health.

References

[1] Flegal KM, Carroll MD, Ogden CL, et al. Prevalence and trends in obesity among U.S. adults, 1999–2000. JAMA 2002;288:1723–7.
[2] Popkin BM. The nutrition transition and its health implications in lower income countries. Public Health Nutr 1998;1:5–21.
[3] Willett WC, Manson JE, Stampfer MJ, et al. Weight, weight change and coronary heart disease in women: risk within the "normal" weight range. JAMA 1995;273(6):461–5.
[4] Allison DB, Fontaine KR, Manson JE, et al. Annual deaths attributable to obesity in the United States. JAMA 1999;282:1530–8.
[5] Fontaine KR, Redden DT, Wang C, et al. Years lost of life due to obesity. JAMA 2003;289: 187–93.
[6] Olshansky SJ, Passaro DJ, Hershow RC, et al. A potential decline in life expectancy in the United States in the 21st century. N Eng J Med 2005;352:1138–45.
[7] Ogden CL, Flegal KM, Carroll MD, et al. Prevalence and trends in overweight among U.S. children and adolescents, 1999–2000. JAMA 2002;288:1728–32.
[8] U.S. Department of Health and Human Services. The Surgeon General's call to action to prevent and decrease overweight and obesity. Rockville (MD): U.S. Department of Health and Human Services, Public Health Service, Office of the Surgeon General; 2001, Available from: U.S. GPO, Washington.
[9] Must A, Jacques PF, Dallal GE, et al. Long-term morbidity and mortality of overweight adolescents: a follow-up of the Harvard Growth Study of 1922 to 1935. N Eng J Med 1992;327:1350–5.
[10] Freedman DS, Dietz WH, Srinivasan SR, et al. The relation of overweight to cardiovascular risk factors among children and adolescents: the Bogalusa Heart Study. Pediatrics 1999; 103:1175–82.

[11] Berenson GS, Srinivasan SR, Bao W, et al. Association between multiple cardiovascular risk factors and atherosclerosis in children and young adults. N End J Med 1998;338: 1650–6.

[12] Pouliot MC, Despres JP, Lemieux S, et al. Waist circumference and abdominal sagittal diameter: best simple anthropometric indices of abdominal visceral adipose tissue accumulation and related cardiovascular risk in men and women. Am J cardiol 1994;73:460–8.

[13] Heart disease and stroke statistics–2008 update. A report from the American Heart Association Statistics Committee and Stroke Statistics Subcommittee. Circulation 2008;117: e25–146.

[14] Calle EE, Thun MJ, Petrelli JM, et al. Body-mass index and mortality in a prospective cohort of US adults. N Eng J Med 1999;341:1097–105.

[15] Yusuf S, Hawken S, Ōunpuu S, et al. Obesity and the risk of myocardial infarction in 27000 participants from 52 countries: a case-control study. Lancet 2005;366:1640–9.

[16] De Koning L, Merchant AT, Pogue J, et al. Waist circumference and waist-to-hip ratio as predictors of cardiovascular events: meta-regression analysis of prospective studies. Eur heart J 2007;28(7):850–6.

[17] Schulte H, Cullen P, Assmann G. Obesity, mortality and cardiovascular disease in the Munster Heart Study (PROCAM). Atherosclerosis 1999;144(1):199–209.

[18] Bogers RP, Bemelmans WJ, Hoogenveen RT, et al. Association of overweight with increased risk of coronary heart disease partly independent of blood pressure and cholesterol levels. Arch Intern Med 2007;167(16):1720–8.

[19] Hubert HB, Feinleib M, McNamara PM, et al. Obesity as an independent risk factor for cardiovascular disease: a 26-year follow-up of participants in the Framingham Heart Study. Circulation 1983;67(5):968–77.

[20] Eisenstein E, Shaw L, Nelson C, et al. Obesity and long-term clinical and economic outcomes in coronary artery disease patients. Obes Res 2002;10:83–91.

[21] Eckel RH. Obesity and heart disease: a statement for healthcare professionals from the Nutrition Committee, American Heart Association. Circulation 1997;96(9):3248–50.

[22] Levy D, Wilson PW. Atherosclerotic cardiovascular disease: an epidemiologic perspective. In: Topol EJ, editor. Text of cardiovascular medicine. Philadelphia: Lippincott-Raven; 1998. p. 13–30.

[23] Chen YT, Vaccarino V, Williams CS, et al. Risk factors for heart failure in the elderly: a prospective community-based study. Am J Med 1999;106:605–12.

[24] He J, Ogden LG, Bazzano LA, et al. Risk factors for congestive heart failure in US men and women: NHANES I epidemiologic follow-up study. Arch Intern Med 2001;161:996–1002.

[25] Kenchaiah S, Evans JC, Levy D, et al. Obesity and the risk of heart failure. N Engl J Med 2002;347(5):305–13.

[26] Alpert MA. Obesity cardiomyopathy: pathophysiology and evolution of the clinical syndrome. Am J Med Sci 2001;321:225–36.

[27] Kasper EK, Hruban RH, Baughman KL. Cardiomyopathy of obesity: a clinicopathologic evaluation of 43 obese patients with heart failure. Am J Cardiol 1992;70:921–4.

[28] Ku CS, Lin SL, Wang DJ, et al. Left ventricular filling in young normotensive obese adults. Am J Cardiol 1994;73:613–5.

[29] Masserli FH. Cardiomyopathy of obesity—a not so Victorian disease. N Engl J Med 1986; 314:378–80.

[30] Wong CY, O'Moore-Sullican T, Fang ZY, et al. Myocardial and vascular dysfunction and exercise capacity in the metabolic syndrome. Am J Cardiol 2005;96:1686–91.

[31] Malavazos AE, Ermetici F, Coman C, et al. Influence of epicardial adipose tissue and adipocytokine levels on cardiac abnormalities in visceral obesity. Int J Cardiol 2007; 121(1):132–4.

[32] Smith HL, Willius FA. Adiposity of the heart. Arch Intern Med 1933;52:811–31.

[33] Iacobellis G, Corradi D, Sharma AM. Epicardial adipose tissue: anatomic, biomolecular and clinical relationship with the heart. Nat clin pract Cardiovasc Med 2005;2:536–43.

[34] Unger RH. Minireview: weapons of lean body mass destruction: the role of ectopic lipids in the metabolic syndrome. Endocrinology 2003;144:5159–65.

[35] Lee Y, Hirose H, Ohneda M, et al. Beta-cell lipotoxicity in the pathogenesis of non-insulin-dependent diabetes mellitus of obese rats: impairment in adipocyte–beta-cell relationships. Proc Natl Acad Sci U S A 1994;91:10878–82.

[36] McGavrock JM, Victor RG, Unger RH, et al. Adiposity of the heart, revisited. Ann Intern Med 2006;144:517–24.

[37] Ezekowitz MD. Atrial fibrillation: the epidemic of the new millennium. Ann Intern Med 1999;131:537–8.

[38] Go AS, Hylek EM, Phillips KA, et al. Prevalence of diagnosed atrial fibrillation in adults: national implication of rhythm management and stroke prevention: the Anticoagulation and Risk Factors in Atrial Fibrillation (ATRIA) study. JAMA 2001;285:2370–5.

[39] Wang TJ, Parise H, Levy D, et al. Obesity and the risk of new-onset atrial fibrillation. JAMA 2004;292:2471–7.

[40] Pritchett AM, Jacobsen SJ, Mahoney DW, et al. Left atrial volume as an index of left atrial size: a population-based study. J Am Coll Cardiol 2003;41:1036–43.

[41] Frost L, Juul Hune L, Vestergaard P. Overweight and obesity as risk factors for atrial fibrillation or flutter: the Danish Diet, Cancer, and Health study. Am J Med 2005;118: 489–95.

[42] Gami AS, Caples SM, Somers VK. Obesity and obstructive sleep apnea. Endocrinol Metab Clin North Am 2003;32:869–94.

[43] Bozkurt B, Deswal A. Obesity as a prognostic factor in chronic symptomatic heart failure. Am Heart J 2005;150:1233–9.

[44] Curtis JP, Selter JG, Wang Y, et al. The obesity paradox. Arch Intern Med 2005;165:55–61.

[45] Lopez-Jimenez F, Jacobson SJ, Reeder GS, et al. Prevalence and secular trends of excess body weight and impact on outcomes after myocardial infarction in the community. Chest 2004;125(4):1205–12.

[46] Uretsky S, Messerli FH, Bangalore S, et al. Obesity paradox in patients with hypertension and coronary artery disease. Am J Med 2007;120:863–70.

[47] Gruberg L, Mercado N, Milo S, et al. Impact of body mass index on the outcome of patients with multivessel disease randomized to either coronary artery bypass grafting or stenting in the ARTS trial: the obesity paradox II? Am J Cardiol 2005;95:439–44.

[48] Nikolsky E, Stone GW, Grines CL, et al. Impact of body mass index on outcomes after primary angioplasty in acute myocardial infarction. Am Heart J 2006;151:168–75.

[49] Curtis JP, Selter JG, Wang Y, et al. The obesity paradox: body mass index and outcomes in patients with heart failure. Arch Intern Med 2005;165(1):55–61.

[50] Romero-Corral A, Montori VM, Somers VK, et al. Association of bodyweight with total mortality and with cardiovascular events in coronary artery disease: a systematic review of cohort studies. Lancet 2006;368:666–78.

[51] Kaplan RC, Heckbert SR, Furburg CD, et al. Predictors of subsequent coronary events, stroke, and death among survivors of first hospitalized myocardial infarction. J Clin Epidemiol 2002;55:654–64.

[52] Grum HS, Whitlow PL, Kip KE. The impact of body mass index on short-term and long-term outcomes inpatients undergoing coronary revascularization. (BARI). J Am Coll Cardiol 2002;39:834–40.

[53] Lissin LW, Gauri AJ, Froelicher VF, et al. The prognostic value of body mass index and standard exercise testing in male veterans with congestive heart failure. J Card Fail 2002; 8:206–15.

[54] King H, Aubert RE, Herman WH. Global burden of diabetes, 1995–2025: prevalence, numerical estimates, and projections. Diabetes Care 1998;21:1414–31.

[55] Mokdad AH, Ford ES, Bowman BA, et al. Prevalence of obesity, diabetes, and obesity-related health risk factors, 2001. JAMA 2003;289:76–9.

[56] Roper NA, Bilous RW, Kelly WF, et al. Excess mortality in a population with diabetes and the impact of material deprivation: longitudinal, population based study. BMJ 2001;332: 1389–93.

[57] Gu K, Cowie CC, Harris MI. Diabetes and decline in heart disease mortality in US adults. JAMA 1999;281:1291–7.

[58] Huxley R, Barzi F, Woodward M. Excess risk of fatal coronary heart disease associated with diabetes in men and women: meta-analysis of 37 prospective cohort studies. BMJ 2006;332:73–8.

[59] National Cholesterol Education Program, Adult Treatment Panel III. Executive summary of the third report of the National Cholesterol Education Program (NCEP) Expert Panel on Detection, Evaluation and Treatment of High Blood Cholesterol in Adults. JAMA 2001; 285(19):2486–98.

[60] Natham DM, Cleary PA, Backlund JY, et al. for the Diabetes Control and Complications Trial/Epidemiology of Diabetes Interventions and Complications (DCCT/EDIC) study research group. Intensive diabetes treatment and cardiovascular disease in patients with type 1 diabetes. N Engl J Med 2005;353:2643–53.

[61] Gaede P, Vedel P, Larsen N, et al. Multifactorial intervention and cardiovascular disease in patients with type 2 diabetes. N Eng J Med 2003;348:383–93.

[62] Pan XR, Li GW, Hu YH, et al. Effects of diet and exercise in preventing NIDDM in people with impaired glucose tolerance. The Da Qing IGT and Diabetes Study. Diabetes Care 1997;20:537–44.

[63] Tuomilehto J, Lindstrom J, Eriksson JG, et al. Finnish Diabetes Prevention Study Group. Prevention of type 2 diabetes mellitus by changes in lifestyle among subjects with impaired glucose tolerence. N Engl J Med 2002;346:393–403.

[64] Knowler WC, Barnett-Connor E, Fowler SE, et al. Reduction in the incidence of type 2 diabetes with lifestyle intervention. N Eng J Med 2002;346:393–403.

[65] Garrison RJ, Kannel WB, Stokes ME, et al. Incidence and precursors of hypertension in young adults: the Framingham offspring study. Prev Med 1987;16:235–51.

[66] El-Atat F, Aneja A, Mcfarlane S, et al. Obesity and hypertension. Endocinol Metab Clin North Am 2003;32:832–54.

[67] Engeli S, Sharma AM. Emerging concepts in the pathophysiology and treatment of obesity-associated hypertension. Curr Opin Cardiol 2002;17:355–9.

[68] Toto RD. Treatment of hypertension in chronic kidney disease. Semin Nephrol 2005;25:435–9.

[69] Lewington S, Clarke R, Qizilbash N, et al. Prospective Studies Collaboration. Age-specific relevance of usual blood pressure to vascular mortality: a meta-analysis of individual data for one million adults in 61 prospective studies. Lancet 2002;360:1903–13.

[70] Stamler J, Stamler R, Neaton JD. Blood pressure systolic and diastolic and cardiovascular risks. US population data. Arch Intern Med 1993;153:598–615.

[71] Frohlich ED, Epstein C, Chobanian AV, et al. The heart in hypertension. N Engl J Med 1992;327:998–1008.

[72] Hall JE, Hildebrandt DA, Kuo J. Obesity hypertension: role of leptin and sympathetic nervous system. Am J Hypertens 2001;14:103S–15S.

[73] He J, Whelton PK. Elevated systolic blood pressure and risk of cardiovascular and renal disease: overview of evidence from observational epidemiologic studies and randomized controlled trials. Am Heart J 1999;138:211–9.

[74] Chobanian AV, Bakris GL, Black HR, et al. The National High Blood Pressure Education Program Coordinating Committee. Seventh report of the Joint National Committee on Prevention, Detection, Evaluation, and Treatment of High Blood Pressure. Hypertension 2003;42:1206–52.

[75] Heart Outcomes Prevention Evaluation Study Investigators. Effects of ramipril on cardio-vascular and microvascular outcomes in people with diabetes mellitus: results of the HOPE study and MICRO-HOPE substudy. Lancet 2000;355:253–9.

[76] Yusuf S, Sleight P, Pogue J, et al. Effects of an angiotensin-converting-enzyme inhibitor, ramipril, on cardiovascular events in high-risk patients. The Heart Outcomes Prevention Evaluation Study Investigators. N Eng J Med 2000;342(3):145–53.

[77] Pedersen TR. Six-year follow-up of the Norwegian Multicenter Study on timolol after acute myocardial infarction. N Eng J Med 1985;313:1055–8.

[78] Tuck ML. Obesity, the sympathetic nervous system, and essential hypertension. Hypertension 1992;19:167–77.

[79] Genest JJ, Martin-Munley SS, McNamara JR, et al. Familial lipoprotein disorders in patients with premature coronary artery disease. Circulation 1992;85(6):2025–33.

[80] Austin MA, Hokanson JE, Edwards KL. Hypertriglyceridemia as a cardiovascular risk factor. Am J Cardiol 1998;81(Suppl):7B–12B.

[81] Garber AM, Alvins AL. Triglyceride concentration and coronary heart disease. Not yet proved of value as a screening test. BMJ 1994;309(6946):2–3.

[82] Austin MA, King MC, Vranizan KM, et al. Atherogenic lipoprotein phenotype. A proposed genetic marker for coronary heart disease risk. Circulation 1990;82(2):495–506.

[83] Anderson TJ, Meredith IT, Charbonneau F, et al. Endothelium-dependent coronary vasomotion relates to the susceptibility of LDL to oxidation in humans. Circulation 1996;93(9):1647–50.

[84] Griffin JH, Fernandez JA, Deguchi H. Plasma lipoproteins, hemostasis and thrombosis. Thromb Haemost 2001;86(1):386–94.

[85] Grundy SM, Cleeman JI, Mez CN, et al. Implications of recent clinical trials for the National Cholesterol Education Program Adult Treatment Panel III guidelines. Circulation 2004;110:227–39.

[86] Nesto RW. Beyond low-density lipoprotein: addressing the atherogenic lipid triad in type 2 diabetes mellitus and metabolic syndrome. Am J Cardiovasc Drugs 2005;5:379–87.

[87] Robins SJ, Rubins HB, Faas FH, et al, for the VA-HIT Study Group. Insulin resistance and cardiovascular events with low HDL cholesterol. The Veterans Affairs HDL Intervention trial (VA-HIT). Diabetes Care 2003;26:1513–7.

[88] Keech A, Simes RJ, Barter P, et al. for the FIELD study investigators. Effects of long-term fenofibrate therapy on cardiovascular events in 9795 people with type 2 diabetes mellitus (the FIELD study) randomized controlled trial. Lancet 2005;366:1849–61.

[89] Goff DC, Gerstein HC, Ginsberg HN, et al. Prevention in cardiovascular disease in persons with type 2 diabetes mellitus: current knowledge and rationale for the Action to Control Cardiovascular Risk in Diabetes (ACCORD) trial. Am J Cardiol 2007; 99(Suppl):4i–20i.

[90] Ford ES, Giles WH, Dietz WH. Prevalence of the metabolic syndrome among US adults: findings from the Third National Health and Nutritional Examination Survey. JAMA 2002;287(3):356–9.

[91] Sattar N, Gaw A, Scherbakova O, et al. Metabolic syndrome with and without C-reactive protein as a predictor of coronary heart disease and diabetes in the West of Scotland Coronary Prevention Study. Circulation 2003;108:414–9.

[92] Isomaa B, Almgren P, Tuomi T, et al. Cardiovascular morbidity and mortality associated with the metabolic syndrome. Diabetes Care 2001;24:683–9.

[93] Hunt KJ, Resendez RG, Williams K, et al. National cholesterol education program versus World Health Organization metabolic syndrome in relation to all-cause and cardiovascular mortality in the San Antonio Heart Study. Circulation 2004;110:1251–7.

[94] Forseca VA. Rationale for the use of insulin sensitizers to prevent cardiovascular events in type 2 diabetes. Am J Med 2007;120:S18–25.

[95] Després J-P, Lamrche B, Mauriége P, et al. Hyperinsulinemia as an independent risk factor for ischemic heart disease. N Engl J Med 1996;334:952–7.

[96] Olefsky JM, Farqunar JW, Reaven GM. Reappraisal of the role of insulin in hypertriglyceridemia. Am J Med 1974;57:551–60.

[97] Miller WM, Nori Janosz KE, Yanez J, et al. Effects of weight loss and pharmacotherapy on inflammatory markers of cardiovascular disease. Expert Rev Cardiovasc Ther 2005;3(4): 743–59.

[98] Juonala M, Viikari JS, Laitinen T, et al. Interrelations between brachial endothelial function and carotid intima-media thickness in young adults: the Cardiovascular Risk in Young Finns study. Circulation 2004;110:2918–23.

[99] Eschwege E, Richard JL, Thibult N, et al. Coronary heart disease mortality in relation with diabetes, blood glucose and plasma insulin levels: the Paris Prospective Study, ten years later. Horm Metab Res Suppl 1985;15:41s–6s.

[100] Fonseca V, Desouza C, Asnani S, et al. Nontraditional risk factors for cardiovascular disease in diabetes. Endocr Rev 2004;25:153–75.

[101] Mazzone T, Meyer PM, Feinstein SB, et al. Effect of pioglitazone compared with glimipiride on carotid-media thickness in type 2 diabetes. JAMA 2006;296:2572–81.

[102] Tenenbaum A, Motro M Fisman EZ. Dual and panperoxisome proliferators-activated receptors (PPAR) co-agonism: the benzafibrate lessons. Cardiovasc Diabetol 2005;4:14–9.

[103] Keane WF, Eknoyan G. Proteinuria, Albuminuria, Risk Assessment, Detection, Elimination (PARADE): a position paper of the National Kidney Foundation. Am J Kidney Dis 1999;33:1004–10.

[104] Yudkin JS. Hyperinsulinemia, insulin resistance, microalbuminuria and the risk of coronary heart disease. Ann Med 1996;28:433–8.

[105] Mykkanen L, Zaccaro DJ, Wagenknecht LE, et al. Microalbuminuria is associated with insulin resistance in nondiabetic subjects: the Insulin Resistance Atherosclerosis Study. Diabetes 1998;47:793–800.

[106] deZeeuw D, Remuzzi G, Parving HH, et al. Albuminuria, a therapeutic target for cardiovascular protection in type 2 diabetic patients with nephropathy. Circulation 2004;110: 921–7.

[107] Grassi G, Seravalle G, Dell'Oro R, et al. Comparative effects of candesartan and hydrochlorothiazide on blood pressure, insulin sensitivity and sympathetic drive in obese hypertensive individuals: results of the CROSS study. J Hypertens 2003;21:1761–9.

[108] Lefebre AM, Laville M, Vega N, et al. Depot-specific differences in adipose tissue gene expression in lean and obese subjects. Diabetes 1998;47:98–103.

[109] Rosito GA, D'Agostino RB, Massaro J, et al. Association between obesity and a prothrombotic state: the Framingham offspring study. Thromb Haemost 2004;91:683–9.

[110] Kohler HP, Grant PJ. Plasminogen-activating inhibitor type 1 and CAD. N Engl J Med 2000;342:1792–801.

[111] Ridker PM, Cushman M, Stamfer MJ, et al. Inflammation, aspirin and the risk of cardiovascular disease in apparently healthy men. N Eng J Med 1997;336:973–9.

[112] Pearson TA, Mensah GA, Alexander RW, et al. American heart association guide for improving cardiovascular health at the community level: a statement for public health practitioners, healthcare providers and health policy makers from the American heart association expert panel on population and prevention science. Circulation 2003;107:645–51.

[113] Ridker PM, for the JUPITTER Study group. Rosuvastatin in the primary prevention of cardiovascular disease among patients with low levels of low-density lipoprotein cholesterol and elevated high-sensitivity C-reactive protein: rationale and design of the JUPITER trial. Circulation 2003;108:2292–7.

[114] McConnell JP, Hoefner DM. Lipoprotein-associated phospholipase A2. Clin Lab Med 2006;26(3):679–97.

[115] Grunstein K, Wilcox I, Yang T-S, et al. Snoring and sleep apnea in men: association with central obesity and hypertension. Int J Obes 1993;17:533–40.

[116] Malhotra A, White DP. Obstructive sleep apnea. Lancet 2002;360(9328):237–45.

[117] Young T, Palta M, Dempsey J, et al. The occurrence of sleep-disordered breathing among middle-aged adults. N Eng J Med 1993;328(17):1230–5.

[118] Blankfield RP, Hudgel DW, Tapolyai AA, et al. Bilateral leg edema, obesity pulmonary hypertension and obstructive sleep apnea. Arch Intern Med 2000;160:2357–62.

[119] Young T, Peppard P, Palta M, et al. Population-based study of sleep-disordered breathing as a risk factor for hypertension. Arch Intern Med 1997;157:1746–52.

[120] Gami AS, Pressman G, Caples SM, et al. Association of atrial fibrillation and obstructive sleep apnea. Circulation 2004;110:364–7.

[121] Shahar E, Whitney CW, Redline S, et al. Sleep-disordered breathing and cardiovascular disease: cross-sectional results of the Sleep Heart Health study. Am J Respir Crit Care Med 2001;163:19–25.

[122] Peker Y, Kraiczi H, Hedner J, et al. An independent association between obstructive sleep apnea and coronary artery disease. Eur Respir J 1999;14(1):179–84.

[123] Dyken ME, Somers VK, Yamanda T, et al. Investigating the relationship between stroke and obstructive sleep apnea. Stroke 1996;27:401–7.

ELSEVIER
SAUNDERS

Endocrinol Metab Clin N Am
37 (2008) 685–711

ENDOCRINOLOGY
AND METABOLISM
CLINICS
OF NORTH AMERICA

An Integrated View of Insulin Resistance and Endothelial Dysfunction

Ranganath Muniyappa, MD, PhD[a],
Micaela Iantorno, MD[b], Michael J. Quon, MD, PhD[b],*

[a]Diabetes Unit, National Center for Complementary and Alternative Medicine,
National Institutes of Health, 10 Center Drive, 10-CRC, Room 4-1741,
Bethesda, MD 20892-1632, USA
[b]Diabetes Unit, National Center for Complementary and Alternative Medicine,
National Institutes of Health, 9 Memorial Drive, Building 9,
Room 1N-105 MSC 0920, Bethesda, MD 20892-0920, USA

Insulin resistance plays a major patho-physiologic role in type 2 diabetes and is tightly associated with major public health problems, including obesity, hypertension, coronary artery disease, dyslipidemias, and a cluster of metabolic and cardiovascular abnormalities that define the metabolic syndrome [1,2]. A global epidemic of obesity is driving the increased incidence and prevalence of insulin resistance and its cardiovascular complications [3]. Insulin regulates glucose homeostasis by promoting glucose disposal in skeletal muscle and adipose tissue and inhibiting gluconeogenesis in liver [4]. In addition to these classical insulin target tissues, insulin has important physiologic functions in the brain, pancreatic beta cells, heart, and vascular endothelium that help coordinate and couple metabolic and cardiovascular homeostasis under healthy conditions [5]. For example, vasodilator actions of insulin to stimulate production of nitric oxide (NO) from vascular endothelium lead to increased blood flow that further enhances glucose uptake in skeletal muscle [6,7]. The time- and dose-response for metabolic and cardiovascular actions of insulin are distinct and tissue-specific [5,8,9]. Insulin resistance is typically defined as decreased sensitivity or responsiveness to metabolic actions of insulin, such as insulin-mediated glucose disposal. However, diminished sensitivity or resistance to the actions

This work was supported by the Intramural Research Program, NCCAM, NIH.
* Corresponding author.
E-mail address: quonm@nih.gov (M.J. Quon).

0889-8529/08/$ - see front matter. Published by Elsevier Inc.
doi:10.1016/j.ecl.2008.06.001

of insulin in vascular endothelium also contributes importantly to the clinical phenotype of insulin-resistant states [5,10,11].

Insulin binding to its cognate receptor at the cell surface activates two major branches of a complex insulin signal transduction network. Metabolic actions of insulin tend to be mediated by phosphatidylinositol 3-kinase (PI3K)-dependent signaling pathways, whereas mitogen-activated protein kinase (MAPK)-dependent insulin signaling typically regulates mitogenesis, growth, and differentiation [12,13]. Insulin-signaling pathways regulating endothelial production of NO are PI3K-dependent and exhibit striking parallels with metabolic insulin-signaling pathways in skeletal muscle and adipose tissue [14]. Insulin resistance is characterized by pathway-selective impairment in PI3K-dependent signaling in both metabolic and vascular insulin target tissues [15,16]. Consequently, glucotoxicity, lipotoxicity, and inflammation that contribute to development of insulin resistance also lead to endothelial dysfunction. Indeed, pathway-specific impairment in PI3K-dependent insulin signaling contributes to reciprocal relationships between insulin resistance and endothelial dysfunction that foster the clustering of metabolic and cardiovascular diseases in insulin-resistant states [14]. This article discusses the implications of pathway-specific insulin resistance in vascular endothelium, effects of endothelial dysfunction on insulin resistance, and therapeutic interventions that may simultaneously improve both metabolic and endothelial function in insulin-resistant conditions.

Nitric oxide and endothelial function

NO, an important determinant of endothelial function, is produced in vascular endothelium by activation of endothelial NO synthase (eNOS) [17]. Classical cholinergic vasodilators (eg, acetylcholine) activate serpentine G protein-coupled receptors on endothelial cells that mediate a rise in intracellular calcium levels. Interaction of calcium/calmodulin with the calmodulin-binding site on eNOS results in increased enzymatic activity. In addition, phosphorylation of eNOS at Ser^{1177} by serine kinases, including Akt, AMPK, and PKA also stimulate production of NO in a calcium-independent manner. This eNOS activity is also regulated by other posttranslational modifications, including acylation (myristoylation and palmitoylation), and S-nitrosylation [18]. Availability of L-arginine (substrate for eNOS) and enzymatic cofactors (nicotinamide adenine dinucleotide phosphate, flavin adenine dinucleotide, flavin mononucleotide, and tetrahydrobiopterin) also play a role in regulating NO production by eNOS [17]. Endothelial-derived NO diffuses into adjacent vascular smooth muscle cells (VSMC), where it activates guanylate cyclase. Increased levels of cyclic guanosine monophosphate then lead to vasorelaxation. In addition to modulating vascular tone, NO attenuates production of proinflammatory cytokines, decreases expression of vascular cell adhesion molecules (VCAM), limits leukocyte recruitment, inhibits VSMC proliferation, opposes apoptosis, attenuates platelet aggregation, and reduces monocyte adhesion to the vascular wall [19]. Inactivation of NO by enhanced production of reactive oxygen species (ROS) in the vasculature can significantly reduce NO bioavailability. This contributes to endothelial dysfunction and promotes the development of atherosclerosis. The term "endothelial dysfunction" refers to a maladapted endothelial phenotype characterized by reduced NO bioavailability, increased oxidative stress, elevated expression of proinflammatory and prothrombotic factors, and abnormal vasoreactivity [20]. Endothelial dysfunction is linked to insulin-resistant states, including diabetes, obesity, and the metabolic syndrome. This increases the susceptibility of patients with these metabolic diseases to cardiovascular complications, including accelerated atherosclerosis, coronary heart disease, and hypertension. Importantly, endothelial dysfunction is independently associated with and predicts cardiac death, myocardial infarction, and stroke [21].

Clinical assessment of endothelial function

Direct assessment of endothelial production of NO in vivo is challenging because of its short-half life (approximately 5 seconds) and low physiologic concentrations (pM range). Therefore, the vasodilator effect of endothelium-derived NO is often used to evaluate endothelial function in human beings (Table 1) [22]. Changes in limb blood flow (assessed by plethysmography) or conduit artery diameter (assessed by ultrasound) in response to intra-arterial infusion of agents that stimulate endothelium-dependent production of NO, such as acetylcholine, are used primarily in research settings to evaluate endothelial function. Another less-invasive method involves shear stress-induced flow-mediated dilatation (FMD) of the brachial artery. High resolution doppler ultrasonography is used to measure changes in arterial diameter and blood flow in the brachial artery in response to shear stress induced by inflating and deflating a blood pressure cuff. Elevated circulating plasma concentrations of biomarkers for inflammation, hemostasis, and oxidative stress are also used as indicators that accompany and promote endothelial dysfunction [22].

Signaling pathways mediating insulin-stimulated production of nitric oxide

One of the key vascular actions of insulin is to stimulate production of the potent vasodilator NO from endothelium. Recent studies have elucidated a complete biochemical insulin-signaling pathway in endothelium regulating production of NO [5,23]. Insulin binding to its receptor (a receptor tyrosine kinase) results in phosphorylation of insulin receptor substrate (IRS)-1, which then binds and activates PI3K. Lipid products of PI3K (PI-3, 4, 5-triphosphate or PIP_3) stimulate phosphorylation and activation of PDK-1 that in turn phosphorylates and activates Akt. Akt directly phosphorylates

Table 1
Current approaches for assessing endothelial function in vivo

Measure of endothelial function	Method	Stimuli
Endothelium-dependent vascular tone		
Coronary arteries	Coronary angiography to follow changes in vessel diameter	Acetylcholine, bradykinin or substance-P
		FMD induced by adenosine or papaverine
Perpheral arteries	High-resolution ultrasonography with Doppler to follow changes in vessel diameter and blood flow;	Shear stress-induced NO production-FMD
	Forearm perfusion technique, where blood flow is measured noninvasively using strain gauge plethysmograph;	Acetylcholine, bradykinin or substance-P
	Applanation tonometry to measure changes in pulse wave form and augmentation index;	β2-agonist
	Peripheral artery tonometry with plethysmograph	Reactive hyperemia
Surrogate markers of endothelial activation		
VCAM-1	Plasma, ELISA	—
ICAM-1	Plasma, ELISA	—
P- and E-selectin	Plasma, ELISA	—
Circulating endothelial progenitor cells	Immunomagnetic separation or flow cytometry	—
von Willebrand factor	Plasma, ELISA	—

Abbreviations: ELISA, enzyme-linked immunosorbent assay; FMD, flow-mediated dilation; ICAM, intercellular adhesion molecule; VCAM, vascular cell adhesion molecules.

eNOS at Ser[1177], resulting in increased eNOS activity and subsequent NO production. Although insulin-induced eNOS activation is calcium-independent [24], insulin stimulates calmodulin binding to eNOS. This requires HSP90 binding to eNOS, which facilitates insulin-stimulated activation of eNOS mediated by phosphorylation of eNOS at Ser[1177] by Akt. The Ras/MAP-kinase branch of insulin-signaling pathways does not contribute significantly to activation of eNOS in response to insulin (Fig. 1) [5].

Signaling pathways mediating insulin-stimulated secretion of endothelin-1, plasminogen activator inhibitor type-1, and adhesion molecules

ET-1, a potent vasoconstrictor synthesized and secreted from vascular endothelium, plays an important role in endothelial dysfunction and may contribute to development of hypertension [25]. Insulin stimulates ET-1 production using MAPK-dependent (but not PI3K-dependent) signaling pathways (see Fig. 1) [26]. Increased endothelial expression of plasminogen activator inhibitor type-1 (PAI-1) and cellular adhesion molecules, ICAM-1, VCAM-1, and E-selectin may contribute to accelerated atherosclerosis in

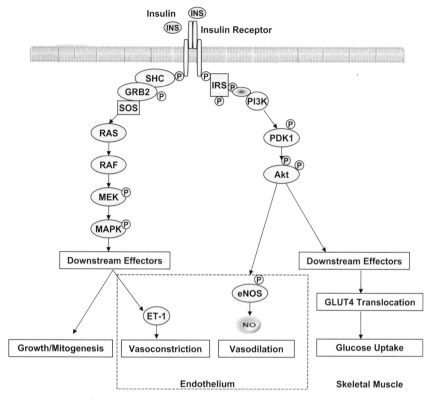

Fig. 1. General features of insulin signal transduction pathways. PI 3-kinase branch of insulin signaling regulates GLUT4 translocation and glucose uptake in skeletal muscle and NO production and vasodilation in vascular endothelium. MAP-kinase branch of insulin signaling generally regulates growth and mitogenesis and controls secretion of endothelin-1 in vascular endothelium. eNOS, endothelial nitric oxide synthase; ET-1, endothelin-1; GLUT, glucose transporter; GRB2, growth factor receptor-bound protein 2. INS, insulin; IRS, insulin receptor substrate; MEK, MAPK kinase; PDK, phosphoinositide-dependent protein kinase.

insulin-resistant states [21]. Insulin stimulates increased expression of PAI-1, VCAM-1 and E-selectin on endothelium using an MAPK-dependent pathway [27,28]. Inhibition of PI3K or Akt increases insulin-induced PAI-1 and expression of adhesion molecules [27]. These findings suggest that insulin-stimulated PI3K/Akt pathways oppose atherothrombotic factors in endothelium by multiple mechanisms, including production of beneficial molecules such as NO and inhibition of pathogenenic molecules, including PAI-1, ICAM-1, VCAM-1, and E-selectin.

Endothelial actions link metabolic effects of insulin

PI3K-dependent insulin signaling pathways in vascular endothelium, skeletal muscle, and adipose tissue regulate vasodilator and metabolic actions of insulin. However, MAPK-dependent insulin signaling pathways tend to promote pro-hypertensive and pro-atherogenic actions of insulin in various tissues. In human beings, intravenous insulin infusion stimulates capillary recruitment, vasodilation, and increased blood flow in a NO-dependent fashion [7]. These actions of insulin occur in distinct stages. First, dilation of terminal arterioles increases the number of perfused capillaries (capillary recruitment) within a few minutes without concomitant changes in total limb blood flow. This is followed by relaxation of larger resistance vessels that increases overall limb blood flow (maximum flow reached after 2 hours) [29]. The overall vasodilator response to insulin is an integration of enhanced capillary recruitment and elevated total blood flow. Local intra-arterial infusion of insulin (arterial plasma levels of approximately 300 pM) results in a 25% increase in capillary blood volume in the deep flexor muscles of the human forearm [30]. Similarly, an hour after a mixed meal, microvascular volume in the human forearm increases by appro-ximately 45% [31]. Thus, physiologic concentrations of insulin rapidly enhance skeletal muscle capillary recruitment. These vascular actions play an important role in augmenting the delivery of insulin and glucose to skel-etal muscle. Glucose delivery to skeletal muscle is dependent on muscle blood flow, as well as vascular capillary surface area and permeability. After a mixed meal, an oral glucose load, or infusion of insulin, recruitment of capillaries expands the capillary surface area and increases muscle blood flow, which together substantially increase glucose and insulin delivery [30–32]. This enhances direct effects of insulin to stimulate glucose uptake and utilization in skeletal muscle. Indeed, the time course for insulin-stimu-lated capillary recruitment approximates the time course for insulin-medi-ated glucose uptake in skeletal muscle [7]. Moreover, inhibitors of NOS that block insulin-mediated capillary recruitment cause a concomitant 40% reduction in glucose disposal [7,33]. Thus, PI3K-dependent metabolic actions of insulin directly promote glucose uptake in skeletal muscle by stim-ulating translocation of insulin responsive glucose transporters (GLUT4). At the same time, PI3K-dependent vascular actions of insulin to increase blood flow and capillary recruitment substantially contribute to promoting glucose disposal under healthy conditions and help to couple metabolic and hemodynamic homeostasis (see Fig. 1).

Role of insulin-stimulated secretion of ET-1 to oppose metabolic actions of insulin

In human beings, peripheral insulin infusion increases both vascular ET-1 production and circulating levels of ET-1 [34]. NO-dependent vasodilator actions of insulin are potentiated by ET-1 receptor blockade in healthy individuals. Conversely, ET-1 infusion decreases insulin-induced increases in blood flow in human beings. In a recent animal study, ET-1 not only diminished insulin-mediated skeletal muscle capillary recruitment, but also decreased skeletal muscle glucose uptake by 50% [35]. In human beings, insulin-stimulated ET-1 production may influence skeletal muscle glucose disposal. For example, ET-1 infusion in human beings induces peripheral insulin resistance [36]. However, NO is known to inhibit ET-1 production and action [37]. Consequently, under healthy conditions, the effects of insulin-stimulated ET-1 on the metabolic actions of insulin are likely to be offset by insulin-stimulated production of NO. In support of this notion, endothelin-antagonism (by ET-1A receptor blocker) in healthy individuals fails to affect insulin-mediated whole body or limb glucose uptake [38]. However, in insulin-resistant states associated with impaired PI3K-dependent insulin signaling pathways, insulin-mediated ET-1 secretion is augmented and blockade of ET-1 receptors significantly improves insulin sensitivity and peripheral glucose uptake in the context of insulin resistance [38,39].

Potential mechanisms mediating reciprocal relationships between endothelial dysfunction and insulin resistance

Endothelial dysfunction per se is associated with and predicts cardiovascular disease. Many established risk factors for coronary artery disease, including dyslipidemia, hypertension, diabetes, obesity, and physical inactivity also increase the risk of developing endothelial dysfunction. Similarly, many risk factors for developing cardiovascular disease also enhance the risk of developing insulin resistance [21]. Thus, endothelial dysfunction and insulin resistance frequently coexist. In cross-sectional studies, endothelial dysfunction is consistently present in patients with insulin resistance [40–42]. This includes relatives of patients with type 2 diabetes and patients with type 2 diabetes themselves [43,44]. Shared causal factors, such as glucotoxicity, lipotoxicity, inflammation, and oxidative stress interact at multiple levels to create reciprocal relationships between insulin resistance and endothelial dysfunction that may help explain the frequent clustering of metabolic and cardiovascular disorders (Fig. 2) [14].

Role of endothelial dysfunction in development of insulin resistance

Cross-sectional studies suggest that endothelial dysfunction independently predicts the incidence of diabetes [45–48]. In a prospective study (Framingham Offspring Study) of the children and spouses of children of the original Framingham Heart Study cohort, circulating plasma markers of endothelial dysfunction (PAI-1 and von Willebrand factor) increases the risk of developing diabetes independent of other risk factors for diabetes, including obesity, insulin resistance, and inflammation [46]. Similarly, in a large, prospective, nested case-controlled study from an ethnically diverse cohort of United States postmenopausal women (Women's Health Initiative Observational Study), higher levels of circulating E-selectin and ICAM-1

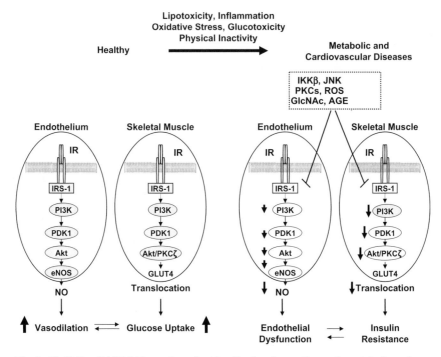

Fig. 2. (*Left*) Parallel PI 3-kinase-dependent insulin-signaling pathways in metabolic and vascular tissues synergistically couple metabolic and vascular physiology under healthy conditions. (*Right*) Parallel impairment in insulin-signaling pathways under pathologic conditions contributes to synergistic coupling of insulin resistance and endothelial dysfunction. AGE, advanced glycation end products; PKC?, a-typical protein kinase C; GlcNAc, N-acetylglucosamine; IKK, inhibitor of Ikβ kinase; JNK, c-jun aminoterminal kinase; PKC, protein kinase C.

were consistently associated with increased risk of developing diabetes [47]. These studies support a potential causal role for endothelial dysfunction in insulin resistance. Rodent models of endothelial dysfunction provide additional important insights into this issue. The central role of endothelium in regulating metabolic actions of insulin is evident by the presence of insulin resistance and hypertension in eNOS knockout mice. These animals also demonstrate microvascular changes, including reduced capillary density (rarefaction) [49,50]. Insulin-mediated glucose disposal is reduced by nearly 40% in these mice, an amount roughly equivalent to the contribution of capillary recruitment in insulin-mediated glucose disposal in healthy rodents. Moreover, these mice also have increased triglyceride and free fatty acid (FFA) levels, decreased energy expenditure, defective beta-oxidation, and impaired mitochondrial function [51]. These findings suggest that endothelium-derived NO has additional and direct metabolic effects on mitochondrial function. Although mice with partial eNOS deficiency (eNOS +/−) are insulin sensitive and normotensive, they develop insulin resistance and hypertension when challenged with a high-fat diet [52]. Thus, partial defects in endothelial function characterized by reduced NO bioavailability are sufficient to cause cardiometabolic abnormalities (insulin resistance and dyslipidemia) under pathogenic conditions (eg, caloric excess, physical inactivity, inflammation), a situation not unlike that observed in human beings.

Role of insulin resistance in the development of endothelial dysfunction

In human beings with metabolic insulin resistance there is simultaneous impairment in insulin's ability to induce vasodilation. Diminished effects of insulin to stimulate blood flow has been demonstrated in obese subjects, type 2 diabetes, and polycystic ovarian syndrome [41,53–55]. Diminished insulin-stimulated blood flow and glucose uptake is also present in patients with various cardiovascular diseases such as essential hypertension, microvascular angina, and heart failure. Nondiabetic offspring of diabetic parents have both insulin resistance and endothelial dysfunction [43,44,56]. Thus, there may be similar genetic and acquired contributions to both insulin resistance and endothelial dysfunction. At the cellular level, a key feature of insulin resistance is the pathway-selective impairment in PI3K-dependent signaling pathways, while other insulin signaling branches, including Ras/MAPK-dependent pathways, are relatively unaffected. This has important pathophysiologic implications because metabolic insulin resistance is typically accompanied by compensatory hyperinsulinemia to maintain euglycemia. In the vasculature and elsewhere, hyperinsulinemia will overdrive unaffected MAPK-dependent pathways, leading to an imbalance between PI3K- and MAPK-dependent functions of insulin. Lipotoxicity, glucotoxicity, and inflammation that contribute to insulin resistant states differentially affect PI3K and MAPK pathways through multiple independent and interdependent mechanisms in the endothelium. The imbalance between PI3K/Akt/eNOS/NO and MAPK/ET-1 vascular actions of insulin provoked by dyslipidemia, hyperglycemia, and inflammatory cytokines may contribute to both impaired vascular and metabolic actions of insulin. That is, compensatory hyperinsulinemia that typically accompanies pathway-selective insulin resistance (in PI3K pathways) activates unopposed MAPK pathways, leading to enhanced pro-hypertensive and atherogenic actions of insulin [14].

Proinflammatory cytokines

Insulin resistance and endothelial dysfunction are characterized by elevated circulating markers of inflammation [14,57]. Visceral fat accumulation may play a key role in the development of the ssystemic proinflammatory state associated with insulin resistance [58]. The most extensively studied proinflammatory cytokine implicated in insulin resistance is tumor necrosis factor (TNF)-α. TNF-α activates of variety of serine kinases, including

JNK, IKKβ, and interleukin (IL)-1β receptor-associated kinase that directly or indirectly increase serine phosphorylation of IRS-1 and -2, leading to decreased insulin-stimulated activation of PI3K/Akt/eNOS in endothelial cells [59–62]. In addition, TNF-α increases ET-1 secretion in a MAPK-dependent fashion [63]. IL-6, another cytokine elevated in insulin resistant states, also inhibits insulin-stimulated increases in eNOS activity and NO production in the endothelium [64]. Similarly, c-reactive protein (CRP), a marker of inflammation, has important biologic actions to inhibit insulin-evoked NO production in endothelial cells through specific inactivation of the PI3K/Akt/eNOS pathway [65,66]. Similar to TNF-α, CRP simultaneously increases endothelial ET-1 production [66]. Systemic infusion of high doses of TNF-α results in the loss of insulin-induced increases in glucose uptake, limb blood flow, and capillary recruitment in rat hind limb [62]. In the presence of TNF-α, insulin constricts skeletal muscle arterioles. However, pretreatment of these arterioles with the nonselective ET-1 receptor antagonist abolishes these vasoconstrictor actions of insulin [67]. In human beings, high local concentrations of TNF-α achieved by intra-arterial infusion simultaneously inhibits both insulin-stimulated glucose uptake and endothelium-dependent vasodilation in the forearm [68]. These findings suggest that TNF-α specifically down-regulates the insulin-dependent PI3K/Akt/eNOS vasodilator pathway without modulating insulin-stimulated ET-1-mediated vasoconstriction. Thus, proinflammatory cytokines may contribute to coupling of metabolic and vascular insulin resistance manifested by impaired insulin signaling and endothelial dysfunction.

Adipokines

Adipocyte-derived hormones, such as leptin and adiponectin, have both metabolic and vascular actions. Adiponectin is an anti-inflammatory peptide whose circulating levels are positively correlated with insulin sensitivity and that may serve to link obesity with insulin resistance [57]. Adiponectin mimics vascular and metabolic actions of insulin, and the interaction between these two hormones may play a part in determining the cardiac, vascular, and metabolic phenotype in insulin-resistant states, such as diabetes, obesity and hypertension. Similar to insulin, adiponectin has vasodilator actions to stimulate NO production in endothelial cells [69]. In addition, adiponectin enhances NO bioavailability by up-regulating eNOS expression and reducing ROS production in endothelial cells [70]. Decreased plasma adiponectin levels are observed in patients with obesity, type 2 diabetes, hypertension, metabolic syndrome, and coronary artery disease [71,72]. Moreover, low plasma adiponectin levels are significantly correlated with endothelial dysfunction [72]. These results suggest that low adiponectin levels may be a useful marker for early-stage atherosclerosis.

Leptin, a key regulator of appetite, body weight and energy balance in the central nervous system acts directly on the vasculature. Similar to insulin, leptin induces endothelium-dependent vasodilation through a PI3K/Akt/eNOS pathway [73]. Like insulin, leptin-evoked vasodilation is opposed by sympathetically-induced vasoconstriction [74]. Angiotensin II and TNF-α stimulate the production of leptin. Consequently, in insulin resistant states, characterized by elevated sympathetic activity, angiotensin II, and TNF-α activity, leptin may potentiate pressor effects of hyperinsulinemia [75]. Therefore, interactions between angiotensin II and insulin with leptin may have deleterious cardiovascular effects in obesity. These actions may contribute to the pathogenesis of hypertension, atherosclerosis, and left ventricular hypertrophy. In fact, in the large, prospective West of Scotland Coronary Prevention Study elevated circulating leptin levels independently predicted increased risk of coronary events [76]. Thus, acute, beneficial vasodilator effects of leptin at low concentrations do not reflect the potentially detrimental effects of chronic elevations in leptin levels observed in the presence of insulin and leptin resistance. Human studies specifically examining interactions between cardiovascular actions of insulin and leptin in normal and pathologic states are needed to fully understand potential beneficial and detrimental effects of leptin on metabolic and cardiovascular physiology.

Resistin, a proinflammatory peptide expressed in human macrophages, mononuclear leukocytes, and bone marrow cells has been implicated in insulin resistance. Recent studies suggest that resistin may adversely impact endothelial function and vascular relaxation by stimulating ET-1 production, inhibiting vasodilator actions of insulin, and decreasing eNOS expression [77,78]. Thus, resistin may participate in the reciprocal relationships between insulin resistance and endothelial dysfunction. In support of this notion, resistin expression in circulating monocytes independently predicts reduced flow-mediated vasodilation in individuals with insulin resistance [79].

Lipotoxicity

Patients with type 2 diabetes mellitus or the metabolic syndrome have a distinctive dyslipidemia characterized by hypertriglyceridemia, elevated blood levels of apolipoprotein B, small, dense low-density lipoprotein cholesterol, and low levels of high-density lipoprotein cholesterol. This contributes to endothelial dysfunction, atherosclerosis, and insulin resistance. Treatment of vascular endothelial cells with FFA impairs insulin-stimulated activation of PI3K, PDK1, Akt, and eNOS [80–82]. Elevated cellular levels of lipid metabolites, such as diacylglycerols, ceramide, and long-chain fatty acyl CoAs activate serine kinases, such as PKC and IKKβ, which cause insulin resistance by increasing serine phosphorylation of IRS-1 [80–82]. In addition, FFAs increase production of ROS [80]. Thus, impaired PI3K signaling reduces eNOS activity, accentuates FFA-evoked oxidative stress, and diminishes NO bioavailability. In support of these findings, raising circulating FFA levels significantly impairs insulin-induced increases in skeletal muscle capillary recruitment with a concomitant decrease in glucose disposal [83]. Insulin's effects on capillary recruitment and glucose uptake are impaired when FFA levels are increased in healthy lean women [84]. Moreover, when FFA levels are lowered in obese women, vasodilator actions of insulin are improved, suggesting that insulin's microvascular and metabolic effects are coupled in response to changes in FFA levels. Indeed, changes in capillary recruitment account for 30% of the association between changes in FFA levels and changes in insulin-mediated glucose uptake [84]. Infusion of a lipid emulsion in conjunction with heparin to elevate circulating FFA concentrations simultaneously decreases glucose uptake and attenuates insulin-induced increases in leg blood flow and NO flux, with significant correlations between FFA-induced changes in glucose uptake and FFA-induced decreases in leg blood flow [85]. Moreover, FFA infusion in human beings accentuates insulin-mediated ET-1 release [86]. The magnitude of this effect is significantly higher in insulin-resistant individuals (when compared with healthy controls). Decreasing forearm lipid oxidation reduces insulin-evoked ET-1 release while simultaneously increasing NO bioavailability and glucose uptake [87]. These studies suggest that in the context of pathway-selective impairment of PI3K signaling induced by elevated FFA levels, insulin stimulates increased ET-1 secretion through an unopposed MAPK signaling that leads to relative vasoconstriction and insulin resistance.

Glucotoxicity

Hyperglycemia associated with impaired glucose tolerance and diabetes causes insulin resistance and endothelial dysfunction by increasing oxidative stress, formation of advanced glycation end products (AGEs), and flux through the hexosamine biosynthetic pathway. In endothelial cells exposed to high glucose concentrations, insulin-stimulated activation of Akt and eNOS is significantly reduced [88]. Hyperglycemia induces increased ROS production, posttranslational O-GlcNacylation, PKC activity, and AGE formation that are known to specifically inhibit the PI3K/Akt/eNOS pathway [5,88]. ROS decreases NO bioavailability, reduces cellular tetrahydrobiopterin levels, and promotes generation of superoxide by eNOS. Glucosamine, a product of the hexosamine biosynthetic pathway, impairs insulin-stimulated glucose uptake in skeletal muscle and production of NO in endothelium in vitro. In vivo, acute intravenous glucosamine administration causes metabolic insulin resistance and impairs insulin-mediated increases in femoral arterial blood flow and capillary recruitment [89]. Local hyperglycemia, achieved by infusing concentrated glucose directly into the brachial artery of healthy human beings, diminishes agonist-induced vasodilation, an effect prevented by intra-arterial administration of ascorbate (an antioxidant) [90]. Acute hyperglycemia consistently impairs endothelial function in individuals with insulin resistance or type 2 diabetes

[91]. Collectively, these data suggest that hyperglycemia impairs insulin action in skeletal and cardiac muscle, as well as in vascular endothelium. Consistent with these findings, activity of Akt and eNOS in vasculature and muscle is significantly attenuated in patients with diabetes when compared with nondiabetics [92]. By contrast, with deleterious effects on the PI3K/Akt/eNOS pathway, hyperglycemia enhances endothelial ET-1 secretion and thereby alters the balance between NO and ET-1 to favor vasoconstriction and endothelial dysfunction. An oral glucose load significantly increases plasma ET-1 in insulin-resistant, but not in healthy, individuals [93]. In addition, selective ET_A receptor blockade in the forearm significantly increases forearm blood flow in patients with type 2 diabetes but not in healthy individuals [94]. Thus, a parallel increase in ET-1 activity and diminished NO bioactivity associated with hyperglycemia and insulin resistance may contribute to abnormal vascular function. This illustrates the altered balance between the vasodilator and vasoconstrictor actions of insulin in insulin resistant states that contributes to reciprocal relationships between insulin resistance and endothelial dysfunction.

Fatness and fitness in insulin resistance and endothelial dysfunction

Increased adiposity and inadequate physical activity are strong and independent predictors of coronary artery disease. Many studies consistently report associations between obesity and endothelial dysfunction. In the largest study, the Framingham Heart Study, body mass index (BMI) independently predicts reduced brachial artery FMD [95]. Furthermore, increased abdominal adiposity (determined by waist-to-hip ratio) is also a strong independent predictor of endothelial dysfunction, even in overweight otherwise healthy adults [96]. Recently, Clerk and colleagues [53] directly measured capillary recruitment using contrast enhanced ultrasonography in the forearm flexor muscles of lean and obese adults before and during a 120-minute euglycemic-hyperinsulinemic glucose clamp. When compared with baseline measurements, insulin significantly increased microvascular blood volume (an index of microvascular recruitment) in the lean group but not in the obese group. These results demonstrate impaired insulin-mediated microvascular function in obesity. Obesity and accompanying changes in local and humoral adipocytokine profiles are frequently associated with insulin resistance. These alterations, coupled with metabolic abnormalities that cause insulin resistance, such as lipotoxicity and glucotoxicity, all contribute importantly to endothelial dysfunction.

Physical inactivity and reduced exercise capacity predicts cardiovascular disease independent of conventional risk factors and is associated with endothelial dysfunction and insulin resistance [97,98]. Interestingly, when rats are segregated and bred based on aerobic exercise capacity, low-capacity runners are characterized by endothelial dysfunction and insulin resistance [99]. In human beings, reduced maximum oxygen consumption ($V_{O2\ max}$), along with impaired mitochondrial function and biogenesis, are associated with insulin-resistance [100]. This is also observed in first-degree relatives of patients with type 2 diabetes [101]. Taken together, these data suggest a genetic component to the relationship between reduced aerobic capacity, endothelial dysfunction, and insulin resistance. In human skeletal muscle, NO-derived from eNOS plays an important role in mitochondrial biogenesis [102]. Moreover, skeletal muscle eNOS activity and capillary density is significantly reduced in insulin-resistant individuals [92,103]. Thus, physical inactivity is accompanied by reduced eNOS and NO activity that may contribute to impaired mitochondrial function. Further studies are required to determine if mitochondrial dysfunction is causally related to endothelial dysfunction or insulin resistance. Long-term inactivity in human beings also results in a significant increase in ET-1-dependent vascular tone in skeletal muscle vascular beds [104]. Thus, physical inactivity is not only associated with impairment in the eNOS and NO pathway but augmented ET-1 secretion. This is consistent with animal studies where deficiency of eNOS promotes ET-1-induced endothelial dysfunction and hypertension [105].

Therapeutic interventions targeting endothelial dysfunction and insulin resistance

Acquired and genetic factors influence metabolic, vascular, and inflammatory homeostasis that involve multiple cellular and physiologic mechanisms to contribute, often simultaneously, to development of insulin resistance and endothelial dysfunction. There are no validated screening tools for assessing endothelial dysfunction in the clinical setting. Therefore, clinical assessment of conventional risk factors and a comprehensive management approach is needed to effectively treat or prevent endothelial dysfunction and insulin resistance. Interventions aimed at improving either insulin resistance or endothelial dysfunction that raise plasma adiponectin levels, block renin angiotensin and endothelin systems, lower oxidative stress, and attenuate inflammation are predicted to have simultaneous beneficial effects on both metabolic and cardiovascular function.

Dietary and lifestyle modifications

Diet, weight loss, and physical exercise decrease insulin resistance and improve endothelial dysfunction (Table 2) [102,106–130]. Calorie restriction alone (25% less than baseline energy requirements) or a combination of calorie restriction and physical exercise for 6 months increases eNOS expression in human skeletal muscle [102]. Calorie restriction and exercise also improves NO-dependent vasodilation, reduces circulating ET-1 levels, and increases adiponectin levels in insulin resistant individuals [119–121]. A Mediterranean-style diet significantly reduces serum concentrations of inflammatory markers, decreases insulin resistance, and improves endothelial function in patients with metabolic syndrome when compared with matched subjects on a control diet [122]. Likewise, a 2-year lifestyle intervention consisting of weight loss, physical exercise, and a Mediterranean-style diet decreases BMI and inflammatory markers while increasing adiponectin levels in a cohort of obese women [123].

Increased physical activity and exercise enhances insulin sensitivity and NO-dependent vasodilatation in both conduit and resistance vessels of individuals characterized by endothelial dysfunction and insulin resistance [124–128]. Exercise increases insulin-stimulated blood flow in athletes, healthy controls, and type 2 diabetic individuals [129,130]. There appears to be a threshold for exercise-induced improvement in endothelial function. Moderate (50% $V_{O2\ max}$), but not low (25% $V_{O2\ max}$) or high intensity (75% $V_{O2\ max}$) exercise for 12 weeks is associated with enhanced acetylcholine-mediated forearm vasodilation [131]. Physical exercise increases forearm skeletal muscle capillary recruitment in healthy individuals and may augment glucose uptake by enhancing nutritive blood flow [31]. The protective effects of exercise on the vasculature do not seem to be dependent on improvement of coexisting cardiovascular risk factors. Regular exercise increases eNOS protein expression and activity via PI3K/Akt-dependent phosphorylation in human vasculature [132]. The salutary effects of exercise on vascular actions of insulin may involve enhanced insulin signaling, accentuated eNOS activity and expression, reduced oxidative and inflammatory stress, enhanced NO availability, restoration of balance between vasocontrictor and vasodilator actions, and increased capillary density.

Pharmacologic interventions

Routinely used pharmacotherapies, such as insulin sensitizers, hypolipidemic agents, or angiotensin II antagonists improve endothelial dysfunction in insulin-resistant individuals (Table 3) [54,106,133–149]. These studies suggest that a combinatorial therapeutic strategy may be more effective in ameliorating endothelial dysfunction frequently observed in insulin-resistant states.

Primary prevention of endothelial dysfunction

It is well established that dysfunctional endothelium contributes to development and progression of atherosclerosis. Consequently, early detection and treatment of endothelial dysfunction may be an attractive strategy for preventing chronic heart diesease. Unfortunately, established validated methods for assessment of endothelial dysfunction for chronic heart disease risk prediction in the clinical setting are not currently available. Current techniques to assess endothelial function (see Table 1), are invasive, expensive, or suffer from lack of high sensitivity, specificity, reproducibility, or clinically defined cut-off values. Therefore, at this time, targeting established

Table 2
Summary of studies involving lifestyle and dietary modifications that target endothelial dysfunction in insulin resistance

Study	Target population	Therapeutic intervention	Treatment duration	Outcome measures	Treatment effect
Life style modification					
Esposito [122]	Metabolic syndrome	Mediterranean-style diet	2 yrs	L-arginine test + adenosine-induced decrease in blood pressure	↑
Esposito [123]	Metabolic syndrome	Mediterranean-style diet + exercise	2 yrs	Adiponectin, CRP, IL-6, IL-18	Adiponectin ↑, CRP ↓, IL-6 ↓, IL-18 ↓
Hamdy [119]	Obesity	Low-calorie diet (500 calories/day negative balance) + exercise, 30 min/wk	6 mos	FMD	↑
Lavrencic [124]	Metabolic syndrome	Bicycle exercise, 3 times/wk	12 wks	FMD	↑
Maiorana [125]	Type 2 diabetes	Circuit training, 3 times/wk	8 wks	FMD	↑
De Filippis [126]	Obesity/type 2 diabetes	Cycle exercise, 45 min, 4 times/wk	8 wks	ACh-induced vasodilation	↑
Sasaki [127]	Obesity/hypertension	Low-calorie diet (800 kcal/d)	2 wks	ACh-induced vasodilation	↑
Meyer [128]	Obesity	Structured exercise 1 h, 3 times/wk)	6 mos	FMD	↑
Antioxidants/nutritional supplements					
Sola [106]	Metabolic syndrome	Lipoic acid, 300 mg/d, orally	4 wks	FMD, IL-6	↑
Heitzer [107]	Type 2 diabetes	Lipoic acid, 0.7 mg/min, intra-arterial	Acute (5 min)	ACh-induced vasodilation	↑
Heitzer [107]	Type 2 diabetes	Vitamin C, 24 mg/min, intra-arterial	Acute (10 min)	ACh-induced vasodilation	↑

Study	Condition	Intervention	Duration	Measure	Result
Chen [108]	Type 2 diabetes	Vitamin C, 800 mg/day, orally	4 wks	ACh-induced vasodilation	↔
Perticone [109]	Obesity	Vitamin C, 24 mg/min, intra-arterial	Acute (5 min)	ACh-induced vasodilation	↑
Lekakis [110]	History of GDM	Vitamin C, 2 g, orally	Acute (120 min)	FMD	↑
Darko [111]	Type 2 diabetes	Vitamin C, 1.5 g/d, orally	3 wks	ACh-induced vasodilation	↔
Regensteiner [112]	Type 2 diabetes	Vit E (1.8 g/d) + Vit C (1.0 g/d), orally	1 wks	FMD	↑
Beckman [113]	Type 2 diabetes	Vit E (800 IU/d) + Vit C (1.0 g/d), orally	6 mos	FMD	↔
Pena [114]	Obesity	Folic acid, 5 mg/d, orally	8 wks	FMD	↔
Title [115]	Type 2 diabetes	Folic acid, 10 mg/d, orally	2 wks	FMD	↑
Regensteiner [112]	Type 2 diabetes	L-arginine, 9 g/d, orally	1 wk	FMD	↑
Heitzer [116]	Type 2 diabetes	BH$_4$, 500 µg/min, intra-arterial	Acute (30 min)	ACh-induced vasodilation	↑
Nystrom [117]	Type 2 diabetes	BH$_4$, 500 µg/min, Intra-arterial	Acute (2 h)	Insulin-induced ΔFMD	↔
Grassi D [118]	Insulin-resistant hypertensives	Dark cocoa (flavanols, 88 mg/d), orally	15 d	FMD	↑

Abbreviations: Ach, acetylcholine; BH$_4$, tetrahydrobiopterin; CRP, c-reactive protein; FMD, flow-mediated dilation; GDM, gestational diabetes mellitus.

Table 3
Summary of studies involving pharmacologic interventions that target endothelial dysfunction in insulin resistance

Study	Target population	Therapeutic intervention	Treatment duration	Outcome measures	Treatment effect
Insulin sensitizers					
Diamanti-Kandarakis [133]	PCOS	Metformin, 1700 mg/d, orally	6 mos	FMD and plasma ET-1	FMD ↑ and plasma ET-1 ↓
Mathers [134]	Type 2 diabetes	Metformin, 1000 mg/d, orally	12 wks	ACh-induced vasodilation	↑
de Aguiar [135]	Metabolic syndrome	Metformin, 1700 mg/d, orally	3 mos	ACh-induced vasodilation	↑
Martens [136]	Type 2 diabetes	Pioglitazone, 30 mg/d, orally	4 wks	FMD	↑
Mittermayer [137]	FFA-induced endothelial dysfunction	Rosiglitazone, 8 mg/d, orally	3 wks	ACh-induced vasodilation	↑
Wang [138]	Metabolic syndrome	Rosiglitazone, 4 mg/d, orally	8 wks	FMD	↑
Esposito [139]	Metabolic syndrome	Rosiglitazone, 20 mg/d, orally	12 mos	FMD, adiponectin, CRP, IL-6, IL-18	FMD ↑, adiponectin ↑, CRP ↓, IL-6 ↓, IL-18 ↓
Hypolipidemic agents					
Ceriello [140]	High-fat and glucose-induced endothelial dysfunction	Atorvastatin, 40 mg/d, orally	4 d	FMD, ICAM-1, nitrotyrosine, IL-6	FMD ↑, ICAM-1 ↓, nitrotyrosine ↓, IL-6 ↓
Economides [141]	Type 2 diabetes	Atorvastatin, 40 mg/d, orally	12 wks	FMD	↑
Shimabukuro [142]	Obesity	Fluvastatin, 20 mg/ d–40 mg/d, orally	12 wks	Peak FBF during reactive hyperemia	↑

Study	Condition	Drug, dose	Duration	Measure	Result
Evans [143]	Type 2 diabetes	Ciprofibrate, 100 mg/d, orally	3 mos	FMD	↑
Avogaro [144]	Type 2 diabetes	Gemfibrozil, 1,200 mg/d, orally	12 wks	FMD	↑
Koh [145]	Metabolic syndrome	Fenofibrate, 200 mg/d, orally	2 mos	FMD	↑
Renin-angiotensin system blockers					
Hermann [54]	Type 2 diabetes	Quinapril, 20 mg/d, orally	2 mos	Insulin-induced Δforearm blood flow	↑
Koh [146]	Metabolic syndrome	Losartan, 100 mg/d, orally	2 mos	FMD	↑
O'Driscoll [147]	Type 2 diabetes	Enalapril, 20 mg/d, orally	4 wks	ACh-induced vasodilation	↑
Combination therapies					
Koh [148]	Metabolic syndrome	Atorvastatin, 10 mg/d + fenofibrate, 200 mg/d	2 mos	FMD	↑
Koh [149]	Type 2 diabetes	Simvastatin 20 mg/d + ramipril 10 mg/d	2 mos	FMD	↑
Ceriello [140]	High-fat and Glucose-induced endothelial dysfunction	Atorvastatin, 40 mg/d + Irbesartan, 300 mg/d	4 d	FMD, ICAM-1, nitrotyrosine, IL-6	FMD ↑, ICAM-1↓, nitrotyrosine ↓, IL-6↓
Sola [106]	Metabolic syndrome	Irbesartan, 150 mg/d + lipoic acid, 300 mg/d	4 wks	FMD	↑

Abbreviations: FBF, forearm blood flow; PCOS, polycystic ovarian syndrome.

and modifiable risk factors for endothelial dysfunction and insulin resistance is the best primary strategy to prevent these conditions.

Summary

Pathway-specific impairment of PI3K-dependent insulin signaling pathways facilitates reciprocal relationships between endothelial dysfunction and insulin resistance that contribute to clustering of metabolic and cardiovascular diseases. Therapeutic interventions that target this pathway-selective impairment simultaneously ameliorate endothelial dysfunction and insulin resistance. Thus, an integrated approach that combines lifestyle modifications with pharmacotherapy to restore balance between vasodilator and vasoconstrictor actions of insulin may promote endothelial health, insulin sensitivity, and reduce the risk of metabolic and cardiovascular diseases.

References

[1] DeFronzo RA, Ferrannini E. Insulin resistance. A multifaceted syndrome responsible for NIDDM, obesity, hypertension, dyslipidemia, and atherosclerotic cardiovascular disease. Diabetes Care 1991;14(3):173–94.

[2] Petersen KF, Dufour S, Savage DB, et al. The role of skeletal muscle insulin resistance in the pathogenesis of the metabolic syndrome. Proc Natl Acad Sci U S A 2007;104(31):12587–94.

[3] Poirier P, Giles TD, Bray GA, et al. Obesity and cardiovascular disease: pathophysiology, evaluation, and effect of weight loss: an update of the 1997 American Heart Association scientific statement on obesity and heart disease from the Obesity Committee of the Council on Nutrition, Physical Activity, and Metabolism. Circulation 2006;113(6):898–918.

[4] Accili D. Lilly lecture 2003: The struggle for mastery in insulin action: from triumvirate to republic. Diabetes 2004;53(7):1633–42.

[5] Muniyappa R, Montagnani M, Koh KK, et al. Cardiovascular actions of insulin. Endocr Rev 2007;28(5):463–91.

[6] Zeng G, Quon MJ. Insulin-stimulated production of nitric oxide is inhibited by Wortmannin. Direct measurement in vascular endothelial cells. J Clin Invest 1996;98(4):894–8.

[7] Vincent MA, Clerk LH, Lindner JR, et al. Microvascular recruitment is an early insulin effect that regulates skeletal muscle glucose uptake in vivo. Diabetes 2004;53(6):1418–23.

[8] Zhang L, Vincent MA, Richards SM, et al. Insulin sensitivity of muscle capillary recruitment in vivo. Diabetes 2004;53(2):447–53.

[9] Vicent D, Ilany J, Kondo T, et al. The role of endothelial insulin signaling in the regulation of vascular tone and insulin resistance. J Clin Invest 2003;111(9):1373–80.

[10] Baron AD, Laakso M, Brechtel G, et al. Mechanism of insulin resistance in insulin-dependent diabetes mellitus: a major role for reduced skeletal muscle blood flow. J Clin Endocrinol Metab 1991;73(3):637–43.

[11] Natali A, Taddei S, Quinones Galvan A, et al. Insulin sensitivity, vascular reactivity, and clamp-induced vasodilatation in essential hypertension. Circulation 1997;96(3):849–55.

[12] Nystrom FH, Quon MJ. Insulin signalling: metabolic pathways and mechanisms for specificity. Cell Signal 1999;11(8):563–74.

[13] Ver MR, Chen H, Quon MJ. Insulin signaling pathways regulating translocation of glut4. Current Medical Chemistry–Immune, Endocrine, and Metabolic Agents 2005;5:159–65.

[14] Kim JA, Montagnani M, Koh KK, et al. Reciprocal relationships between insulin resistance and endothelial dysfunction: molecular and pathophysiological mechanisms. Circulation 2006;113(15):1888–904.

[15] Cusi K, Maezono K, Osman A, et al. Insulin resistance differentially affects the pi 3-kinase- and map kinase-mediated signaling in human muscle. J Clin Invest 2000;105(3):311–20.

[16] Jiang ZY, Lin YW, Clemont A, et al. Characterization of selective resistance to insulin signaling in the vasculature of obese zucker (fa/fa) rats. J Clin Invest 1999;104(4):447–57.

[17] Dudzinski DM, Michel T. Life history of enos: partners and pathways. Cardiovasc Res 2007;75(2):247–60.

[18] Fleming I, Busse R. Molecular mechanisms involved in the regulation of the endothelial nitric oxide synthase. Am J Physiol Regul Integr Comp Physiol 2003;284(1):R1–12.

[19] Herman AG, Moncada S. Therapeutic potential of nitric oxide donors in the prevention and treatment of atherosclerosis. Eur Heart J 2005;26(19):1945–55.

[20] Drexler H. Endothelial dysfunction: clinical implications. Prog Cardiovasc Dis 1997;39(4): 287–324.

[21] Bonetti PO, Lerman LO, Lerman A. Endothelial dysfunction: a marker of atherosclerotic risk. Arterioscler Thromb Vasc Biol 2003;23(2):168–75.

[22] Barac A, Campia U, Panza JA. Methods for evaluating endothelial function in humans. Hypertension 2007;49(4):748–60.

[23] Vincent MA, Montagnani M, Quon MJ. Molecular and physiologic actions of insulin related to production of nitric oxide in vascular endothelium. Curr Diab Rep 2003;3(4): 279–88.

[24] Montagnani M, Chen H, Barr VA, et al. Insulin-stimulated activation of enos is independent of Ca2+ but requires phosphorylation by Akt at ser(1179). J Biol Chem 2001;276(32): 30392–8.

[25] Marasciulo FL, Montagnani M, Potenza MA. Endothelin-1: the yin and yang on vascular function. Curr Med Chem 2006;13(14):1655–65.

[26] Potenza MA, Marasciulo FL, Chieppa DM, et al. Insulin resistance in spontaneously hypertensive rats is associated with endothelial dysfunction characterized by imbalance between NO and ET-1 production. Am J Physiol Heart Circ Physiol 2005;289(2):H813–22.

[27] Montagnani M, Golovchenko I, Kim I, et al. Inhibition of phosphatidylinositol 3-kinase enhances mitogenic actions of insulin in endothelial cells. J Biol Chem 2002;277(3):1794–9.

[28] Mukai Y, Wang CY, Rikitake Y, et al. Phosphatidylinositol 3-kinase/protein kinase Akt negatively regulates plasminogen activator inhibitor type 1 expression in vascular endothelial cells. Am J Physiol Heart Circ Physiol 2007;292(4):H1937–42.

[29] Baron AD. Hemodynamic actions of insulin. Am J Physiol 1994;267(2 Pt 1):E187–202.

[30] Coggins M, Lindner J, Rattigan S, et al. Physiologic hyperinsulinemia enhances human skeletal muscle perfusion by capillary recruitment. Diabetes 2001;50(12):2682–90.

[31] Vincent MA, Clerk LH, Lindner JR, et al. Mixed meal and light exercise each recruit muscle capillaries in healthy humans. Am J Physiol Endocrinol Metab 2006;290(6):E1191–7.

[32] Gudbjornsdottir S, Sjostrand M, Strindberg L, et al. Direct measurements of the permeability surface area for insulin and glucose in human skeletal muscle. J Clin Endocrinol Metab 2003;88(10):4559–64.

[33] Vincent MA, Barrett EJ, Lindner JR, et al. Inhibiting nos blocks microvascular recruitment and blunts muscle glucose uptake in response to insulin. Am J Physiol Endocrinol Metab 2003;285(1):E123–9.

[34] Cardillo C, Nambi SS, Kilcoyne CM, et al. Insulin stimulates both endothelin and nitric oxide activity in the human forearm. Circulation 1999;100(8):820–5.

[35] Ross RM, Kolka CM, Rattigan S, et al. Acute blockade by endothelin-1 of haemodynamic insulin action in rats. Diabetologia 2007;50(2):443–51.

[36] Ahlborg G, Lindstrom J. Insulin sensitivity and big et-1 conversion to et-1 after eta- or etb-receptor blockade in humans. J Appl Physiol 2002;93(6):2112–21.

[37] Kelly LK, Wedgwood S, Steinhorn RH, et al. Nitric oxide decreases endothelin-1 secretion through the activation of soluble guanylate cyclase. Am J Physiol Lung Cell Mol Physiol 2004;286(5):L984–91.

[38] Lteif A, Vaishnava P, Baron AD, et al. Endothelin limits insulin action in obese/insulin-resistant humans. Diabetes 2007;56(3):728–34.

[39] Ahlborg G, Shemyakin A, Bohm F, et al. Dual endothelin receptor blockade acutely improves insulin sensitivity in obese patients with insulin resistance and coronary artery disease. Diabetes Care 2007;30(3):591–6.

[40] Williams SB, Cusco JA, Roddy MA, et al. Impaired nitric oxide-mediated vasodilation in patients with non-insulin-dependent diabetes mellitus. J Am Coll Cardiol 1996;27(3):567–74.

[41] Paradisi G, Steinberg HO, Hempfling A, et al. Polycystic ovary syndrome is associated with endothelial dysfunction. Circulation 2001;103(10):1410–5.

[42] Steinberg HO, Chaker H, Leaming R, et al. Obesity/insulin resistance is associated with endothelial dysfunction. Implications for the syndrome of insulin resistance. J Clin Invest 1996;97(11):2601–10.

[43] Goldfine AB, Beckman JA, Betensky RA, et al. Family history of diabetes is a major determinant of endothelial function. J Am Coll Cardiol 2006;47(12):2456–61.

[44] Tesauro M, Rizza S, Iantorno M, et al. Vascular, metabolic, and inflammatory abnormalities in normoglycemic offspring of patients with type 2 diabetes mellitus. Metabolism 2007;56(3):413–9.

[45] Meigs JB, Hu FB, Rifai N, et al. Biomarkers of endothelial dysfunction and risk of type 2 diabetes mellitus. JAMA 2004;291(16):1978–86.

[46] Meigs JB, O'Donnell CJ, Tofler GH, et al. Hemostatic markers of endothelial dysfunction and risk of incident type 2 diabetes: the Framingham Offspring Study. Diabetes 2006;55(2):530–7.

[47] Song Y, Manson JE, Tinker L, et al. Circulating levels of endothelial adhesion molecules and risk of diabetes in an ethnically diverse cohort of women. Diabetes 2007;56(7):1898–904.

[48] Donahue RP, Rejman K, Rafalson LB, et al. Sex differences in endothelial function markers before conversion to pre-diabetes: does the clock start ticking earlier among women? The Western New York study. Diabetes Care 2007;30(2):354–9.

[49] Duplain H, Burcelin R, Sartori C, et al. Insulin resistance, hyperlipidemia, and hypertension in mice lacking endothelial nitric oxide synthase. Circulation 2001;104(3):342–5.

[50] Kubis N, Richer C, Domergue V, et al. Role of microvascular rarefaction in the increased arterial pressure in mice lacking for the endothelial nitric oxide synthase gene (enos3pt-/-). J Hypertens 2002;20(8):1581–7.

[51] Le Gouill E, Jimenez M, Binnert C, et al. Endothelial nitric oxide synthase (enos) knockout mice have defective mitochondrial beta-oxidation. Diabetes 2007;56(11):2690–6.

[52] Cook S, Hugli O, Egli M, et al. Partial gene deletion of endothelial nitric oxide synthase predisposes to exaggerated high-fat diet-induced insulin resistance and arterial hypertension. Diabetes 2004;53(8):2067–72.

[53] Clerk LH, Vincent MA, Jahn LA, et al. Obesity blunts insulin-mediated microvascular recruitment in human forearm muscle. Diabetes 2006;55(5):1436–42.

[54] Hermann TS, Li W, Dominguez H, et al. Quinapril treatment increases insulin-stimulated endothelial function and adiponectin gene expression in patients with type 2 diabetes. J Clin Endocrinol Metab 2006;91(3):1001–8.

[55] Rask-Madsen C, Ihlemann N, Krarup T, et al. Insulin therapy improves insulin-stimulated endothelial function in patients with type 2 diabetes and ischemic heart disease. Diabetes 2001;50(11):2611–8.

[56] Balletshofer BM, Rittig K, Enderle MD, et al. Endothelial dysfunction is detectable in young normotensive first-degree relatives of subjects with type 2 diabetes in association with insulin resistance. Circulation 2000;101(15):1780–4.

[57] Koh KK, Han SH, Quon MJ. Inflammatory markers and the metabolic syndrome: insights from therapeutic interventions. J Am Coll Cardiol 2005;46(11):1978–85.

[58] Hotamisligil GS. Inflammation and metabolic disorders. Nature 2006;444(7121):860–7.

[59] Gustafson B, Hammarstedt A, Andersson CX, et al. Inflamed adipose tissue: a culprit underlying the metabolic syndrome and atherosclerosis. Arterioscler Thromb Vasc Biol 2007;27(11):2276–83.

[60] Anderson HD, Rahmutula D, Gardner DG. Tumor necrosis factor-alpha inhibits endothelial nitric-oxide synthase gene promoter activity in bovine aortic endothelial cells. J Biol Chem 2004;279(2):963–9.

[61] Eringa EC, Stehouwer CD, van Nieuw Amerongen GP, et al. Vasoconstrictor effects of insulin in skeletal muscle arterioles are mediated by erk1/2 activation in endothelium. Am J Physiol Heart Circ Physiol 2004;287(5):H2043–8.

[62] Zhang L, Wheatley CM, Richards SM, et al. TNF-alpha acutely inhibits vascular effects of physiological but not high insulin or contraction. Am J Physiol Endocrinol Metab 2003; 285(3):E654–60.

[63] Sury MD, Frese-Schaper M, Muhlemann MK, et al. Evidence that n-acetylcysteine inhibits TNF-alpha-induced cerebrovascular endothelin-1 upregulation via inhibition of mitogen- and stress-activated protein kinase. Free Radic Biol Med 2006;41(9):1372–83.

[64] Andreozzi F, Laratta E, Procopio C, et al. Interleukin-6 impairs the insulin signaling pathway, promoting production of nitric oxide in human umbilical vein endothelial cells. Mol Cell Biol 2007;27(6):2372–83.

[65] Schwartz R, Osborne-Lawrence S, Hahner L, et al. C-reactive protein downregulates endothelial NO synthase and attenuates reendothelialization in vivo in mice. Circ Res 2007; 100(10):1452–9.

[66] Xu JW, Morita I, Ikeda K, et al. C-reactive protein suppresses insulin signaling in endothelial cells—role of syk tyrosine kinase. Mol Endocrinol 2006;21(2):564–73.

[67] Eringa EC, Stehouwer CD, Walburg K, et al. Physiological concentrations of insulin induce endothelin-dependent vasoconstriction of skeletal muscle resistance arteries in the presence of tumor necrosis factor-alpha dependence on c-jun n-terminal kinase. Arterioscler Thromb Vasc Biol 2006;26(2):274–80.

[68] Rask-Madsen C, Dominguez H, Ihlemann N, et al. Tumor necrosis factor-alpha inhibits insulin's stimulating effect on glucose uptake and endothelium-dependent vasodilation in humans. Circulation 2003;108(15):1815–21.

[69] Chen H, Montagnani M, Funahashi T, et al. Adiponectin stimulates production of nitric oxide in vascular endothelial cells. J Biol Chem 2003;278(45):45021–6.

[70] Motoshima H, Wu X, Mahadev K, et al. Adiponectin suppresses proliferation and superoxide generation and enhances enos activity in endothelial cells treated with oxidized LDL. Biochem Biophys Res Commun 2004;315(2):264–71.

[71] Lau DC, Dhillon B, Yan H, et al. Adipokines: molecular links between obesity and atheroslcerosis. Am J Physiol Heart Circ Physiol 2005;288(5):H2031–41.

[72] Shimabukuro M, Higa N, Asahi T, et al. Hypoadiponectinemia is closely linked to endothelial dysfunction in man. J Clin Endocrinol Metab 2003;88(7):3236–40.

[73] Vecchione C, Maffei A, Colella S, et al. Leptin effect on endothelial nitric oxide is mediated through Akt-endothelial nitric oxide synthase phosphorylation pathway. Diabetes 2002; 51(1):168–73.

[74] Rahmouni K, Correia ML, Haynes WG, et al. Obesity-associated hypertension: new insights into mechanisms. Hypertension 2005;45(1):9–14.

[75] Skurk T, van Harmelen V, Blum WF, et al. Angiotensin II promotes leptin production in cultured human fat cells by an erk1/2-dependent pathway. Obes Res 2005;13(6):969–73.

[76] Wallace AM, McMahon AD, Packard CJ, et al. Plasma leptin and the risk of cardiovascular disease in the West of Scotland Coronary Prevention Study (WOSCOPS). Circulation 2001;104(25):3052–6.

[77] Verma S, Li SH, Wang CH, et al. Resistin promotes endothelial cell activation: further evidence of adipokine-endothelial interaction. Circulation 2003;108(6):736–40.

[78] Shen YH, Zhang L, Gan Y, et al. Up-regulation of pten (phosphatase and tensin homolog deleted on chromosome ten) mediates p38 mapk stress signal-induced inhibition of insulin signaling. A cross-talk between stress signaling and insulin signaling in resistin-treated human endothelial cells. J Biol Chem 2006;281(12):7727–36.

[79] Lupattelli G, Marchesi S, Ronti T, et al. Endothelial dysfunction in vivo is related to monocyte resistin mRNA expression. J Clin Pharm Ther 2007;32(4):373–9.

[80] Du X, Edelstein D, Obici S, et al. Insulin resistance reduces arterial prostacyclin synthase and enos activities by increasing endothelial fatty acid oxidation. J Clin Invest 2006; 116(4):1071–80.

[81] Kim F, Tysseling KA, Rice J, et al. Free fatty acid impairment of nitric oxide production in endothelial cells is mediated by IKKbeta. Arterioscler Thromb Vasc Biol 2005;25(5): 989–94.

[82] Wang XL, Zhang L, Youker K, et al. Free fatty acids inhibit insulin signaling-stimulated endothelial nitric oxide synthase activation through upregulating pten or inhibiting Akt kinase. Diabetes 2006;55(8):2301–10.

[83] Clerk LH, Rattigan S, Clark MG. Lipid infusion impairs physiologic insulin-mediated capillary recruitment and muscle glucose uptake in vivo. Diabetes 2002;51(4):1138–45.

[84] de Jongh RT, Serne EH, Ijzerman RG, et al. Free fatty acid levels modulate microvascular function: relevance for obesity-associated insulin resistance, hypertension, and microangiopathy. Diabetes 2004;53(11):2873–82.

[85] Steinberg HO, Paradisi G, Hook G, et al. Free fatty acid elevation impairs insulin-mediated vasodilation and nitric oxide production. Diabetes 2000;49(7):1231–8.

[86] Piatti PM, Monti LD, Conti M, et al. Hypertriglyceridemia and hyperinsulinemia are potent inducers of endothelin-1 release in humans. Diabetes 1996;45(3):316–21.

[87] Monti LD, Setola E, Fragasso G, et al. Metabolic and endothelial effects of trimetazidine on forearm skeletal muscle in patients with type 2 diabetes and ischemic cardiomyopathy. Am J Physiol Endocrinol Metab 2006;290(1):E54–9.

[88] Du XL, Edelstein D, Dimmeler S, et al. Hyperglycemia inhibits endothelial nitric oxide synthase activity by posttranslational modification at the Akt site. J Clin Invest 2001; 108(9):1341–8.

[89] Wallis MG, Smith ME, Kolka CM, et al. Acute glucosamine-induced insulin resistance in muscle in vivo is associated with impaired capillary recruitment. Diabetologia 2005;48(10): 2131–9.

[90] Beckman JA, Goldfine AB, Gordon MB, et al. Ascorbate restores endothelium-dependent vasodilation impaired by acute hyperglycemia in humans. Circulation 2001;103(12): 1618–23.

[91] Calles-Escandon J, Cipolla M. Diabetes and endothelial dysfunction: a clinical perspective. Endocr Rev 2001;22(1):36–52.

[92] Kashyap SR, Roman LJ, Lamont J, et al. Insulin resistance is associated with impaired nitric oxide synthase activity in skeletal muscle of type 2 diabetic subjects. J Clin Endocrinol Metab 2005;90(2):1100–5.

[93] Desideri G, Ferri C, Bellini C, et al. Effects of ace inhibition on spontaneous and insulin-stimulated endothelin-1 secretion: in vitro and in vivo studies. Diabetes 1997;46(1):81–6.

[94] Cardillo C, Campia U, Bryant MB, et al. Increased activity of endogenous endothelin in patients with type II diabetes mellitus. Circulation 2002;106(14):1783–7.

[95] Benjamin EJ, Larson MG, Keyes MJ, et al. Clinical correlates and heritability of flow-mediated dilation in the community: the Framingham Heart Study. Circulation 2004; 109(5):613–9.

[96] Williams IL, Chowienczyk PJ, Wheatcroft SB, et al. Effect of fat distribution on endothelial-dependent and endothelial-independent vasodilatation in healthy humans. Diabetes Obes Metab 2006;8(3):296–301.

[97] Van Gaal LF, Mertens IL, De Block CE. Mechanisms linking obesity with cardiovascular disease. Nature 2006;444(7121):875–80.

[98] Hamburg NM, McMackin CJ, Huang AL, et al. Physical inactivity rapidly induces insulin resistance and microvascular dysfunction in healthy volunteers. Arterioscler Thromb Vasc Biol 2007;27(12):2650–6.

[99] Wisloff U, Najjar SM, Ellingsen O, et al. Cardiovascular risk factors emerge after artificial selection for low aerobic capacity. Science 2005;307(5708):418–20.

[100] Mootha VK, Lindgren CM, Eriksson KF, et al. Pgc-1alpha-responsive genes involved in oxidative phosphorylation are coordinately downregulated in human diabetes. Nat Genet 2003;34(3):267–73.

[101] Befroy DE, Petersen KF, Dufour S, et al. Impaired mitochondrial substrate oxidation in muscle of insulin-resistant offspring of type 2 diabetic patients. Diabetes 2007;56(5):1376–81.

[102] Civitarese AE, Carling S, Heilbronn LK, et al. Calorie restriction increases muscle mitochondrial biogenesis in healthy humans. PLoS Med 2007;4(3):e76.

[103] Mather K, Verma S. Function determines structure in the vasculature: lessons from insulin resistance. Am J Physiol Regul Integr Comp Physiol 2005;289(2):R305–6.

[104] Thijssen DH, Ellenkamp R, Kooijman M, et al. A causal role for endothelin-1 in the vascular adaptation to skeletal muscle deconditioning in spinal cord injury. Arterioscler Thromb Vasc Biol 2007;27(2):325–31.

[105] Quaschning T, Voss F, Relle K, et al. Lack of endothelial nitric oxide synthase promotes endothelin-induced hypertension: lessons from endothelin-1 transgenic/endothelial nitric oxide synthase knockout mice. J Am Soc Nephrol 2007;18(3):730–40.

[106] Sola S, Mir MQ, Cheema FA, et al. Irbesartan and lipoic acid improve endothelial function and reduce markers of inflammation in the metabolic syndrome: results of the irbesartan and lipoic acid in endothelial dysfunction (island) study. Circulation 2005;111(3):343–8.

[107] Heitzer T, Finckh B, Albers S, et al. Beneficial effects of alpha-lipoic acid and ascorbic acid on endothelium-dependent, nitric oxide-mediated vasodilation in diabetic patients: relation to parameters of oxidative stress. Free Radic Biol Med 2001;31(1):53–61.

[108] Chen H, Karne RJ, Hall G, et al. High-dose oral vitamin C partially replenishes vitamin C levels in patients with type 2 diabetes and low vitamin C levels but does not improve endothelial dysfunction or insulin resistance. Am J Physiol Heart Circ Physiol 2006;290(1): H137–45.

[109] Perticone F, Ceravolo R, Candigliota M, et al. Obesity and body fat distribution induce endothelial dysfunction by oxidative stress: protective effect of vitamin C. Diabetes 2001; 50(1):159–65.

[110] Lekakis JP, Anastasiou EA, Papamichael CM, et al. Short-term oral ascorbic acid improves endothelium-dependent vasodilatation in women with a history of gestational diabetes mellitus. Diabetes Care 2000;23(9):1432–4.

[111] Darko D, Dornhorst A, Kelly FJ, et al. Lack of effect of oral vitamin C on blood pressure, oxidative stress and endothelial function in type II diabetes. Clin Sci (Lond) 2002;103(4): 339–44.

[112] Regensteiner JG, Popylisen S, Bauer TA, et al. Oral l-arginine and vitamins E and C improve endothelial function in women with type 2 diabetes. Vasc Med 2003;8(3):169–75.

[113] Beckman JA, Goldfine AB, Gordon MB, et al. Oral antioxidant therapy improves endothelial function in type 1 but not type 2 diabetes mellitus. Am J Physiol Heart Circ Physiol 2003;285(6):H2392–8.

[114] Pena AS, Wiltshire E, Gent R, et al. Folic acid does not improve endothelial function in obese children and adolescents. Diabetes Care 2007;30(8):2122–7.

[115] Title LM, Ur E, Giddens K, et al. Folic acid improves endothelial dysfunction in type 2 diabetes—an effect independent of homocysteine-lowering. Vasc Med 2006;11(2):101–9.

[116] Heitzer T, Krohn K, Albers S, et al. Tetrahydrobiopterin improves endothelium-dependent vasodilation by increasing nitric oxide activity in patients with type II diabetes mellitus. Diabetologia 2000;43(11):1435–8.

[117] Nystrom T, Nygren A, Sjoholm A. Tetrahydrobiopterin increases insulin sensitivity in patients with type 2 diabetes and coronary heart disease. Am J Physiol Endocrinol Metab 2004;287(5):E919–25.

[118] Grassi D, Necozione S, Lippi C, et al. Cocoa reduces blood pressure and insulin resistance and improves endothelium-dependent vasodilation in hypertensives. Hypertension 2005; 46(2):398–405.

[119] Hamdy O, Ledbury S, Mullooly C, et al. Lifestyle modification improves endothelial function in obese subjects with the insulin resistance syndrome. Diabetes Care 2003; 26(7):2119–25.

[120] Maeda S, Jesmin S, Iemitsu M, et al. Weight loss reduces plasma endothelin-1 concentration in obese men. Exp Biol Med (Maywood) 2006;231(6):1044–7.

[121] Hotta K, Funahashi T, Arita Y, et al. Plasma concentrations of a novel, adipose-specific protein, adiponectin, in type 2 diabetic patients. Arterioscler Thromb Vasc Biol 2000; 20(6):1595–9.

[122] Esposito K, Marfella R, Ciotola M, et al. Effect of a Mediterranean-style diet on endothelial dysfunction and markers of vascular inflammation in the metabolic syndrome: a randomized trial. JAMA 2004;292(12):1440–6.

[123] Esposito K, Pontillo A, Di Palo C, et al. Effect of weight loss and lifestyle changes on vascular inflammatory markers in obese women: a randomized trial. JAMA 2003; 289(14):1799–804.

[124] Lavrencic A, Salobir BG, Keber I. Physical training improves flow-mediated dilation in patients with the polymetabolic syndrome. Arterioscler Thromb Vasc Biol 2000;20(2): 551–5.

[125] Maiorana A, O'Driscoll G, Cheetham C, et al. The effect of combined aerobic and resistance exercise training on vascular function in type 2 diabetes. J Am Coll Cardiol 2001; 38(3):860–6.

[126] De Filippis E, Cusi K, Ocampo G, et al. Exercise-induced improvement in vasodilatory function accompanies increased insulin sensitivity in obesity and type 2 diabetes mellitus. J Clin Endocrinol Metab 2006;91(12):4903–10.

[127] Sasaki S, Higashi Y, Nakagawa K, et al. A low-calorie diet improves endothelium-dependent vasodilation in obese patients with essential hypertension. Am J Hypertens 2002;15(4 Pt 1):302–9.

[128] Meyer AA, Kundt G, Lenschow U, et al. Improvement of early vascular changes and cardiovascular risk factors in obese children after a six-month exercise program. J Am Coll Cardiol 2006;48(9):1865–70.

[129] Dela F, Larsen JJ, Mikines KJ, et al. Insulin-stimulated muscle glucose clearance in patients with NIDDM. Effects of one-legged physical training. Diabetes 1995;44(9):1010–20.

[130] Hardin DS, Azzarelli B, Edwards J, et al. Mechanisms of enhanced insulin sensitivity in endurance-trained athletes: effects on blood flow and differential expression of glut 4 in skeletal muscles. J Clin Endocrinol Metab 1995;80(8):2437–46.

[131] Goto C, Higashi Y, Kimura M, et al. Effect of different intensities of exercise on endothelium-dependent vasodilation in humans: role of endothelium-dependent nitric oxide and oxidative stress. Circulation 2003;108(5):530–5.

[132] Hambrecht R, Adams V, Erbs S, et al. Regular physical activity improves endothelial function in patients with coronary artery disease by increasing phosphorylation of endothelial nitric oxide synthase. Circulation 2003;107(25):3152–8.

[133] Diamanti-Kandarakis E, Alexandraki K, Protogerou A, et al. Metformin administration improves endothelial function in women with polycystic ovary syndrome. Eur J Endocrinol 2005;152(5):749–56.

[134] Mather KJ, Verma S, Anderson TJ. Improved endothelial function with metformin in type 2 diabetes mellitus. J Am Coll Cardiol 2001;37(5):1344–50.

[135] de Aguiar LG, Bahia LR, Villela N, et al. Metformin improves endothelial vascular reactivity in first-degree relatives of type 2 diabetic patients with metabolic syndrome and normal glucose tolerance. Diabetes Care 2006;29(5):1083–9.

[136] Martens FM, Visseren FL, de Koning EJ, et al. Short-term pioglitazone treatment improves vascular function irrespective of metabolic changes in patients with type 2 diabetes. J Cardiovasc Pharmacol 2005;46(6):773–8.

[137] Mittermayer F, Schaller G, Pleiner J, et al. Rosiglitazone prevents free fatty acid-induced vascular endothelial dysfunction. J Clin Endocrinol Metab 2007;92(7):2574–80.

[138] Wang TD, Chen WJ, Lin JW, et al. Effects of rosiglitazone on endothelial function, c-reactive protein, and components of the metabolic syndrome in nondiabetic patients with the metabolic syndrome. Am J Cardiol 2004;93(3):362–5.

[139] Esposito K, Ciotola M, Carleo D, et al. Effect of rosiglitazone on endothelial function and inflammatory markers in patients with the metabolic syndrome. Diabetes Care 2006;29(5): 1071–6.

[140] Ceriello A, Assaloni R, Da Ros R, et al. Effect of atorvastatin and irbesartan, alone and in combination, on postprandial endothelial dysfunction, oxidative stress, and inflammation in type 2 diabetic patients. Circulation 2005;111(19):2518–24.

[141] Economides PA, Caselli A, Tiani E, et al. The effects of atorvastatin on endothelial function in diabetic patients and subjects at risk for type 2 diabetes. J Clin Endocrinol Metab 2004; 89(2):740–7.

[142] Shimabukuro M, Higa N, Asahi T, et al. Fluvastatin improves endothelial dysfunction in overweight postmenopausal women through small dense low-density lipoprotein reduction. Metabolism 2004;53(6):733–9.

[143] Evans M, Anderson RA, Graham J, et al. Ciprofibrate therapy improves endothelial function and reduces postprandial lipemia and oxidative stress in type 2 diabetes mellitus. Circulation 2000;101(15):1773–9.

[144] Avogaro A, Miola M, Favaro A, et al. Gemfibrozil improves insulin sensitivity and flow-mediated vasodilatation in type 2 diabetic patients. Eur J Clin Invest 2001;31(7):603–9.

[145] Koh KK, Han SH, Quon MJ, et al. Beneficial effects of fenofibrate to improve endothelial dysfunction and raise adiponectin levels in patients with primary hypertriglyceridemia. Diabetes Care 2005;28(6):1419–24.

[146] Koh KK, Quon MJ, Han SH, et al. Additive beneficial effects of losartan combined with simvastatin in the treatment of hypercholesterolemic, hypertensive patients. Circulation 2004;110(24):3687–92.

[147] O'Driscoll G, Green D, Maiorana A, et al. Improvement in endothelial function by angiotensin-converting enzyme inhibition in non-insulin-dependent diabetes mellitus. J Am Coll Cardiol 1999;33(6):1506–11.

[148] Koh KK, Quon MJ, Han SH, et al. Additive beneficial effects of fenofibrate combined with atorvastatin in the treatment of combined hyperlipidemia. J Am Coll Cardiol 2005;45(10): 1649–53.

[149] Koh KK, Quon MJ, Han SH, et al. Vascular and metabolic effects of combined therapy with ramipril and simvastatin in patients with type 2 diabetes. Hypertension 2005;45(6): 1088–93.

ELSEVIER
SAUNDERS

Endocrinol Metab Clin N Am
37 (2008) 713–731

ENDOCRINOLOGY
AND METABOLISM
CLINICS
OF NORTH AMERICA

Mitochondrial Dysfunction in Type 2 Diabetes and Obesity

Kurt Højlund, MD, PhD[a,*], Martin Mogensen, MSc[b],
Kent Sahlin, PhD[b,c],
Henning Beck-Nielsen, MD, DMSc[a]

[a]Diabetes Research Center, Department of Endocrinology, Odense University Hospital,
Kloevervaenget 6, 3 DK-5000 Odense C, Denmark
[b]Institute of Sports Science and Clinical Biomechanics, University of Southern Denmark,
Campusvej 55, DK-5230 Odense, Denmark
[c]Swedish School of Sport and Health Sciences, GIH, Box 5626, S-11486 Stockholm, Sweden

Type 2 diabetes mellitus (T2D) is the most common metabolic disease, currently affecting approximately 170 million people worldwide [1]. The development of T2D is the result of a complex interaction between genetic and environmental factors [2], the latter being evidenced by a rapid decrease in age at onset under the influence of a Western lifestyle and marked by physical inactivity, increased caloric intake, and obesity. T2D and obesity are characterized by insulin resistance in major metabolic tissues such as skeletal muscle, liver, and fat cells. In T2D, failure of the pancreatic β-cells to compensate for this abnormality causes hyperglycemia [3]. In T2D and obesity, an elevated risk of cardiovascular disease causes increased morbidity and mortality and decreased quality of life, and places a substantial economic burden on our health system. A better understanding of the complex pathogenesis of insulin resistance in T2D and obesity is therefore of major importance to improve preventive and therapeutic strategies.

Skeletal muscle accounts for most insulin-stimulated glucose disposal in humans in vivo [4] and is correspondingly the predominant site of peripheral insulin resistance in T2D and obesity [4–8]. At the cellular level, insulin resistance in skeletal muscle is characterized by impaired insulin stimulation of glucose transport and glycogen synthesis [4–8]. Indeed, a number of abnormalities explaining these defects have been reported in skeletal muscle

This work was supported by the Danish Medical Research Council, the Novo Nordisk Research Foundation, and the Danish Diabetes Association.

* Corresponding author.
E-mail address: k.hojlund@dadlnet.dk (K. Højlund).

biopsy samples obtained from insulin-resistant subjects [8]. Thus, attenuated insulin signaling to glucose transport through insulin receptor substrate 1 (IRS-1) and phosphatidylinositol 3-kinase (PI3K) [5,7,9,10] and impaired insulin activation of glycogen synthase [5–7,11,12] (the rate-limiting enzyme in glycogen synthesis) represent well-established biochemical defects in muscle in T2D and obesity (Fig. 1). Despite extensive research of insulin signaling in skeletal muscle, however, the primary molecular events leading to insulin resistance remain largely unknown.

In addition to impaired insulin-stimulated glucose transport and glycogen synthesis, perturbations in the capacity of skeletal muscle to oxidize glucose and lipids under different physiologic conditions seem to play a role for insulin resistance [13,14]. Markers of fatty acid metabolism in skeletal muscle correlate strongly with insulin sensitivity in obesity [15], and measurements of the respiratory quotient across the tissue bed of the leg in patients who have T2D and in obese subjects have provided evidence that during fasting conditions, glucose oxidation is increased, whereas reliance on lipid oxidation is decreased [16,17]. Conversely, insulin-mediated stimulation of glucose oxidation and suppression of lipid oxidation are impaired in patients who have T2D and in obese subjects [13,14,17]. This impaired ability to switch between lipid and glucose oxidation in response to insulin and fasting has been described as "metabolic inflexibility" of skeletal muscle, and may be a major determinant of skeletal muscle insulin resistance [13,14]. A reduced reliance on lipid oxidation during fasting conditions is likely a key mechanism by which excess amounts of triglyceride and lipid

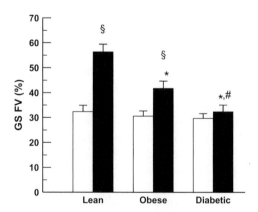

Fig. 1. Impaired insulin activation of muscle glycogen synthase in T2D and obesity. Glycogen synthase activity is given as percent fractional velocity (GS FV) at the basal state (*white bars*) and the insulin-stimulated state (*black bars*) of euglycemic-hyperinsulinemic clamp in lean, obese, and type 2 diabetic subjects. Data are mean ± SEM. *$P<.01$ versus lean subjects; #$P<.05$ versus obese subjects; §$P<.001$ versus basal. (*From* Højlund K, Frystyk J, Levin K, et al. Reduced plasma adiponectin concentrations may contribute to impaired insulin activation of glycogen synthase in skeletal muscle of patients with type 2 diabetes. Diabetologia 2006;49:1287; with permission.)

metabolites accumulate within skeletal muscle [14]. In humans, there is a strong inverse relationship between intramyocellular lipid content (IMCL) and insulin sensitivity [18,19], and an increased amount of muscle lipids is another key marker of insulin resistance in T2D and obesity [18–21]. Increased levels of specific lipid metabolites such as long-chain acyl coenzyme A, diacylglycerol, and ceramides have been linked to impaired insulin signaling due to activation of serine/threonine kinase (eg, protein kinase C), leading to inhibitory serine phosphorylation of proximal components in the insulin signaling cascade and glycogen synthase and, therefore, to insulin resistance [8,22–24].

Recent work, including transcriptomic and proteomic profiling of skeletal muscle, has pointed to impaired mitochondrial oxidative metabolism as a potential mechanism explaining the abnormalities in lipid and glucose metabolism and insulin signaling observed in insulin-resistant subjects. This article focuses on the current evidence for a link between mitochondrial dysfunction and insulin resistance in humans who have T2D and obesity.

Markers of impaired oxidative capacity in insulin resistance

Being the major site of fuel oxidation, the mitochondrion has gained increasing interest in T2D research over the last 5 years. Several earlier studies have been suggestive of an association between decreased muscle oxidative capacity and insulin resistance in T2D and obesity. Thus, muscle citrate synthase (CS) activity, which correlates strongly with mitochondrial content, oxidative capacity, and maximal oxygen consumption ($\dot{V}o_2max$), has been reported to be reduced in T2D [25,26] and obesity [27]. Moreover, studies of key metabolic enzymes in muscle have demonstrated (1) an increased ratio of glycolytic relative to mitochondrial oxidative capacity in patients who have T2D and in obese women and (2) a significant correlation between the ratio of glycolytic to oxidative enzyme capacity and insulin resistance [28,29]. The higher glycolytic-to-oxidative enzyme capacity is, at least in part, explained by an altered fiber-type composition in skeletal muscle of insulin-resistant individuals. Thus, in skeletal muscle of obese subjects, of patients who have T2D [30–33], and their first-degree relatives (FDRs) [34], a higher proportion of the glycolytic type 2X fibers or a lower proportion of the oxidative, type 1 fibers have been reported. Furthermore, Vo_2max, which is a measure of physical fitness and often correlated with muscle oxidative capacity, is reduced in patients who have T2D [35], in FDRs [36,37], and in obese women who have polycystic ovary syndrome (PCOS) [38]. These data suggest that an altered fiber-type composition and reduced Vo_2max represent early markers of impaired mitochondrial oxidative metabolism and insulin resistance in human skeletal muscle. Mitochondria in skeletal muscle of patients who have T2D and, to some extent, of obese subjects are smaller and show an altered morphology [20,26]. Moreover, a significant inverse relationship between muscle oxidative enzyme capacity and IMCL has been demonstrated in patients who have T2D and in obese subjects [20], and single-fiber analysis showed that lower oxidative enzyme capacity and increased lipid content in skeletal muscle of type 2 diabetic and obese subjects were present within each fiber type [20]. These data indicate that in addition to an altered fiber-type composition, other factors should be sought to explain reduced reliance on lipid oxidation, impaired mitochondrial oxidative capacity, and insulin resistance in T2D and obesity. There is evidence that environmental factors associated with insulin resistance, such as physical inactivity and aging, contribute to impaired mitochondrial oxidative capacity [39–41]. Furthermore, in recent years, an increasing number of studies have pointed to potential novel mechanisms underlying the association between mitochondrial dysfunction and insulin resistance in human skeletal muscle. These findings are reviewed in the following sections.

Transcriptomic evidence of impaired mitochondrial biogenesis

Transcriptional profiling has proved to be a powerful tool to identify novel genes and biologic pathways of potential interest in the pathogenesis of complex disorders such as insulin resistance. Several research groups have applied DNA microarrays to determine changes in muscle gene expression in patients who have T2D and in high-risk individuals who have insulin resistance [42–46]. Despite differences in the type of Affymetrix Gene Chip (Affymetrix, Santa Clara, California) used, number of probes on the chip, sample size, study design, subject ethnicity, and data analysis, collectively, these studies have shown only modest differences in muscle transcripts between patients who have insulin resistance with or without T2D and healthy control subjects. Thus, in most of these studies, no single gene remained differentially expressed after correction for multiple testing [42–45]. Nevertheless, these studies have shown similar changes in gene expression pattern that point to abnormalities in mitochondrial oxidative phosphorylation (OXPHOS).

In the first published study by Sreekumar and coworkers [44], microarray analysis of muscle gene expression in poorly controlled obese patients who had T2D compared with obese control subjects showed a down-regulation of gene transcripts involved in muscle mitochondrial energy metabolism, including several subunits of the respiratory complexes I through V and the tricarboxylic acid cycle. Intensive insulin treatment of these poorly controlled diabetic subjects for 10 days normalized glucose levels and reversed most of these transcriptional changes, indicating that they were secondary to hyperglycemia. Only changes in single gene expression before correction for multiple testing were reported, however, and no pathway analysis was performed to confirm the data [44].

A major breakthrough in identifying a relationship between insulin resistance and impaired mitochondrial biogenesis in human skeletal muscle was the simultaneous publication of two microarray studies in 2003 [42,43].

These studies of muscle transcripts in humans who had T2D and prediabetes in Mexican American [42] and Caucasian populations [43] led to the same conclusions. In the study of Mexican Americans, muscle transcript levels were analyzed in patients who had T2D, glucose-tolerant FDRs, and healthy control subjects [42]. Functional annotation using gene ontology terms revealed a coordinated down-regulation of genes coding for proteins involved in mitochondrial function and ATP synthesis in patients who had T2D and FDRs. Many of the down-regulated OXPHOS genes were known to be coordinately regulated by the nuclear respiratory factors (NRFs) and cofactor PGC-1α [47]. In an independent cohort made up of patients who had T2D, FDRs, and healthy controls, the investigators were able to demonstrate a reduced mRNA expression of NRF-1 in patients who had T2D, and a reduced mRNA expression of PGC-1α and PGC-1β in patients who had T2D and FDRs using quantitative real-time polymerase chain reaction (RT-PCR) analysis [42]. It was suggested that this gene expression pattern may be an early, if not primary, phenotype in diabetes development, which precedes the onset of hyperglycemia.

In the Caucasian study population, muscle gene expression was studied in patients who had T2D, in subjects who had impaired glucose tolerance, and in healthy control subjects [43]. In this study, the sample size was sufficient to demonstrate a difference in insulin-stimulated glucose disposal between diabetic and nondiabetic subjects. Moreover, a novel method to analyze data (called gene-set enrichment analysis) was used [48]. This analysis included the a priori definition of 149 sets of genes [43]. Using this approach, a set of genes involved in mitochondrial OXPHOS whose expression was coordinately down-regulated in human diabetic muscle was identified. The investigators showed that a large subset of these OXPHOS genes is coregulated by PGC-1α in different insulin-sensitive tissues in rodents. Furthermore, they demonstrated a significant correlation between this subset of OXPHOS genes and Vo_2max in the study population, whereas no relationship between fiber-type composition and OXPHOS gene expression was found [43].

More recently, Skov and colleagues [46] used DNA microarrays to compare muscle transcripts in insulin-resistant obese women who had PCOS and in matched obese women. Using two different approaches for global pathway analysis, the investigators observed a consistent down-regulation of OXPHOS gene expression in PCOS patients. Quantitative RT-PCR analysis validated the findings and showed that decreased expression of PGC-1α could play a role for these abnormalities (Fig. 2). The women who had PCOS were weight-matched to the control group and had normal plasma glucose levels, providing evidence that transcriptional down-regulation of OXPHOS genes may be an early marker of insulin resistance independent of obesity and hyperglycemia.

Taken together, these studies of muscle gene expression in patients who have T2D and in high-risk individuals suggest that genes involved in mitochondrial oxidative metabolism are coordinately down-regulated and that

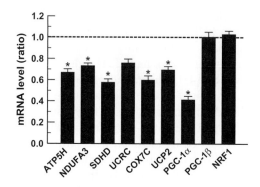

Fig. 2. Decreased expression of OXPHOS genes and PGC-1α in skeletal muscle of insulin-resistant women who have PCOS. Relative expression of nine selected genes in skeletal muscle of PCOS patients versus control subjects determined by quantitative RT-PCR. Down-regulated genes in PCOS patients have mRNA levels below 1.0 (*dotted line*), and up-regulated genes have mRNA levels above 1.0. Data are means ± SEM. *$P < .05$ PCOS versus control subjects. (*From* Skov V, Glintborg D, Knudsen S, et al. Reduced expression of nuclear-encoded genes involved in mitochondrial oxidative metabolism in skeletal muscle of insulin-resistant women with polycystic ovary syndrome. Diabetes 2007;56:2352; with permission. Copyright © 2007, American Diabetes Association. Reprinted with permission from *The American Diabetes Association.*)

reduced expression of PGC-1α could play a key role for these transcriptional changes and represent an early event in the pathogenesis of insulin resistance in human skeletal muscle. Exactly how PGC-1α is regulated in human skeletal muscle remains to be clarified. The gene expression of this transcription cofactor increases in response to acute exercise and endurance training [49,50] and decreases in response to physical inactivity and increasing age [51,52]. A detailed description of the potential molecular mechanisms by which PGC-1α activity and expression are regulated is given elsewhere [49]; however, one of its critical upstream regulators in skeletal muscle seems to be AMP-activated protein kinase (AMPK), which antagonizes a decrease in the cellular energy status (ATP depletion) by increasing its activity [49,53]. There is experimental evidence that AMPK induces the expression and activity of PGC-1α by phosphorylation [54]. Somewhat surprisingly, most studies of the AMPK system in human skeletal muscle in vivo have failed to demonstrate lower protein content or activity of AMPK in patients who have T2D, in obese subjects, and in women who have PCOS [55–59]. Thus, although it may be too early to rule out a role for AMPK dysregulation in insulin resistance, these data emphasize that the role of other potential regulators of PGC-1α in insulin resistance and impaired mitochondrial biogenesis needs to be investigated.

Proteomic evidence of mitochondrial dysfunction

It is likely that expression of muscle mRNA does not accurately reflect the abundance or activity of proteins and it certainly gives no information regarding their posttranslational modification. The authors [60] recently applied quantitative proteomics in human skeletal muscle to identify protein markers of T2D in the fasting state. Eight potential markers of T2D in skeletal muscle were identified by mass spectrometry (MS) and indicated increased cellular stress and perturbations in ATP (re)synthesis. Thus, in patients who have T2D, two heat shock proteins (GRP78 and HSP90beta) were up-regulated, whereas the protein content of creatine kinase B and ATP synthase β-subunit was reduced. ATP synthase β-subunit was one of the first OXPHOS proteins shown to be tightly regulated by PGC-1α [47]; the authors' data, therefore, were supported by simultaneous reports of transcriptional down-regulation of OXPHOS and PGC-1α in insulin resistance and T2D [42,43,46]. Phosphorylation appeared to play a key role for most of the protein markers identified in this proteomic study. As a novel finding, the authors demonstrated that the catalytic β-subunit of ATP synthase is phosphorylated, most likely at multiple sites in vivo. This finding has been confirmed in several subsequent studies of mammalian tissues and cells [61–64], suggesting a potential role for phosphorylation of the catalytic β-subunit of ATP synthase in the regulation of ATP synthesis in vivo. In patients who have T2D, one of the most phosphorylated forms was down-regulated and correlated inversely with plasma glucose (Fig. 3). These data indicate that alterations in the regulation of ATP synthesis and cellular stress proteins may contribute to the pathogenesis of insulin resistance in T2D.

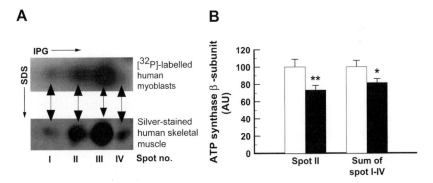

Fig. 3. Decreased phosphorylation and protein content of ATP synthase β-subunit in skeletal muscle of patients who have T2D. (A) Enlarged regions of images of two-dimensional gels showing four spots in human skeletal muscle (silver staining) identified as ATP synthase β-subunit by MS, and the phosphorylation of the same protein spots in [^{32}P]-labeled human myoblasts indicating multisite phosphorylation of ATP synthase β-subunit. (B) Down-regulation of a specific phosphoisoform (Spot II) and the sum of spots (Sum of spot I-IV) identified as ATP synthase β-subunit in skeletal muscle of patients who have T2D (black bars) versus control subjects (white bars). **$P = .01$ and *$P < .05$ versus control subjects. (Adapted from Højlund K, Wrzesinski K, Larsen PM, et al. Proteome analysis reveals phosphorylation of ATP synthase beta-subunit in human skeletal muscle and proteins with potential roles in type 2 diabetes. J Biol Chem 2003;278:10439; with permission.)

More recently, Hittel and coworkers [65] performed a proteome analysis of cytosolic proteins extracted from skeletal muscle obtained from obese women and lean control subjects. This study showed an increased protein level of three glycolytic enzymes (aldolase A, glyceraldehyde-phosphate dehydrogenase, and adenylate kinase 1) in obese women [65]. Although mitochondrial proteins were not evaluated in this study, these results support earlier reports of an increased glycolytic-to-oxidative enzyme capacity in skeletal muscle in T2D and obesity [28,29]. A recent reanalysis of public datasets of skeletal muscle gene expression in insulin-resistant individuals [42,43] also showed an up-regulation of genes implicated in glycolytic metabolism [66].

Considering the extensive use of human vastus lateralis muscle in studies of insulin resistance, it is surprising that this includes only two proteomic studies. In both studies, protein separation by two-dimensional gel electrophoresis and protein identification by matrix-assisted laser desorption ionization time-of-flight MS and tandem MS/MS were used [60,65]. Using this approach, the most comprehensive assessment of the human muscle proteome reported only 107 different proteins, mainly high-abundant structural or metabolic proteins [67]. This finding indicates that proteome analysis of human skeletal muscle has been more challenging than expected, most likely due to the high abundance of cytoskeletal and contractile proteins combined with a lower dynamic range and restricted intervals of pI and mW associated with the two-dimensional gel approach. In a recent study, however, the authors [68] were able to identify approximately 1000 different proteins in human vastus lateralis muscle using a combination of one-dimensional gel electrophoresis and high-performance liquid chromatography–electrospray ionization-MS/MS. More than 200 (22%) of these proteins were functionally annotated to the mitochondrion, including 55 of 88 known subunits of the respiratory complexes I through V. These data hold promise for global assessment of quantitative changes in the muscle proteome in future studies of insulin resistance and T2D. Moreover, an increasing number of kinases, phosphatases, and phosphoproteins, including several subunits in the respiratory complexes I through V, have been identified within the last 5 years [63,69]. Thus, it is expected that future characterization of the mitochondrial proteome and phosphoproteome in human skeletal muscle and changes associated with insulin resistance and T2D will highly increase our insight into the mechanisms underlying the mitochondrial dysfunction associated with these conditions.

Mitochondrial content versus mitochondrial function

Within the past 5 years, several studies have provided further support for the hypothesis of a link between mitochondrial dysfunction and insulin resistance in human skeletal muscle. With magnetic resonance spectroscopy (MRS), mitochondrial oxidative capacity and IMCL content can be measured noninvasively in the same muscle in vivo [70]. Applying these techniques, decreased basal rates of mitochondrial ATP production and substrate oxidation (by way of the tricarboxylic acid cycle) and lower mitochondrial density in skeletal muscle were found to be associated with increased IMCL content in lean, insulin-resistant FDRs compared with matched insulin-sensitive subjects who did or did not have a family history of T2D [71–73]. More recently, MRS techniques were used to determine IMCL content and in vivo mitochondrial function by measuring phosphocreatine recovery half-time (PCr half-time) immediately after exercise [74]. The PCr half-time was 45% longer in muscle of overweight patients who had T2D compared with weight-matched control subjects. No difference in IMCL content was observed, however, indicating a disassociation between IMCL and mitochondrial dysfunction, at least in overweight/obese subjects who did or did not have T2D. The PCr half-time correlated with hemoglobin A_{1c} in the diabetic group and with fasting plasma glucose in the entire group, supporting other studies and indicating a role for hyperglycemia in mitochondrial dysfunction [33,44,60,75]. These noninvasive studies have not clarified whether mitochondrial dysfunction in human skeletal of insulin resistant subjects is caused by a lower mitochondrial content, a functional impairment of mitochondria, or both. Microarray studies of muscle from patients who have T2D and from high-risk individuals suggest that the reduction in mitochondrial activity in vivo primarily reflects a lower content of mitochondria [42,43,46]. On the other hand, an altered phosphorylation of ATP synthase β-subunit in muscle of patients who have T2D emphasizes that impaired functionality of mitochondria should also be considered [60,69].

In a study by Kelley and colleagues [26], decreased ETC activity measured as the activity of $NADH:O_2$ oxidoreductase in a mitochondrial fraction was observed in type 2 diabetic and obese subjects compared with lean subjects. ETC activity that was corrected for mitochondrial content (CS activity), however, did not differ significantly across the groups, implicating a greater role for mitochondrial content than function in mitochondrial dysfunction. In another study from the same research group [76], ETC activity was measured as the activity of succinate oxidase in the total, subsarcolemmal, and intermyofibrillar subpopulations of muscle mitochondria. Total ETC activity, mitochondrial DNA (mtDNA) content, and the ratio between these measures were reduced similarly in type 2 diabetic and obese subjects relative to lean subjects. These results provided some evidence for a reduced functional capacity of mitochondria in T2D and obesity. Strikingly, ETC activity in the subsarcolemmal mitochondria was lower in muscle of type 2 diabetic subjects compared not only with lean (sevenfold) both also with obese (twofold) subjects [76]. Nevertheless, it was not examined whether the latter was caused by a lower content or functional capacity of subsarcolemmal mitochondria.

The functionality of the mitochondrion can be assessed by measuring respiration in isolated mitochondria or in permeabilized muscle fibers from human skeletal muscle biopsy samples under controlled conditions without the influence of circulating hormones and substrates [77]. By using different substrate combinations, different enzymatic pathways can be included and excluded. By relating the mitochondrial respiration to CS activity or to mtDNA, the respiratory capacity per mitochondrion can be assessed. Very recently, the authors [33] reported a significant decreased respiratory function per mitochondrion in obese T2D patients compared with obese healthy subjects. This finding was evident in fully coupled isolated mitochondria using pyruvate and malate (state 3 respiration) as substrates, and in permeabilized uncoupled mitochondria using NADH and cytochrome c (maximal respiration through the electron transport chain [ETC]) as substrates (Fig. 4). A decreased respiration per mitochondrion suggests an intrinsic inhibition or damage to some of the involved mitochondrial pathways. In a study of mitochondria in saponin-permeabilized muscle fibers, ADP-stimulated state 3 respiration using glutamate or glutamate plus succinate as substrates was lower in patients who had T2D than in healthy controls [78]. In contrast to the authors' results, the differences disappeared when respiration was normalized for mtDNA or CS activity, and the investigators concluded that mitochondrial function is normal in T2D. The conflicting results of these studies could be explained by differences in study design, methodology, and the substrates used. Although it is clear that the lack of difference in the latter study could be due to a type II error, it must be admitted that the sample size needed to confirm the small difference

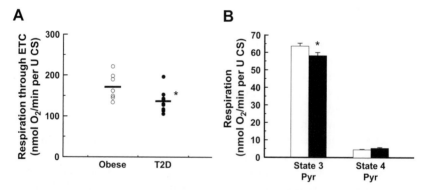

Fig. 4. Decreased respiration in isolated mitochondria from human skeletal muscle of obese patients who have T2D compared with obese control subjects. (*A*) Maximal respiration through the ETC in permeabilized isolated mitochondria using NADH and cytochrome c as substrates. The mean value for each group is indicated by a line. (*B*) State 3 and state 4 respiration in isolated mitochondria with pyruvate plus malate (Pyr) as substrates. Data represent mean ± SEM from diabetic patients (*black bars*) and control subjects (*white bars*). Measures of respiration were divided by CS activity (U CS) in the mitochondrial suspension to correct for mitochondrial content. *$P<.05$ versus control subjects. (*From* Mogensen M, Sahlin K, Fernström M, et al. Mitochondrial respiration is decreased in skeletal muscle of patients with type 2 diabetes. Diabetes 2007;56:1595; with permission. Copyright © 2007, American Diabetes Association. Reprinted with permission from *The American Diabetes Association*.)

in the authors' study with sufficient power is about twofold higher than the one used. Thus, further studies are warranted to clarify whether and how mitochondrial dysfunction differs between obese subjects who have and do not have T2D.

Is mitochondrial dysfunction a primary defect?

One important question that remains to be answered is whether mitochondrial dysfunction is the cause or consequence of insulin resistance. Direct studies of oxidative enzyme capacity, mitochondrial morphology, and single-fiber analysis in skeletal muscle of FDRs are unavailable. As noted earlier, however, a number of studies have demonstrated that mitochondrial dysfunction and insulin resistance coexist at an early point in the development of T2D and therefore provide support for the hypothesis that mitochondrial dysfunction may represent a primary defect. Thus, transcriptional profiling of skeletal muscle has indicated impaired mitochondrial biogenesis in normoglycemic high-risk individuals, independent of obesity and hyperglycemia [42,46], and studies using MRS have shown lower rates of mitochondrial ATP production and substrate oxidation and reduced mitochondrial density in lean FDRs who have severe insulin resistance [71–73]. More recently, it was shown that metabolic inflexibility in substrate switching between whole-body fat oxidation and carbohydrate oxidation was associated with a lower mitochondrial content in muscle of sedentary young men who have a family history of T2D [79].

In contrast to these studies of human muscle, recent studies of tissue-specific knockout mice have reported that OXPHOS-deficient muscle in vitro shows an increased or normal glucose use in response to insulin [80,81]. Although these findings do not fully exclude the possibility of a primary defect in mitochondrial function in human skeletal muscle, none of the present human studies proves a cause-and-effect relationship between mitochondrial dysfunction and insulin resistance. It is possible that intact insulin signaling is required for maintenance of muscle mitochondria and that insulin resistance, therefore, results in mitochondrial dysfunction rather than the reverse [82]. In support of this idea, it has been found that insulin infusion for longer than 4 hours increased ATP production in mitochondria isolated from muscle of healthy subjects, whereas in patients who had T2D, no effect of insulin infusion was observed [83]. In healthy subjects, the increase in ATP production was accompanied by increased expression of OXPHOS genes and CS and cytochrome c oxidase activity. Consistently, insulin caused an increase in muscle transcripts of several OXPHOS genes in healthy subjects [84]. More recently, MRS studies have reported a 60% to 90% increase in muscle ATP synthesis in response to insulin infusion in healthy young and old subjects, whereas no or only a minor increase was seen in patients who had T2D or in FDRs who had severe insulin resistance, respectively [85,86]. Lipid infusion in healthy subjects also impaired this response, suggesting that primary and secondary mechanisms may work to impair this effect of insulin in vivo [87]. These studies provide evidence for an effect of insulin on mitochondrial function and indicate that this effect is impaired in muscle from type 2 diabetic subjects and high-risk individuals and could be a potential intrinsic defect. Based on these findings, it could be hypothesized that impaired insulin regulation of mitochondrial function is yet another mechanism contributing to the pathogenesis of T2D and that mitochondrial dysfunction is the consequence of this insulin resistance. On the other hand, resistance to the effect of insulin could also be due to an intrinsic defect in one or several of these mitochondrial genes or proteins.

Reversal of mitochondrial dysfunction

Numerous factors are known to influence mitochondrial function. Some of these factors, including age, obesity, fiber-type distribution, and physical activity, have also been related to insulin resistance and T2D. Physical activity has been shown to have a positive influence on T2D by increasing insulin sensitivity and inducing weight loss. Muscular adaptations in relation to increased physical fitness include an increased muscle and lipid oxidative capacity mainly caused by an increased mitochondrial volume [41]. It has been argued that a potential lower level of physical activity in T2D patients and obese subjects is the major cause of impaired mitochondrial oxidative metabolism in muscle [78,88]. If this is true, it is obvious that increased physical activity and weight loss should be the first steps taken to reduce the risk of cardiovascular disease and T2D in insulin-resistant subjects. Two recent studies of patients who had T2D and obesity have demonstrated that a combined intervention of physical activity and weight loss improves insulin sensitivity and mitochondrial function, the latter primarily by increasing mitochondrial content [75,89]. In these studies, the effect of exercise training per se was not examined. Moreover, because no control subjects participated, it remains to be determined whether mitochondrial function in insulin-resistant subjects is normalized or just improved. There is evidence that obese subjects who have early-onset T2D show resistance to exercise training with respect to insulin sensitivity [90] and that this may also apply to mitochondrial function in T2D and obesity.

A number of recent studies suggest that pharmacologic treatment should be considered in addition to increased physical activity and weight loss to achieve the goals of normal mitochondrial function and insulin sensitivity. Thus, treatment with pioglitazone for 12 weeks increased CS activity, mtDNA copy number, PGC-1α mRNA, and expression of genes required for fatty acid oxidation in subcutaneous fat of patients who had T2D [91]. In another study, treatment with rosiglitazone for 8 weeks increased expression of PGC-1α and activity of oxidative enzymes in skeletal muscle of patients who had T2D [92]. Using gene expression profiling and biologic pathway analysis, an increased expression of OXPHOS genes and PGC-1α in skeletal muscle of women who had PCOS in response to treatment with pioglitazone for 16 weeks was found [93]. These changes were seen together with improved insulin sensitivity and a twofold increase in plasma adiponectin in the same cohort [59]. The fact that these effects of thiazolidinediones (TZD) on muscle mitochondria are secondary to activation of peroxisome proliferator-activated receptor (PPAR)γ in adipocytes and to a subsequent increase in plasma adiponectin is supported by the finding of a strong association between plasma adiponectin and mtDNA copy number in human muscle [94]; however, a potential direct effect of TZD on muscle cannot be excluded. There is experimental evidence that recombinant adiponectin promotes AMPK activity [95] and that AMPK may increase mitochondrial biogenesis [96,97]. In a single study, treatment with rosiglitazone increased AMPK activity in muscle in T2D and obesity, but plasma adiponectin was not measured [98]. In contrast, the twofold increase in plasma adiponectin seen in women who have PCOS after treatment with pioglitazone was not caused by a simultaneous increase in AMPK activity [59]. Thus, further studies are warranted to delineate the molecular mechanisms by which TZD improves mitochondrial function in muscle of insulin-resistant individuals.

Taken together, the current data suggest that the combination of increased physical activity, weight loss, and pharmacologic treatment with insulin sensitizers can improve and perhaps normalize mitochondrial function and hence insulin sensitivity in people who have T2D or obesity.

Tissue-specific abnormalities in mitochondrial biogenesis

The studies reviewed in the previous sections have provided evidence that decreased mitochondrial oxidative metabolism is an early abnormality of human skeletal muscle, which is worsened by environmental factors such as obesity, physical inactivity, and ageing. In addition, expression of several genes in the ETC was shown to be down-regulated in visceral fat and, to a lesser extent, subcutaneous fat from women who have T2D independent of obesity [99]. These data indicate a link between mitochondrial dysfunction and disturbed production of adipokines and therefore the low-grade inflammatory state observed in insulin-resistant subjects. It is also known that mitochondrial function and ATP synthesis play a critical role in glucose-mediated insulin secretion [24]. Accordingly, a reduced insulin secretion in response to glucose was reported to be associated with impaired mitochondrial ATP synthesis in β-cells isolated from patients who had T2D [100]; however, the mitochondrial density volume and protein expression of OXPHOS subunits including uncoupling protein 2 were significantly higher in diabetic β-cells [100]. Moreover, a recent microarray-based study demonstrated an increased expression of OXPHOS genes and PGC-1α in the liver of patients who had T2D [101]. These latter studies clearly indicate that disturbances in mitochondrial function and biogenesis are tissue specific and not always in the same direction. The same paradoxic roles for PGC-1α

in muscle, liver, and β-cells are seen in animal models of diabetes [49,53], suggesting that the identification of factors upstream of PGC-1α and other transcriptional regulators of mitochondrial biogenesis would help to explain the tissue-specific abnormalities in OXPHOS genes and their role in the pathogenesis of insulin resistance and T2D.

Summary

There is accumulating evidence for a link between mitochondrial dysfunction and insulin resistance in human skeletal muscle, even before the development of obesity and hyperglycemia (Fig. 5). Most data indicate that mitochondrial dysfunction is primarily due to a reduced content of

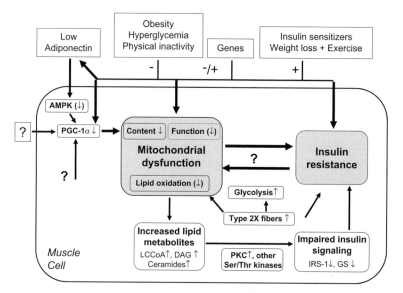

Fig. 5. Potential mechanisms involved in mitochondrial dysfunction in human skeletal muscle. Mitochondrial dysfunction in insulin-resistant individuals involves a lower content and probably a reduced functionality of muscle mitochondria and is caused by genetic and environmental factors. It can, at least in part, be reversed by insulin sensitizers and the combination of weight loss and exercise, and could be mediated by reversal of the low adiponectin levels or decreased PGC-1α function and activity seen in insulin-resistant individuals. The factors inside and outside the muscle cell that regulate PGC-1α are at present unclear, but a role for AMPK has been suggested. An increased amount of the type 2X muscle fibers contributes to mitochondrial dysfunction by increasing the glycolytic relative to the oxidative enzyme capacity. Mitochondrial dysfunction likely causes decreased lipid oxidation and subsequent accumulation of lipid metabolites (DAG, long-chain coenzyme A [LCCoA], and ceramides), which in turn activates certain protein kinase C (PKC) isoforms and serine/threonine (Ser/Thr) kinases and leads to inhibitory Ser phosphorylation of proximal and distal components of the insulin signaling cascade (IRS-1 and glycogen synthase [GS]). This sequence of events is believed to contribute to impaired insulin-stimulated glucose uptake and glycogen synthesis and, therefore, to insulin resistance. The cause-and-effect relationship between mitochondrial dysfunction and insulin resistance, however, remains to be established.

muscle mitochondria, whereas a role for a decreased functional capacity of mitochondria warrants further studies. Combined intervention of physical activity, weight loss, and treatment with insulin sensitizers improves mito- chondrial function in subjects who have T2D and obesity, showing that at least to some extent, this defect can be reversed. Future studies are needed to address the question whether mitochondrial dysfunction is a primary defect in the pathogenesis of insulin resistance and T2D. The tissue-specific expression of OXPHOS genes suggests that factors upstream of PGC-1α should be searched to identify a potential primary defect.

References

[1] Zimmet P, Alberti KG, Shaw J. Global and societal implications of the diabetes epidemic. Nature 2001;414:782–7.

[2] Beck-Nielsen H, Vaag A, Poulsen P, et al. Metabolic and genetic influence on glucose metabolism in type 2 diabetic subjects—experiences from relatives and twin studies. Best Pract Res Clin Endocrinol Metab 2003;17:445–67.

[3] Kahn SE. The relative contributions of insulin resistance and beta-cell dysfunction to the pathophysiology of type 2 diabetes. Diabetologia 2003;46:3–19.

[4] Shulman GI, Rothman DL, Jue T, et al. Quantitation of muscle glycogen synthesis in normal subjects and subjects with non-insulin-dependent diabetes by 13C nuclear magnetic resonance spectroscopy. N Engl J Med 1990;322:223–8.

[5] Cusi K, Maezono K, Osman A, et al. Insulin resistance differentially affects the PI 3-kinase- and MAP kinase-mediated signaling in human muscle. J Clin Invest 2000;105:311–20.

[6] Damsbo P, Vaag A, Hother-Nielsen O, et al. Reduced glycogen synthase activity in skeletal muscle from obese patients with and without type 2 (non-insulin-dependent) diabetes mellitus. Diabetologia 1991;34:239–45.

[7] Højlund K, Staehr P, Hansen BF, et al. Increased phosphorylation of skeletal muscle glycogen synthase at NH2-terminal sites during physiological hyperinsulinemia in type 2 diabetes. Diabetes 2003;52:1393–402.

[8] Højlund K, Beck-Nielsen H. Impaired glycogen synthase activity and mitochondrial dysfunction in skeletal muscle. Markers or mediators of insulin resistance in type 2 diabetes. Curr Diabetes Rev 2006;2:375–95.

[9] Krook A, Bjornholm M, Galuska D, et al. Characterization of signal transduction and glucose transport in skeletal muscle from type 2 diabetic patients. Diabetes 2000;49:284–92.

[10] Bjornholm M, Kawano Y, Lehtihet M, et al. Insulin receptor substrate-1 phosphorylation and phosphatidylinositol 3-kinase activity in skeletal muscle from NIDDM subjects after in vivo insulin stimulation. Diabetes 1997;46:524–7.

[11] Højlund K, Frystyk J, Levin K, et al. Reduced plasma adiponectin concentrations may contribute to impaired insulin activation of glycogen synthase in skeletal muscle of patients with type 2 diabetes. Diabetologia 2006;49:1283–91.

[12] Pratipanawatr T, Cusi K, Ngo P, et al. Normalization of plasma glucose concentration by insulin therapy improves insulin-stimulated glycogen synthesis in type 2 diabetes. Diabetes 2002;51:462–8.

[13] Kelley DE, Mandarino LJ. Fuel selection in human skeletal muscle in insulin resistance: a reexamination. Diabetes 2000;49:677–83.

[14] Kelley DE. Skeletal muscle fat oxidation: timing and flexibility are everything. J Clin Invest 2005;115:1699–702.

[15] Simoneau JA, Veerkamp JH, Turcotte LP, et al. Markers of capacity to utilize fatty acids in human skeletal muscle: relation to insulin resistance and obesity and effects of weight loss. FASEB J 1999;13:2051–60.

[16] Kelley DE, Simoneau JA. Impaired free fatty acid utilization by skeletal muscle in non-insulin-dependent diabetes mellitus. J Clin Invest 1994;94:2349–56.

[17] Kelley DE, Goodpaster B, Wing RR, et al. Skeletal muscle fatty acid metabolism in association with insulin resistance, obesity, and weight loss. Am J Physiol 1999;277: E1130–41.

[18] Pan DA, Lillioja S, Kriketos AD, et al. Skeletal muscle triglyceride levels are inversely related to insulin action. Diabetes 1997;46:983–8.

[19] Phillips DI, Caddy S, Ilic V, et al. Intramuscular triglyceride and muscle insulin sensitivity: evidence for a relationship in nondiabetic subjects. Metabolism 1996;45:947–50.

[20] He J, Watkins S, Kelley DE. Skeletal muscle lipid content and oxidative enzyme activity in relation to muscle fiber type in type 2 diabetes and obesity. Diabetes 2001;50:817–23.

[21] Levin K, Daa Schroeder H, Alford FP, et al. Morphometric documentation of abnormal intramyocellular fat storage and reduced glycogen in obese patients with type II diabetes. Diabetologia 2001;44:824–33.

[22] Krebs M, Roden M. Molecular mechanisms of lipid-induced insulin resistance in muscle, liver and vasculature. Diabetes Obes Metab 2005;7:621–32.

[23] Adams JM II, Pratipanawatr T, Berria R, et al. Ceramide content is increased in skeletal muscle from obese insulin-resistant humans. Diabetes 2004;53:25–31.

[24] Lowell BB, Shulman GI. Mitochondrial dysfunction and type 2 diabetes. Science 2005;307: 384–7.

[25] Kruszynska YT, Mulford MI, Baloga J, et al. Regulation of skeletal muscle hexokinase II by insulin in nondiabetic and NIDDM subjects. Diabetes 1998;47:1107–13.

[26] Kelley DE, He J, Menshikova EV, et al. Dysfunction of mitochondria in human skeletal muscle in type 2 diabetes. Diabetes 2002;51:2944–50.

[27] Kim JY, Hickner RC, Cortright RL, et al. Lipid oxidation is reduced in obese human skeletal muscle. Am J Physiol Endocrinol Metab 2000;279:E1039–44.

[28] Simoneau JA, Kelley DE. Altered glycolytic and oxidative capacities of skeletal muscle contribute to insulin resistance in NIDDM. J Appl Physiol 1997;83:166–71.

[29] Simoneau JA, Colberg SR, Thaete FL, et al. Skeletal muscle glycolytic and oxidative enzyme capacities are determinants of insulin sensitivity and muscle composition in obese women. FASEB J 1995;9:273–8.

[30] Marin P, Andersson B, Krotkiewski M, et al. Muscle fiber composition and capillary density in women and men with NIDDM. Diabetes Care 1994;17:382–6.

[31] Lillioja S, Young AA, Culter CL, et al. Skeletal muscle capillary density and fiber type are possible determinants of in vivo insulin resistance in man. J Clin Invest 1987;80:415–24.

[32] Oberbach A, Bossenz Y, Lehmann S, et al. Altered fiber distribution and fiber-specific glycolytic and oxidative enzyme activity in skeletal muscle of patients with type 2 diabetes. Diabetes Care 2006;29:895–900.

[33] Mogensen M, Sahlin K, Fernström M, et al. Mitochondrial respiration is decreased in skeletal muscle of patients with type 2 diabetes. Diabetes 2007;56:1592–9.

[34] Nyholm B, Qu Z, Kaal A, et al. Evidence of an increased number of type IIb muscle fibers in insulin-resistant first-degree relatives of patients with NIDDM. Diabetes 1997;46:1822–8.

[35] Østergård T, Jessen N, Schmitz O, et al. The effect of exercise, training, and inactivity on insulin sensitivity in diabetics and their relatives: what is new? Appl Physiol Nutr Metab 2007;32:541–8.

[36] Nyholm B, Mengel A, Nielsen S, et al. Insulin resistance in relatives of NIDDM patients: the role of physical fitness and muscle metabolism. Diabetologia 1996;39:813–22.

[37] Thamer C, Stumvoll M, Niess A, et al. Reduced skeletal muscle oxygen uptake and reduced beta-cell function. Diabetes Care 2003;26:2126–32.

[38] Orio F Jr, Giallauria F, Palomba S, et al. Cardiopulmonary impairment in young women with polycystic ovary syndrome. J Clin Endocrinol Metab 2006;91:2967–71.

[39] Petersen KF, Befroy D, Dufour S, et al. Mitochondrial dysfunction in the elderly: possible role in insulin resistance. Science 2003;300:1140–2.

[40] Barazonni R. Skeletal muscle mitochondrial protein metabolism and function in ageing and type 2 diabetes. Curr Opin Clin Nutr Metab Care 2004;7:97–102.

[41] Hood DA, Irrcher I, Ljubicic V, et al. Coordination of metabolic plasticity in skeletal muscle. J Exp Biol 2006;209:2265–75.

[42] Patti ME, Butte AJ, Crunkhorn S, et al. Coordinated reduction of genes of oxidative metabolism in humans with insulin resistance and diabetes: potential role of PGC1 and NRF1. Proc Natl Acad Sci U S A 2003;100:8466–71.

[43] Mootha VK, Lindgren CM, Eriksson KF, et al. PGC-1alpha-responsive genes involved in oxidative phosphorylation are coordinately downregulated in human diabetes. Nat Genet 2003;34:267–73.

[44] Sreekumar R, Halvatsiotis P, Schimke JC, et al. Gene expression profile in skeletal muscle of type 2 diabetes and the effect of insulin treatment. Diabetes 2002;51:1913–20.

[45] Yang X, Pratley RE, Tokraks S, et al. Microarray profiling of skeletal muscle tissues from equally obese, non-diabetic insulin-sensitive and insulin-resistant Pima Indians. Diabetologia 2002;45:1584–93.

[46] Skov V, Glintborg D, Knudsen S, et al. Reduced expression of nuclear-encoded genes involved in mitochondrial oxidative metabolism in skeletal muscle of insulin-resistant women with polycystic ovary syndrome. Diabetes 2007;56:2349–55.

[47] Wu Z, Puigserver P, Andersson U, et al. Mechanisms controlling mitochondrial biogenesis and respiration through the thermogenic coactivator PGC-1. Cell 1999;98:115–24.

[48] Subramanian A, Tamayo P, Mootha VK, et al. Gene set enrichment analysis: a knowledge-based approach for interpreting genome-wide expression profiles. Proc Natl Acad Sci U S A 2005;102:15545–50.

[49] Finck BN, Kelly DP. PGC-1 coactivators: inducible regulators of energy metabolism in health and disease. J Clin Invest 2006;116:615–22.

[50] Lin J, Handschin C, Spiegelman BM. Metabolic control through the PGC-1 family of transcription coactivators. Cell Metab 2005;1:361–70.

[51] Timmons JA, Norrbom J, Scheele C, et al. Expression profiling following local muscle inactivity in humans provides new perspective on diabetes-related genes. Genomics 2006;87:165–72.

[52] Ling C, Poulsen P, Carlsson E, et al. Multiple environmental and genetic factors influence skeletal muscle PGC-1alpha and PGC-1beta gene expression in twins. J Clin Invest 2004;114:1518–26.

[53] Handschin C, Spiegelman BM. Peroxisome proliferator-activated receptor gamma coactivator 1 coactivators, energy homeostasis, and metabolism. Endocr Rev 2006;27:728–35.

[54] Jäger S, Handschin C, St-Pierre J, et al. AMP-activated protein kinase (AMPK) action in skeletal muscle via direct phosphorylation of PGC-1alpha. Proc Natl Acad Sci U S A 2007;104:12017–22.

[55] Musi N, Fujii N, Hirshman MF, et al. AMP-activated protein kinase (AMPK) is activated in muscle of subjects with type 2 diabetes during exercise. Diabetes 2001;50:921–7.

[56] Højlund K, Mustard KJ, Staehr P, et al. AMPK activity and isoform protein expression are similar in muscle of obese subjects with and without type 2 diabetes. Am J Physiol Endocrinol Metab 2004;286:E239–44.

[57] Wojtaszewski JF, Birk JB, Frosig C, et al. 5'AMP activated protein kinase expression in human skeletal muscle: effects of strength training and type 2 diabetes. J Physiol 2005;564:563–73.

[58] Steinberg GR, Smith AC, Van Denderen BJ, et al. AMP-activated protein kinase is not down-regulated in human skeletal muscle of obese females. J Clin Endocrinol Metab 2004;89:4575–80.

[59] Højlund K, Glintborg D, Andersen NR, et al. Impaired insulin-stimulated phosphorylation of Akt and AS160 in skeletal muscle of women with polycystic ovary syndrome is reversed by pioglitazone treatment. Diabetes 2007 Oct 31 [Epub ahead of print].

[60] Højlund K, Wrzesinski K, Larsen PM, et al. Proteome analysis reveals phosphorylation of ATP synthase beta-subunit in human skeletal muscle and proteins with potential roles in type 2 diabetes. J Biol Chem 2003;278:10436–42.

[61] Arrell DK, Elliott ST, Kane LA, et al. Proteomic analysis of pharmacological preconditioning: novel protein targets converge to mitochondrial metabolism pathways. Circ Res 2006; 99:706–14.

[62] Bijur GN, Jope RS. Rapid accumulation of Akt in mitochondria following phosphatidylinositol 3-kinase activation. J Neurochem 2003;87:1427–35.

[63] Hopper RK, Carroll S, Aponte AM, et al. Mitochondrial matrix phosphoproteome: effect of extra mitochondrial calcium. Biochemistry 2006;45:2524–36.

[64] Schulenberg B, Aggeler R, Beechem JM, et al. Analysis of steady-state protein phosphorylation in mitochondria using a novel fluorescent phosphosensor dye. J Biol Chem 2003; 278:27251–5.

[65] Hittel DS, Hathout Y, Hoffman EP, et al. Proteome analysis of skeletal muscle from obese and morbidly obese women. Diabetes 2005;54:1283–8.

[66] Ptitsyn A, Hulver M, Cefalu W, et al. Unsupervised clustering of gene expression data points at hypoxia as possible trigger for metabolic syndrome. BMC Genomics 2006;7:318.

[67] Gelfi C, De Palma S, Cerretelli P, et al. Two-dimensional protein map of human vastus lateralis muscle. Electrophoresis 2003;24:286–95.

[68] Højlund K, Yi Z, Hwang H, et al. Characterization of the human skeletal muscle proteome by one-dimensional gel electrophoresis and HPLC-ESI-MS/MS. Mol Cell Proteomics 2007 Oct 1 [Epub ahead of print].

[69] Pagliarini DJ, Dixon JE. Mitochondrial modulation: reversible phosphorylation takes center stage? Trends Biochem Sci 2006;31:26–34.

[70] Morino K, Petersen KF, Shulman GI. Molecular mechanisms of insulin resistance in humans and their potential links with mitochondrial dysfunction. Diabetes 2006; 55(Suppl 2):S9–15.

[71] Petersen KF, Dufour S, Befroy D, et al. Impaired mitochondrial activity in the insulin-resistant offspring of patients with type 2 diabetes. N Engl J Med 2004;350:664–71.

[72] Befroy DE, Petersen KF, Dufour S, et al. Impaired mitochondrial substrate oxidation in muscle of insulin-resistant offspring of type 2 diabetic patients. Diabetes 2007;56:1376–81.

[73] Morino K, Petersen KF, Dufour S, et al. Reduced mitochondrial density and increased IRS-1 serine phosphorylation in muscle of insulin-resistant offspring of type 2 diabetic parents. J Clin Invest 2005;115:3587–93.

[74] Schrauwen-Hinderling VB, Kooi ME, Hesselink MK, et al. Impaired in vivo mitochondrial function but similar intramyocellular lipid content in patients with type 2 diabetes mellitus and BMI-matched control subjects. Diabetologia 2007;50:113–20.

[75] Toledo FG, Menshikova EV, Ritov VB, et al. Effects of physical activity and weight loss on skeletal muscle mitochondria and relationship with glucose control in type 2 diabetes. Diabetes 2007;56:2142–7.

[76] Ritov VB, Menshikova EV, He J, et al. Deficiency of subsarcolemmal mitochondria in obesity and type 2 diabetes. Diabetes 2005;54:8–14.

[77] Tonkonogi M, Sahlin K. Rate of oxidative phosphorylation in isolated mitochondria from human skeletal muscle: effect of training status. Acta Physiol Scand 1997;161:345–53.

[78] Boushel R, Gnaiger E, Schjerling P, et al. Patients with type 2 diabetes have normal mitochondrial function in skeletal muscle. Diabetologia 2007;50:790–6.

[79] Ukropcova B, Sereda O, de Jonge L, et al. Family history of diabetes links impaired substrate switching and reduced mitochondrial content in skeletal muscle. Diabetes 2007; 56:720–7.

[80] Wredenberg A, Freyer C, Sandström ME, et al. Respiratory chain dysfunction in skeletal muscle does not cause insulin resistance. Biochem Biophys Res Commun 2006;350:202–7.

[81] Pospisilik JA, Knauf C, Joza N, et al. Targeted deletion of AIF decreases mitochondrial oxidative phosphorylation and protects from obesity and diabetes. Cell 2007;131:476–91.

[82] Short KR, Nair KS, Stump CS. Impaired mitochondrial activity and insulin-resistant offspring of patients with type 2 diabetes. N Engl J Med 2004;350:2419–21.

[83] Stump CS, Short KR, Bigelow ML, et al. Effect of insulin on human skeletal muscle mitochondrial ATP production, protein synthesis, and mRNA transcripts. Proc Natl Acad Sci U S A 2003;100:7996–8001.

[84] Rome S, Clément K, Rabasa-Lhoret R, et al. Microarray profiling of human skeletal muscle reveals that insulin regulates ∼800 genes during a hyperinsulinemic clamp. J Biol Chem 2003;278:18063–8.

[85] Petersen KF, Dufour S, Shulman GI. Decreased insulin-stimulated ATP synthesis and phosphate transport in muscle of insulin-resistant offspring of type 2 diabetic parents. PLoS Med 2005;2:e233.

[86] Szendroedi J, Schmid AI, Chmelik M, et al. Muscle mitochondrial ATP synthesis and glucose transport/phosphorylation in type 2 diabetes. PLoS Med 2007;4:e154.

[87] Brehm A, Krssak M, Schmid AI, et al. Increased lipid availability impairs insulin-stimulated ATP synthesis in human skeletal muscle. Diabetes 2006;55:136–40.

[88] Hawley JA, Lessard SJ. Mitochondrial function: use it or lose it. Diabetologia 2007;50: 699–702.

[89] Toledo FG, Watkins S, Kelley DE. Changes induced by physical activity and weight loss in the morphology of intermyofibrillar mitochondria in obese men and women. J Clin Endocrinol Metab 2006;91:3224–7.

[90] Burns N, Finucane FM, Hatunic M, et al. Early-onset type 2 diabetes in obese white subjects is characterised by a marked defect in beta cell insulin secretion, severe insulin resistance and a lack of response to aerobic exercise training. Diabetologia 2007;50:1500–8.

[91] Bogacka I, Xie H, Bray GA, et al. Pioglitazone induces mitochondrial biogenesis in human subcutaneous adipose tissue in vivo. Diabetes 2005;54:1392–9.

[92] Mensink M, Hesselink MK, Russell AP, et al. Improved skeletal muscle oxidative enzyme activity and restoration of PGC-1 alpha and PPAR beta/delta gene expression upon rosiglitazone treatment in obese patients with type 2 diabetes mellitus. Int J Obes (Lond) 2007;31:1302–10.

[93] Skov V, Glintborg D, Knudsen S, et al. Pioglitazone enhances mitochondrial biogenesis and ribosomal protein biosynthesis in skeletal muscle in polycystic ovary syndrome. PloS ONE 2008;3:e2466.

[94] Civitarese AE, Ukropcova B, Carling S, et al. Role of adiponectin in human skeletal muscle bioenergetics. Cell Metab 2006;4:75–87.

[95] Kadowaki T, Yamauchi T. Adiponectin and adiponectin receptors. Endocr Rev 2005;26: 439–51.

[96] Bergeron R, Ren JM, Cadman KS, et al. Chronic activation of AMP kinase results in NRF-1 activation and mitochondrial biogenesis. Am J Physiol Endocrinol Metab 2001; 281:E1340–6.

[97] Zong H, Ren JM, Young LH, et al. AMP kinase is required for mitochondrial biogenesis in skeletal muscle in response to chronic energy deprivation. Proc Natl Acad Sci U S A 2002; 99:15983–7.

[98] Bandyopadhyay GK, Yu JG, Ofrecio J, et al. Increased malonyl-CoA levels in muscle from obese and type 2 diabetic subjects lead to decreased fatty acid oxidation and increased lipogenesis; thiazolidinedione treatment reverses these defects. Diabetes 2006;55:2277–85.

[99] Dahlman I, Forsgren M, Sjögren A, et al. Downregulation of electron transport chain genes in visceral adipose tissue in type 2 diabetes independent of obesity and possibly involving tumor necrosis factor-alpha. Diabetes 2006;55:1792–9.

[100] Anello M, Lupi R, Spampinato D, et al. Functional and morphological alterations of mitochondria in pancreatic beta cells from type 2 diabetic patients. Diabetologia 2005;48:282–9.

[101] Misu H, Takamura T, Matsuzawa N, et al. Genes involved in oxidative phosphorylation are coordinately upregulated with fasting hyperglycaemia in livers of patients with type 2 diabetes. Diabetologia 2007;50:268–77.

ELSEVIER
SAUNDERS

Endocrinol Metab Clin N Am
37 (2008) 733–751

ENDOCRINOLOGY
AND METABOLISM
CLINICS
OF NORTH AMERICA

Lessons from Extreme Human Obesity: Monogenic Disorders

Sayali A. Ranadive, MD[a], Christian Vaisse, MD, PhD[b],*

[a]Department of Pediatrics, Division of Endocrinology, University of California San Francisco, 513 Parnassus Avenue, Room S672D, San Francisco, CA 94143-0434, USA
[b]Department of Medicine and Diabetes Center, University of California San Francisco, 513 Parnassus Avenue, Room HSW1113, San Francisco, CA 94143-0573, USA

The prevalence of common obesity in the United States has dramatically increased over the past 30 years [1]. This rise is largely attributed to the increased caloric richness of the common diet and the decreased physical activity in most individuals' lives. However, obesity is a multifactorial disease that is influenced by genetic and environmental factors. An inherited component to body weight accounts for 40% to 70% of an individual's predisposition to obesity [2]. Therefore, weight gain is caused by dietary and lifestyle choices on a background of genetic susceptibility. Most genes that contribute to this predisposition are still unknown, but the discovery and characterization of single gene defects that cause severe human obesity has provided some insight into the hereditary nature of body weight.

As indicated in Box 1, *monogenic obesity* is defined as obesity resulting from a mutation or deficiency of a single gene.

The known monogenic forms of obesity can be divided into three broad categories. The first category is obesity caused by mutations in genes that have a physiologic role in the hypothalamic leptin–melanocortin system of energy balance. Specifically, obesity caused by leptin, leptin receptor, melanocortin-4 receptor (MC4R), proopiomelanocortin (POMC), and prohormone convertase 1/3 (PC1/3) mutations are addressed. Because these disorders are well characterized and extensively reviewed by others [3–5], they are summarized here only to highlight key clinical points.

This work was supported by the National Institutes of Health RO1 DK60540 and DK068152 Awards, American Heart Association Established Investigator Award (to Dr. Vaisse). Dr. Ranadive was supported by the National Institutes of Health (T32) Award.
 * Corresponding author.
 E-mail address: vaisse@medicine.ucsf.edu (C. Vaisse).

0889-8529/08/$ - see front matter © 2008 Published by Elsevier Inc.
doi:10.1016/j.ecl.2008.07.003

endo.theclinics.com

Box 1. Useful definitions

Monogenic obesity: obesity explained by mutation in a single gene

Early-onset obesity: not clearly defined in the literature. Generally considered as abnormal weight gain occurring in children less than 10 years of age. In this article, referred to as the onset of rapid weight gain before the age of 2 years.

Common obesity: obesity that is most frequently encountered in the general population and is not associated with any developmental syndromes.

The World Health Organization body mass index classification in adults

Overweight: body mass index (BMI) between 25 and 29.99 kg/m^2

Obese: BMI greater than 30 kg/m^2

Obese class I: BMI between 30 and 34.99 kg/m^2

Obese class II (preferable to the term *severe obesity*): BMI between 35 and 39.99 kg/m^2

Obese class III (preferable to the term *morbid obesity*): BMI greater than 40 kg/m^2

Centers for Disease Control and Prevention body mass index classification in children aged 2 to 20 years

At-risk for overweight: BMI greater than or equal to the 85th percentile on BMI-for-age curves

Overweight: BMI greater than or equal to the 95th percentile on BMI-for-age curves

The term *obese* is not defined in children. However, for the purposes of discussion and recruitment for research studies, a child who has a BMI greater than the 97th percentile on BMI-for-age chart can be considered obese, and one with a BMI greater than the 99th percentile can be considered severely obese.

For most recent CDC BMI percentile curves, go to http://www.cdc.gov/growthcharts.

The second category is obesity resulting from mutations in the three genes necessary for development of the hypothalamus: *SIM1*, *BDNF*, and *NTRK2*. These genes have important roles during hypothalamic development and lead to severe obesity when mutated. These conditions further support the concept that the hypothalamus is critical for energy homeostasis, but the exact mechanisms through which these gene defects lead to obesity are not yet understood.

The third category is obesity presenting as part of a complex syndrome caused by mutations in genes whose functional relationship to obesity is also unclear. This article focuses on three of these syndromes: Bardet-Biedl (BBS), Alström, and Carpenter's, the origins of which have recently been ascribed to the dysfunction of the primary cilium. Consideration of these syndromes emphasizes the ongoing discovery of new molecular mechanisms underlying the pathogenesis of obesity.

Obesity caused by gene mutations that affect the leptin–melanocortin system

Naturally occurring mutations in mice that cause severe obesity led to the discovery and understanding of a neuronal system that regulates long-term energy homeostasis in mammals [6]. Thereafter, the occurrence in humans of severe obesity-causing mutations affecting the same pathways as in mice has validated that this system of energy balance is conserved across species, and is in fact crucial to the maintenance of body weight in humans. Referred to as the *leptin-melanocortin system*, this specific network of neurons, centered in the hypothalamus, integrates information about peripheral energy stores relayed primarily by the hormone leptin. The effective output is a change in food intake behavior and basal energy expenditure. Fig. 1 briefly summarizes the current understanding of this system as it pertains to this discussion of monogenic obesity. A detailed description of all molecules and pathways implicated in energy balance is beyond the scope of this review [7–10].

Leptin

Severe early-onset obesity, extremely low serum leptin levels, and successful treatment with exogenous leptin distinguish congenital leptin deficiency from all other monogenic causes of obesity. This condition is a rare autosomal recessive disorder resulting from homozygous mutations in the leptin gene. Only 12 individuals in the world have been reported to have congenital leptin deficiency, all homozygous for one of two known mutations [11]. Two cousins from a consanguineous Pakistani family, homozygous for a frameshift mutation (ΔG133) that leads to a truncated, unsecreted leptin molecule, were first reported in 1997 [12]. Since then, three Turkish patients homozygous for a missense mutation (R105Y) [13] and six patients from four unrelated Pakistani families with the ΔG133 mutation have been described [14,15].

All reported patients share the clinical phenotype of severe obesity, hyperphagia, and serum leptin levels that are disproportionately low for their degree of fat mass. These patients are of normal birth weight, but their dramatic weight gain begins in the first 3 months of life and continues so that they weigh more than 20 kg by 1 year of age and more than 50 kg by 5 years of age [12]. Patients who have a leptin deficiency also have impressive adiposity with greater than 50% body fat, whereas normal children have 15% to 25% body fat [12].

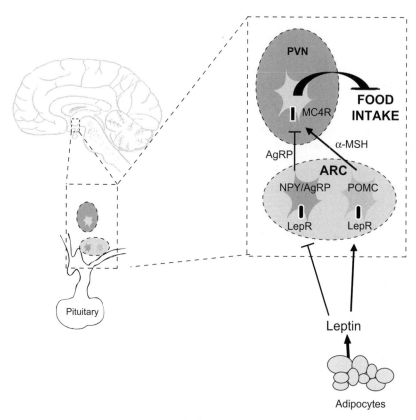

Fig. 1. Leptin–melanocortin system of energy balance. Hormones such as leptin convey information about the body's energy stores to the brain. Leptin is secreted by adipocytes in proportion to the body's fat mass. Leptin binds to its receptors on two populations of neurons in the
arcuate nucleus of the hypothalamus (ARC): the orexigenic agouti-related peptide (AgRP)/neu-
ropeptide Y -expressing neurons and the anorexigenic POMC-expressing neurons. These groups
of neurons have projections to the paraventricular nucleus of the hypothalamus and to other
regions of the brain. The paraventricular nucleus of the hypothalamus (PVN) has a dense
neuronal population that expresses MC4R. When leptin binds its receptor (LepR) on POMC
neurons, α-melanocyte-stimulating hormone (α-MSH), a cleavage product of the POMC transcript, is released. Activation of MC4R in the PVN by α-MSH relays a satiety signal and causes
a decrease in food intake. AgRP is an antagonist of MC4R, and competes with α-MSH to bind
MC4R. Binding of AgRP to MC4R leads to increased food intake. Leptin activates POMC
neurons and inhibits AgRP neurons. Therefore, by activating its receptors on these two neuronal populations, leptin acts in a concerted way to increase MC4R activation by α-MSH and decrease its antagonism by AgRP, to cause a decrease in food intake. Mutations in genes with
critical roles in the Leptin–melanocortin system cause early-onset and severe obesity. Autosomal recessive mutations in leptin, LepR, POMC and PC1/3, and autosomal dominant MC4R
mutations have been described.

Aside from their striking weight phenotype, these patients come to clinical attention for their lack of pubertal development [13–15]. The absent or delayed puberty results from hypogonadotropic hypogonadism and highlights leptin's importance in the onset of puberty [16]. Abnormal T-cell number and function, which may present as frequent respiratory infections [17], also occurs in congenital leptin deficiency and is explained by leptin's role in proliferation of CD4+ T cells and release of cytokines from T-helper-1 cells. Additionally, leptin regulates prohormone convertase 1/3 (PC1/3), which is necessary for the synthesis of thyrotropin-releasing hormone (TRH) and growth hormone–releasing hormone (GHRH). This role may explain the thyroid and growth hormone dysfunction reported in some of these patients [18]. Because congenital leptin deficiency is so rare, extensive laboratory evaluation to uncover the hormonal and immunologic deficiencies associated with it can only be recommended if the degree of obesity and clinical presentation suggest this disorder.

Daily subcutaneous administration of recombinant human leptin to children who have congenital leptin deficiency results in dramatic weight loss, reduction in fat mass, resumed pubertal progression, and improved thyroid and immune function [14,15]. However, this is an exceptionally rare but remarkable example of effective treatment of obesity arising from an understanding of its physiologic basis. Furthermore, no similar benefit is seen from giving supraphysiologic doses of leptin to obese patients who are not leptin deficient [19]. Thus, congenital leptin deficiency is unique because it can be diagnosed based on a serum leptin level that is extremely low for the patient's fat mass, and daily administration of leptin can successfully treat the disorder.

However, direct sequencing of the leptin gene is still the mainstay of diagnosis because a mutation could arise that does not affect synthesis or secretion of leptin but impairs receptor binding or other downstream function. If a mutation such as this were to occur, the patient would have the clinical phenotype, but a serum leptin level that, similar to other forms of obesity, is proportional to the patient's fat mass rather than diagnostically low.

Leptin receptor

The first report of leptin receptor deficiency was that of a homozygous mutation in three sisters from a consanguineous Algerian family [20]. Much like the patients who had congenital leptin deficiency, these three patients who had no functional leptin receptor had severe, early-onset obesity. They had normal birth weight, rapid weight gain starting before 6 months of age, and weights greater than 15 kg at 1 year of age. When evaluated during adolescence, their BMIs were 50 to 70 kg/m^2, their body fat was greater than 65%, and they lacked pubertal changes because of hypogonadotropic hypogonadism. Impaired growth hormone and thyrotropin secretion were subtle findings only evident through dynamic testing [20].

Recently, eight more individuals who had homozygous or compound heterozygous leptin receptor mutations were identified in a highly consanguineous cohort of severely obese and hyperphagic patients. Functional studies of these mutant receptors showed complete or partial loss of receptor signaling in response to leptin [11]. The clinical features of severe obesity, hypogonadotropic hypogonadism, and impaired immune function were consistent with previous reports by Clement and colleagues [20], and as expected, leptin levels were elevated proportional to fat mass.

Leptin and leptin receptor deficiencies are extraordinarily uncommon. The obesity resulting from these conditions is incomparable in severity and associated with hypogonadism. If encountered in the clinical setting, a serum leptin level can help differentiate between the conditions. Although with leptin deficiency the leptin levels are typically low, serum leptin in leptin receptor deficiency reflects BMI and fat mass, as in common obesity and all other forms of monogenic obesity. The fact that serum leptin levels in leptin receptor deficiency are not any higher than would be predicted by the degree of obesity emphasizes an important point. It shows that leptin synthesis occurs normally independent of a functional leptin receptor. Therefore, no feedback occurs from leptin receptor signaling on the secretion of leptin from adipocytes [21].

Proopiomelanocortin

POMC is the precursor to five biologically active proteins made in the anterior pituitary or hypothalamus and skin. POMC has a prominent role in the leptin–melanocortin system in that *POMC*-expressing neurons are targets of leptin signaling, and α–melanocyte-stimulating hormone (α-MSH) is the POMC cleavage product that activates MC4R. PC1/3 and PC2 are necessary for the proteolytic cleavage of POMC to each of the active peptides (see Fig. 1; Fig. 2).

The unique feature of complete POMC deficiency is that patients present in the newborn period with adrenal insufficiency. Their profound hypocortisolism is caused by lack of the POMC substrate for adrenocorticotropic hormone (ACTH) synthesis in the anterior pituitary. Similar to patients who have panhypopituitarism, ongoing glucocorticoid replacement is required to prevent adrenal crises. The second salient feature of complete POMC deficiency that subsequently presents is the hyperphagia and severe obesity resulting from lack of MC4R activation by α-MSH. These patients have normal birth weight, onset of rapid weight gain before 6 months of age, and weights exceeding 15 kg by 1 year and 25 kg by 3 years.

The first two patients who had complete POMC deficiency were described in 1998. One patient was compound heterozygous for two nonsense mutations, and the other was homozygous for a base pair substitution that disrupted translation of the entire POMC protein [22]. Three more patients who had homozygous or compound heterozygous *POMC* mutations causing congenital POMC deficiency were described in 2003 [23]. The sixth

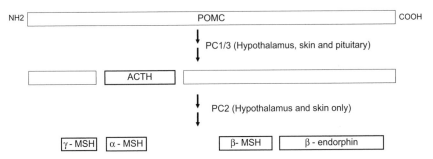

Fig. 2. Processing of POMC. POMC is processed by PC1/3 and PC2 into five biologically active proteins. In the corticotropes of the anterior pituitary, PC1/3 is expressed, but PC2 is not. Therefore, adrenocorticotropic hormone (ACTH) is the only biologically active POMC-derived peptide synthesized in the anterior pituitary. PC1/3 and PC2 are expressed in the melanotropes of the hypothalamus and skin. Thus, POMC is sequentially processed into α-, β-, and γ-MSH and β-endorphin in these tissues. The phenotype of POMC deficiency is explained by the tissue-specific lack of these cleavage products.

case was reported in a Turkish patient who had a homozygous frameshift loss of function mutation with severe obesity and ACTH deficiency, but dark hair [24]. Red hair, because of lack of α-MSH activating MC1R in melanocytes, was initially reported as part of the clinical spectrum of congenital POMC deficiency. However, this finding is not essential for diagnosis, because the Turkish patient who had complete POMC deficiency, and possibly his deceased similarly affected brother, had dark hair [24].

Prohormone convertase 1/3

PCs are a family of serine endoproteases that cleave inactive hormone precursors into biologically active secreted peptides. Of the seven proteins in this family, only PC1/3 and PC2 are selectively expressed in neuroendocrine tissues and involved in the regulated secretory pathway of hormone biosynthesis [25]. Substrates for PC1/3 and PC2 include proTRH, proinsulin, proglucagon, proGHRH, POMC, pro–neuropeptide Y, and pro–cocaine-amphetamine–related transcript [18]. Thus, PC1/3 and PC2 are required for proper synthesis of many peptides involved in energy homeostasis. Moreover, the catalytic activities of PC1/3 and PC2 are tissue-specific, as seen in the example of POMC being processed differentially to ACTH in the pituitary, and α-, β-, and γ-MSH in the hypothalamus (see Fig. 2). Another example of the tissue-specificity of PC1/3 and PC2 is the cleavage of proglucagon to glucagon in the pancreatic α-cell, and to GLP-2 in the intestinal L cell.

Three cases of *PC1/3* mutations that cause severe obesity have been reported [26–29]. All three patients had hyperphagia and early-onset obesity believed to result from improper processing of POMC to α-MSH in hypothalamic neurons. Two of the patients had reported weights of more than 35 kg at

3 years of age. These patients also had mild hypocortisolism caused by partial ACTH deficiency that was not as severe as in the patients who had complete POMC deficiency. All three patients also had malabsorption caused by small bowel dysfunction, although with considerably variable severity. Improper processing of proglucagon in the intestinal cells to GLP-2, which has trophic effects on small bowel epithelium, may contribute to poor integrity of the small bowel mucosa in these patients. Abnormalities of glucose homeostasis, namely postprandial hyperglycemia and subsequent reactive hypoglycemia, were noted in two of the three patients. This effect reflects abnormal processing of proinsulin to insulin in pancreatic β-cells [26,27]. Other findings, such as hypogonadotropic hypogonadism in one patient and central hypothyroidism in another, may be attributed to impaired proTRH and proGHRH processing by PC1/3.

These patients came to clinical attention because of reactive hypoglycemia in one case and intractable neonatal diarrhea in the other two, rather than because of severe obesity. Only three cases of PC1/3 deficiency are known, the variability in their clinical phenotype is considerable, and obesity is not the distinguishing feature. Therefore, heterozygous *PC1/3* mutations are currently extremely rare in the differential diagnosis of monogenic obesity. A better understanding of the various roles of PC1/3 in different tissues would improve the ability to clinically detect subtle deficiencies in its function. Currently, measuring proinsulin and insulin levels after a glucose load to show a high proinsulin-to-insulin ratio is the only laboratory evaluation available to determine PC1/3 deficiency.

Melanocortin-4 receptor

In 1998, two groups simultaneously reported the first two cases of severe obesity and hyperphagia caused by *MC4R* mutations [30,31]. Since then, MC4R has emerged as the most specialized and crucial molecule for body weight regulation in the leptin–melanocortin system. First, *MC4R* mutations are inherited in an autosomal dominant fashion, with marked obesity resulting from only one affected allele. Second, aside from severe obesity and hyperphagia, MC4R deficiency has no other physical, hormonal, or developmental consequence, making the function of this receptor very specific for energy balance. And third, mutations in *MC4R* are the most common cause of monogenic obesity known. Compared with the autosomal recessive mutations in genes for leptin, leptin receptor, POMC, and PC1/3 that together total only 32 reported cases of severe obesity in the world, the global prevalence of *MC4R* mutations is approximately 2.5% in severely obese individuals [32–35]. In a large cohort of obese patients and nonobese controls, Lubrano-Berthelier and colleagues [36] recently confirmed that the prevalence of heterozygous, obesity-causing *MC4R* mutations was 2.6% (2.83% in children who had early-onset obesity and 2.35% in adults who had later-onset obesity).

MC4R mutations segregate with obesity in the families of the probands, and are dominantly inherited with variable penetrance and expressivity. Therefore, the obesity phenotype of heterozygous *MC4R* mutation carriers can range from severely obese to lean. Functional studies of obesity-associated *MC4R* mutations show that more severely impaired receptor function in vitro correlates with earlier age of obesity onset and higher BMI. The in vitro studies also show that each mutation impairs receptor function differently through affecting membrane expression, response to agonist, and constitutive activity to a variable degree [36]. The obesity phenotype of *MC4R* mutations is therefore determined not only through variable penetrance and expressivity but also through allelic heterogeneity that contributes to different pathogenic mechanisms. Although no effective therapy for obesity caused by *MC4R* mutations currently exists, hope exists that ongoing research will provide a better understanding of the mechanisms through which *MC4R* mutations cause obesity and will lead to successful treatment options.

Heterozygous carriers of leptin, leptin receptor, and proopiomelanocortin mutations

Most obesity-causing *MC4R* mutations are heterozygous and dominantly inherited. Fewer than 10 cases of homozygous or compound heterozygous *MC4R* mutations have been reported [33,37,38]. These individuals, lacking both alleles of *MC4R*, are significantly more obese than the heterozygotes, and are comparable to patients who have leptin, leptin receptor, and POMC deficiency.

Some evidence exists that an intermediate-weight phenotype may exist for heterozygous carriers of mutations in genes for leptin, leptin receptor, and POMC, implicating these genes in the susceptibility to common obesity. Farooqi and colleagues [39] evaluated 13 heterozygous carriers of the leptin ΔG133 mutation and found that serum leptin levels were significantly lower, whereas BMI and body fat mass were significantly higher in the heterozygotes than in controls. However, interindividual variability in leptin measurements and the small sample-size make these results difficult to interpret. Heterozygous carriers of leptin receptor mutations were not severely obese, but had increased fat mass to the same extent as heterozygote leptin mutation carriers [11].

Significantly higher BMIs were reported in the heterozygous relatives of a patient with POMC deficiency [24], and screening cohorts of severely obese patients has shown heterozygous mutations in *POMC* that do not occur in controls [40–42]. These heterozygous *POMC* mutations segregate with obesity in the probands' families and cause hyperphagia and obesity without any other clinical manifestations, such as adrenal insufficiency. Thus, like heterozygous *MC4R* mutations, heterozygous *POMC* mutations may be a more common cause of monogenic obesity. The heterozygous carriers of *PC1/3* mutations do not have an obvious phenotype, which is not surprising given the overlap of substrate specificity and functional redundancy between PC1/3 and PC2.

Obesity caused by gene mutations that affect neurodevelopment

Three genes, *SIM1*, *BDNF*, and *NTRK2* have been shown through mouse models to be important in hypothalamic development. Recently, mutations in these genes have also been implicated in the development of obesity in mice and humans. The mechanisms through which these genes regulate body weight are unknown. Abnormal development of the hypothalamus, postnatal impairment of the function of these genes, or both may be responsible for the obesity phenotype.

SIM1

In 2000, Holder and colleagues [43] described a girl who had early-onset, severe obesity, hyperphagia, increased linear growth, and normal energy expenditure. Her rapid weight gain began at 3 months of age, so that she was almost 20 kg by 2 years of age and more than 40 kg by 5 years. Her obesity was not associated with any developmental abnormalities, syndromic features, or endocrine dysfunction. This patient had a de novo translocation that disrupted one of her *SIM1* alleles on chromosome 6q [43].

Mice missing one copy of *Sim1* have the same phenotype as the patient, early-onset obesity with hyperphagia, normal energy expenditure, and increased linear growth, and also have a decrease in the total number of paraventricular nucleus (PVN) neurons [44,45]. Because the PVN is the location of *MC4R*-expressing neurons that are critical for energy balance, abnormal development of the PVN is hypothesized to cause obesity in *Sim1* heterozygous mice and *SIM1* haploinsufficient patients.

More recent evidence shows that SIM1 may have an ongoing, postdevelopmental role in energy balance, and specifically that it may function downstream of MC4R to control food intake [46–48]. However, the molecular pathways downstream of MC4R that regulate food intake are far from understood, and further studies are necessary to determine the exact role of SIM1 in these pathways.

Additional evidence for the role of SIM1 in the development of obesity is provided by patients who are obese because of interstitial deletions of chromosome 6q that involve the *SIM1* locus (6q16.2) [49–51], and from significant linkage of childhood obesity related traits to the chromosomal region (6q22.31-q23.2) that contains *SIM1* [52].

Therefore, haploinsufficiency of *SIM1* has been shown to relate to severe, early-onset obesity in one patient who has the translocation, and implicated in the cause of obesity in patients who have interstitial deletions of chromosome 6 that include the *SIM1* locus.

Finally, rare point mutations in *SIM1* were also shown to be significantly associated with obesity in a large screen of obese patients and matched controls [53]. The extent of this association between rare *SIM1* mutations and obesity was comparable only to that between *MC4R* mutations and obesity in this study. In vitro studies of these *SIM1* mutations are needed to determine the functional significance and confirm the role of these rare mutations in the development of obesity.

Brain-derived neurotrophic factor and tropomyosin-related kinase B

BDNF (brain-derived neurotrophic factor) and its receptor TRKB (tropomyosin-related kinase B) regulate proliferation, survival, and differentiation of neurons during development, and neuronal plasticity in the adult nervous system [54–56]. Specific to energy balance, BDNF and TRKB modulate the development and postnatal plasticity of hypothalamic neurons, but both have also been shown to be important for memory, behavior, and cognitive development [30,55,56]. Partial deficiency of Bdnf and TrkB in mouse models causes hyperphagia and obesity [57–59]. Bdnf decreases food intake in mice [58,60,61], likely through acting downstream of Mc4r [57].

The first human case of severe obesity caused by haploinsufficiency of *BDNF* was reported last year [62]. The patient was an 8-year-old girl who presented with hyperphagia and obesity. Her weight exceeded 20 kg at 2 years of age. She also had impaired cognition, memory, and nociception, and hyperactivity. The patient had a de novo paracentric inversion on chromosome 11 that included the *BDNF* locus. Although the inversion may disrupt other unknown genes contributing to the patient's phenotype, the marked similarity of this patient's presentation to that of a patient who had a mutation in *NTRK2*, the gene that encodes TRKB (see below), supports the hypothesis that her phenotype results from haploinsufficiency of *BDNF* [62]. As in *SIM1* haploinsufficiency, this patient's obesity may result from a lack of BDNF during hypothalamic development, or from its impaired postnatal role in MC4R signaling and control of food intake.

One human case of a heterozygous de novo mutation in *NTRK2* has been reported [63]. The 8-year-old boy presented with hyperphagia and early-onset obesity of a similar magnitude to the patient who had *BDNF* haploinsufficiency. He also had developmental delays, stereotyped behaviors, and impairment in memory, learning, and nociception. Functional studies of his missense mutation showed significantly decreased BDNF-induced receptor autophosphorylation and activation of downstream signaling molecules [63,64]. The authors also found reduced neurite outgrowth and cell survival in response to BDNF in cells transfected with the mutant receptor [64], suggesting that postdevelopmental neuronal plasticity is also affected by *NTRK2* mutations.

Screening of a cohort of individuals who had severe, early-onset obesity, and developmental delay showed three other rare mutations in *NTRK2*

(I98V, P660L and T821A) that were not present in controls, but in vitro studies of these mutations did not show a significant difference in receptor function compared with wild-type [64].

Although the exact role of SIM1, BDNF, and TRKB in the development of obesity has not been clearly delineated, their involvement in hypothalamic development and their postnatal function possibly downstream of MC4R is suggested by evidence from mouse models.

Obesity associated with a pleiotropic developmental syndrome

Several pleiotropic syndromes exist with obesity as a predominant phenotype in association with findings such as mental retardation, congenital organ defects, limb or facial dysmorphisms, and endocrine dysfunction. Prader-Willi syndrome is the most common, characterized by neonatal hypotonia and failure to thrive, and subsequent obesity caused by intense hyperphagia, along with developmental delay, mental retardation, hypogonadism, and small hands and feet. The genetic basis of these syndromes is complex. Although the genes or chromosomal regions implicated in the origin of many of these syndromes are known, their relationship to the development of obesity is unclear. Many monogenic obesity-associated syndromes have been reviewed elsewhere [5,65,66], and therefore are not addressed. Instead, this article focuses on three syndromes with multiple phenotypic similarities in addition to obesity, for which pathogenesis was recently linked to dysfunction of the primary cilium.

The primary cilium is an organelle extending from almost all eukaryotic cells. Its architecture differs from that of the more common motile cilium in that its axoneme is made up of 9 microtubule doublets only (9 + 0), without the additional central doublet present in motile cilia (9 + 2) [67]. Primary cilia are attached to the cell at the basal body and are important for chemo- and mechanosensation of the environment and transduction of intracellular signaling. Many important signaling pathways, such as hedgehog signaling and the Wnt pathway, localize to the primary cilium [68]. Because protein synthesis does not occur in cilia, a mechanism called *intraflagellar transport* (IFT) is required to carry proteins necessary for ciliary maintenance and function into and out of the cilia [67].

Bardet-Biedl syndrome

BBS is characterized by clinical findings of retinal degeneration, postaxial polydactyly, obesity, and structural or functional defects of the kidney. Other associated findings include anosmia, mental retardation, hepatic fibrosis, male hypogonadism or undescended testes, female urogenital tract abnormalities, type 2 diabetes mellitus, hypertension, cardiac abnormalities, Hirschsprung's disease, situs inversus, and predisposition to malignancies [69–71]. Obesity in patients who have BBS ranges from mild to severe, and is reversible with caloric restriction and exercise. Rapid weight gain in the first year of life is associated with hyperphagia. No difference in resting metabolic rates have been observed between patients who have BBS and matched obese controls, but lower levels of spontaneous physical activity in patients who have BBS have been reported [72].

BBS is rare and genetically heterogeneous. Mutations in 12 genes, *BBS1–12*, have been identified that contribute to the development of the phenotype [73]. The functions of these genes are not well delineated but are somehow linked to the primary cilium [74].

Nachury and colleagues [73] recently showed that 7 of the 12 BBS-causing genes encode highly conserved proteins that are necessary for primary cilia function. These proteins form a complex, called the *BBSome*, and associate with another factor, Rab8GTP, to facilitate transport of proteins to the primary cilium.

Despite exciting advances in the understanding of BBS pathogenesis and its relationship to ciliary function, the origin of obesity associated with this syndrome is still largely unclear. Dysfunction of cilia in specific neurons could explain obesity caused by hyperphagia and impaired satiety, because Davenport and colleagues [75] showed that deletion of cilia from neurons throughout the central nervous system, and specifically from POMC-expressing neurons, causes obesity in mice. This finding is the first evidence that even a novel mechanism of pathogenesis such as primary ciliary dysfunction may relate to the hypothalamic regulation of food intake in causing obesity. However, this evidence is preliminary and further research is needed. Although it is well established that hypothalamic POMC neurons are critical for signaling satiety, how disruption of ciliary function in these neurons affects their role in energy balance is not.

Alström syndrome

Alström syndrome is another rare syndrome that shares many pleiotropic clinical findings with BBS, namely retinal degeneration, early-onset obesity, type 2 diabetes mellitus, and perceptive hearing loss. It is an autosomal recessive disorder caused by mutations in the *ALMS1* gene. It is also associated with cardiomyopathy, liver and kidney dysfunction, and delayed puberty. The pathogenesis of Alström syndrome has also been linked to dysfunction of the primary cilium, in that the ALMS1 protein localizes to the centrosome and ciliary basal body, and likely has a role in the formation or maintenance of primary cilia. Li and colleagues [76] show that ALMS1 has an important role in cilia formation in kidney cells. Human mutations in *ALMS1* known to cause Alström syndrome result in truncated ALMS1 proteins. These truncated proteins are able to support normal cilia formation but may cause a subtle and undetermined alteration in ciliary function that leads to the development of the Alström phenotype. Residual function of mutant ALMS1 in Alström syndrome explains the lack of a more severe developmental phenotype.

Carpenter's syndrome

Carpenter's syndrome is a pleiotropic disorder with the following features: craniosynostosis affecting primarily metopic and sagittal sutures, polydactyly, soft-tissue syndactyly, and obesity. Other associated findings include brachydactyly, molar agenesis, genu valgum, hypogenitalism, congenital heart defects, umbilical hernia, and learning disability. The disorder has an autosomal recessive inheritance and was recently described to be caused by a homozygous nonsense mutation *L145X* in *RAB23* in five affected individuals from three families [77]. Evaluation of additional patients who had Carpenter's syndrome identified four other mutations in *RAB23*. Similar nonsense mutations in the mouse *Rab23* gene lead to a far more severe phenotype of neural tube defect, causing exencephaly and embryonic lethality.

Rab23 is from Rab family of small GTPases that regulate intracellular trafficking of membrane-associated proteins. Rab23 negatively regulates the Sonic hedgehog signaling pathway [78–81]. Yoshimura and colleagues [82] recently showed that Rab23 is one of three Rab GTPases (Rab8a, Rab17, and Rab23) involved in the formation of the primary cilium.

The phenotype of Carpenter's syndrome shares findings of limb deformities (polysyndactyly and brachydactyly) with other syndromes that result from impaired hedgehog signaling. However, findings of craniosynostosis and obesity have not been previously associated with the hedgehog pathway. Given the evidence that obesity in BBS and Alström syndrome is associated with dysfunction of the primary cilium, and given that hedgehog signaling occurs on the primary cilium in many cell types, it is possible to implicate ciliary dysfunction that disrupts hedgehog signaling in the pathogenesis of Carpenter's syndrome.

Summary

Several lessons can be gleaned from the study of extreme human obesity. First, the long-term regulation of body weight in humans is centered in the hypothalamus. Within the hypothalamus, the leptin–melanocortin system is critical for energy balance, because disruption of these pathways that sense peripheral energy stores and signal satiety leads to the most severe forms of human obesity. Furthermore, MC4R is the most specialized molecule for body weight maintenance within this system because MC4R deficiency has no other clinical phenotype.

Second, the monogenic causes of obesity identified thus far account for less than 5% of severe obesity, and are in themselves very heterogeneous. BBS, for example, can result from alterations in at least 12 different genes, and obesity caused by *MC4R* mutations can result from different mechanisms that affect receptor function. Furthermore, novel mechanisms are emerging as important for pathogenicity of obesity, such as abnormal hypothalamic development, alterations in neuronal plasticity, and dysfunction of the primary cilium. Therefore, the currently characterized monogenic forms of obesity can be viewed as the "tip of the iceberg," providing clues that the pathogenic mechanisms underlying common obesity is equally heterogeneous.

Third, treatment of congenital leptin deficiency with leptin is a rare but powerful example of successful therapy arising from an understanding of the molecular pathogenesis. Thus, further research to understand the pathogenic mechanisms underlying obesity is required for the development of similarly rational and effective treatments. However, this research is slow and challenging because of the great genetic heterogeneity of the disorder.

Fourth, the lack of specific therapies to treat the various genetic causes of obesity highlights a dichotomy in the approach to an obese patient. Although currently a patient experiences no direct benefit in knowing the genetic basis of his disease, it is important from a research perspective to further explore the genetic cause of this phenotype. Only through elucidating the molecular mechanisms underlying obesity can this devastating condition be rationally approached and effectively treated.

Acknowledgments

The authors would like to thank Jimmy Chen for his contribution to the artwork.

References

[1] Ogden CL, Flegal KM, Carroll MD, et al. Prevalence and trends in overweight among US children and adolescents, 1999–2000. JAMA 2002;288(14):1728–32.
[2] Barsh GS, Farooqi IS, O'Rahilly S. Genetics of body-weight regulation. Nature 2000; 404(6778):644–51.
[3] Farooqi S, O'Rahilly S. Genetics of obesity in humans. Endocr Rev 2006;27(7):710–8.
[4] Bell CG, Walley AJ, Froguel P. The genetics of human obesity. Nat Rev Genet 2005;6(3): 221–34.
[5] Farooqi IS. Genetic and hereditary aspects of childhood obesity. Best Pract Res Clin Endocrinol Metab 2005;19(3):359–74.
[6] Ellacott KL, Cone RD. The role of the central melanocortin system in the regulation of food intake and energy homeostasis: lessons from mouse models. Philos Trans R Soc Lond B Biol Sci 2006;361(1471):1265–74.
[7] Cone RD. Anatomy and regulation of the central melanocortin system. Nat Neurosci 2005; 8(5):571–8.
[8] Butler AA. The melanocortin system and energy balance. Peptides 2006;27(2):281–90.
[9] Niswender KD, Baskin DG, Schwartz MW. Insulin and its evolving partnership with leptin in the hypothalamic control of energy homeostasis. Trends Endocrinol Metab 2004;15(8): 362–9.
[10] Coll AP, Farooqi IS, O'Rahilly S. The hormonal control of food intake. Cell 2007;129(2): 251–62.
[11] Farooqi IS, Wangensteen T, Collins S, et al. Clinical and molecular genetic spectrum of congenital deficiency of the leptin receptor. N Engl J Med 2007;356(3):237–47.

[12] Montague CT, Farooqi IS, Whitehead JP, et al. Congenital leptin deficiency is associated with severe early-onset obesity in humans. Nature 1997;387(6636):903–8.

[13] Strobel A, Issad T, Camoin L, et al. A leptin missense mutation associated with hypogonadism and morbid obesity. Nat Genet 1998;18(3):213–5.

[14] Gibson WT, Farooqi IS, Moreau M, et al. Congenital leptin deficiency due to homozygosity for the Delta133G mutation: report of another case and evaluation of response to four years of leptin therapy. J Clin Endocrinol Metab 2004;89(10):4821–6.

[15] Farooqi IS, Matarese G, Lord GM, et al. Beneficial effects of leptin on obesity, T cell hyporesponsiveness, and neuroendocrine/metabolic dysfunction of human congenital leptin deficiency. J Clin Invest 2002;110(8):1093–103.

[16] Friedman JM, Halaas JL. Leptin and the regulation of body weight in mammals. Nature 1998;395(6704):763–70.

[17] Farooqi IS, O'Rahilly S. Monogenic human obesity syndromes. Recent Prog Horm Res 2004;59:409–24.

[18] Nillni EA. Regulation of prohormone convertases in hypothalamic neurons: implications for prothyrotropin-releasing hormone and proopiomelanocortin. Endocrinology 2007; 148(9):4191–200.

[19] Heymsfield SB, Greenberg AS, Fujioka K, et al. Recombinant leptin for weight loss in obese and lean adults: a randomized, controlled, dose-escalation trial. JAMA 1999;282(16): 1568–75.

[20] Clement K, Vaisse C, Lahlou N, et al. A mutation in the human leptin receptor gene causes obesity and pituitary dysfunction. Nature 1998;392(6674):398–401.

[21] Lahlou N, Clement K, Carel JC, et al. Soluble leptin receptor in serum of subjects with complete resistance to leptin: relation to fat mass. Diabetes 2000;49(8):1347–52.

[22] Krude H, Biebermann H, Luck W, et al. Severe early-onset obesity, adrenal insufficiency and red hair pigmentation caused by POMC mutations in humans. Nat Genet 1998;19(2):155–7.

[23] Krude H, Biebermann H, Schnabel D, et al. Obesity due to proopiomelanocortin deficiency: three new cases and treatment trials with thyroid hormone and ACTH4-10. J Clin Endocrinol Metab 2003;88(10):4633–40.

[24] Farooqi IS, Drop S, Clements A, et al. Heterozygosity for a POMC-null mutation and increased obesity risk in humans. Diabetes 2006;55(9):2549–53.

[25] Rouille Y, Duguay SJ, Lund K, et al. Proteolytic processing mechanisms in the biosynthesis of neuroendocrine peptides: the subtilisin-like proprotein convertases. Front Neuroendocrinol 1995;16(4):322–61.

[26] O'Rahilly S, Gray H, Humphreys PJ, et al. Brief report: impaired processing of prohormones associated with abnormalities of glucose homeostasis and adrenal function. N Engl J Med 1995;333(21):1386–90.

[27] Jackson RS, Creemers JW, Ohagi S, et al. Obesity and impaired prohormone processing associated with mutations in the human prohormone convertase 1 gene. Nat Genet 1997; 16(3):303–6.

[28] Jackson RS, Creemers JW, Farooqi IS, et al. Small-intestinal dysfunction accompanies the complex endocrinopathy of human proprotein convertase 1 deficiency. J Clin Invest 2003; 112(10):1550–60.

[29] Farooqi IS, Volders K, Stanhope R, et al. Hyperphagia and early-onset obesity due to a novel homozygous missense mutation in prohormone convertase 1/3. J Clin Endocrinol Metab 2007;92(9):3369–73.

[30] Vaisse C, Clement K, Guy-Grand B, et al. A frameshift mutation in human MC4R is associated with a dominant form of obesity. Nat Genet 1998;20(2):113–4.

[31] Yeo GS, Farooqi IS, Aminian S, et al. A frameshift mutation in MC4R associated with dominantly inherited human obesity. Nat Genet 1998;20(2):111–2.

[32] Hainerova I, Larsen LH, Holst B, et al. Melanocortin 4 receptor mutations in obese Czech children: studies of prevalence, phenotype development, weight reduction response, and functional analysis. J Clin Endocrinol Metab 2007;92(9):3689–96.

[33] Farooqi IS, Keogh JM, Yeo GS, et al. Clinical spectrum of obesity and mutations in the melanocortin 4 receptor gene. N Engl J Med 2003;348(12):1085–95.

[34] Zakel UA, Wudy SA, Heinzel-Gutenbrunner M, et al. [Prevalence of melanocortin 4 receptor (MC4R) mutations and polymorphisms in consecutively ascertained obese children and adolescents from a pediatric health care utilization population]. Klin Padiatr 2005;217(4):244–9 [in German].

[35] Wang CL, Liang L, Wang HJ, et al. Several mutations in the melanocortin 4 receptor gene are associated with obesity in Chinese children and adolescents. J Endocrinol Invest 2006; 29(10):894–8.

[36] Lubrano-Berthelier C, Dubern B, Lacorte JM, et al. Melanocortin 4 receptor mutations in a large cohort of severely obese adults: prevalence, functional classification, genotype-phenotype relationship, and lack of association with binge eating. J Clin Endocrinol Metab 2006;91(5):1811–8.

[37] Lubrano-Berthelier C, Le Stunff C, Bougneres P, et al. A homozygous null mutation delineates the role of the melanocortin-4 receptor in humans. J Clin Endocrinol Metab 2004;89(5): 2028–32.

[38] Dubern B, Bisbis S, Talbaoui H, et al. Homozygous null mutation of the melanocortin-4 receptor and severe early-onset obesity. J Pediatr 2007;150(6):613–7, 617 e611.

[39] Farooqi IS, Keogh JM, Kamath S, et al. Partial leptin deficiency and human adiposity. Nature 2001;414(6859):34–5.

[40] Challis BG, Pritchard LE, Creemers JW, et al. A missense mutation disrupting a dibasic pro-hormone processing site in pro-opiomelanocortin (POMC) increases susceptibility to early-onset obesity through a novel molecular mechanism. Hum Mol Genet 2002;11(17):1997–2004.

[41] Biebermann H, Castaneda TR, van Landeghem F, et al. A role for beta-melanocyte-stimulating hormone in human body-weight regulation. Cell Metab 2006;3(2):141–6.

[42] Lee YS, Challis BG, Thompson DA, et al. A POMC variant implicates beta-melanocyte-stimulating hormone in the control of human energy balance. Cell Metab 2006;3(2):135–40.

[43] Holder JL Jr, Butte NF, Zinn AR. Profound obesity associated with a balanced translocation that disrupts the SIM1 gene. Hum Mol Genet 2000;9(1):101–8.

[44] Michaud JL, Rosenquist T, May NR, et al. Development of neuroendocrine lineages requires the bHLH-PAS transcription factor SIM1. Genes Dev 1998;12(20):3264–75.

[45] Michaud JL, Boucher F, Melnyk A, et al. Sim1 haploinsufficiency causes hyperphagia, obesity and reduction of the paraventricular nucleus of the hypothalamus. Hum Mol Genet 2001;10(14):1465–73.

[46] Kublaoui BM, Holder JL Jr, Tolson KP, et al. SIM1 overexpression partially rescues agouti yellow and diet-induced obesity by normalizing food intake. Endocrinology 2006;147(10): 4542–9.

[47] Kublaoui BM, Holder JL Jr, Gemelli T, et al. Sim1 haploinsufficiency impairs melanocortin-mediated anorexia and activation of paraventricular nucleus neurons. Mol Endocrinol 2006; 20(10):2483–92.

[48] Holder JL Jr, Zhang L, Kublaoui BM, et al. Sim1 gene dosage modulates the homeostatic feeding response to increased dietary fat in mice. Am J Physiol Endocrinol Metab 2004; 287(1):E105–13.

[49] Villa A, Urioste M, Bofarull JM, et al. De novo interstitial deletion q16.2q21 on chromosome 6. Am J Med Genet 1995;55(3):379–83.

[50] Gilhuis HJ, van Ravenswaaij CM, Hamel BJ, et al. Interstitial 6q deletion with a Prader-Willi-like phenotype: a new case and review of the literature. Eur J Paediatr Neurol 2000; 4(1):39–43.

[51] Faivre L, Cormier-Daire V, Lapierre JM, et al. Deletion of the SIM1 gene (6q16.2) in a patient with a Prader-Willi-like phenotype. J Med Genet 2002;39(8):594–6.

[52] Meyre D, Lecoeur C, Delplanque J, et al. A genome-wide scan for childhood obesity-associated traits in French families shows significant linkage on chromosome 6q22.31-q23.2. Diabetes 2004;53(3):803–11.

[53] Ahituv N, Kavaslar N, Schackwitz W, et al. Medical sequencing at the extremes of human body mass. Am J Hum Genet 2007;80(4):779–91.

[54] Tapia-Arancibia L, Rage F, Givalois L, et al. Physiology of BDNF: focus on hypothalamic function. Front Neuroendocrinol 2004;25(2):77–107.

[55] Huang EJ, Reichardt LF. Neurotrophins: roles in neuronal development and function. Annu Rev Neurosci 2001;24:677–736.

[56] Huang EJ, Reichardt LF. Trk receptors: roles in neuronal signal transduction. Annu Rev Biochem 2003;72:609–42.

[57] Xu B, Goulding EH, Zang K, et al. Brain-derived neurotrophic factor regulates energy balance downstream of melanocortin-4 receptor. Nat Neurosci 2003;6(7):736–42.

[58] Kernie SG, Liebl DJ, Parada LF. BDNF regulates eating behavior and locomotor activity in mice. EMBO J 2000;19(6):1290–300.

[59] Lyons WE, Mamounas LA, Ricaurte GA, et al. Brain-derived neurotrophic factor-deficient mice develop aggressiveness and hyperphagia in conjunction with brain serotonergic abnormalities. Proc Natl Acad Sci U S A 1999;96(26):15239–44.

[60] Pelleymounter MA, Cullen MJ, Wellman CL. Characteristics of BDNF-induced weight loss. Exp Neurol 1995;131(2):229–38.

[61] Rios M, Fan G, Fekete C, et al. Conditional deletion of brain-derived neurotrophic factor in the postnatal brain leads to obesity and hyperactivity. Mol Endocrinol 2001;15(10):1748–57.

[62] Gray J, Yeo GS, Cox JJ, et al. Hyperphagia, severe obesity, impaired cognitive function, and hyperactivity associated with functional loss of one copy of the brain-derived neurotrophic factor (BDNF) gene. Diabetes 2006;55(12):3366–71.

[63] Yeo GS, Connie Hung CC, Rochford J, et al. A de novo mutation affecting human TrkB associated with severe obesity and developmental delay. Nat Neurosci 2004;7(11):1187–9.

[64] Gray J, Yeo G, Hung C, et al. Functional characterization of human NTRK2 mutations identified in patients with severe early-onset obesity. Int J Obes (Lond) 2007;31(2):359–64.

[65] Mutch DM, Clement K. Unraveling the genetics of human obesity. PLoS Genet 2006;2(12):1956–63.

[66] O'Rahilly S, Farooqi IS, Yeo GS, et al. Minireview: human obesity-lessons from monogenic disorders. Endocrinology 2003;144(9):3757–64.

[67] Davenport JR, Yoder BK. An incredible decade for the primary cilium: a look at a once-forgotten organelle. Am J Physiol Renal Physiol 2005;289(6):F1159–69.

[68] Singla V, Reiter JF. The primary cilium as the cell's antenna: signaling at a sensory organelle. Science 2006;313(5787):629–33.

[69] Kulaga HM, Leitch CC, Eichers ER, et al. Loss of BBS proteins causes anosmia in humans and defects in olfactory cilia structure and function in the mouse. Nat Genet 2004;36(9):994–8.

[70] Lorda-Sanchez I, Ayuso C, Ibanez A. Situs inversus and hirschsprung disease: two uncommon manifestations in Bardet-Biedl syndrome. Am J Med Genet 2000;90(1):80–1.

[71] Tobin JL, Beales PL. Bardet-Biedl syndrome: beyond the cilium. Pediatr Nephrol 2007;22(7):926–36.

[72] Grace C, Beales P, Summerbell C, et al. Energy metabolism in Bardet-Biedl syndrome. Int J Obes Relat Metab Disord 2003;27(11):1319–24.

[73] Nachury MV, Loktev AV, Zhang Q, et al. A core complex of BBS proteins cooperates with the GTPase Rab8 to promote ciliary membrane biogenesis. Cell 2007;129(6):1201–13.

[74] Ansley SJ, Badano JL, Blacque OE, et al. Basal body dysfunction is a likely cause of pleiotropic Bardet-Biedl syndrome. Nature 2003;425(6958):628–33.

[75] Davenport JR, Watts AJ, Roper VC, et al. Disruption of intraflagellar transport in adult mice leads to obesity and slow-onset cystic kidney disease. Curr Biol 2007;17(18):1586–94.

[76] Li G, Vega R, Nelms K, et al. A role for Alstrom syndrome protein, alms1, in kidney ciliogenesis and cellular quiescence. PLoS Genet 2007;3(1):9–20.

[77] Jenkins D, Seelow D, Jehee FS, et al. RAB23 mutations in carpenter syndrome imply an unexpected role for hedgehog signaling in cranial-suture development and obesity. Am J Hum Genet 2007;80(6):1162–70.

[78] Eggenschwiler JT, Espinoza E, Anderson KV. Rab23 is an essential negative regulator of the mouse Sonic hedgehog signalling pathway. Nature 2001;412(6843):194–8.

[79] Evans TM, Ferguson C, Wainwright BJ, et al. a negative regulator of hedgehog signaling, localizes to the plasma membrane and the endocytic pathway. Traffic 2003;4(12):869–84.

[80] Eggenschwiler JT, Bulgakov OV, Qin J, et al. Mouse Rab23 regulates hedgehog signaling from smoothened to Gli proteins. Dev Biol 2006;290(1):1–12.

[81] Huangfu D, Liu A, Rakeman AS, et al. Hedgehog signalling in the mouse requires intraflagellar transport proteins. Nature 2003;426(6962):83–7.

[82] Yoshimura S, Egerer J, Fuchs E, et al. Functional dissection of Rab GTPases involved in primary cilium formation. J Cell Biol 2007;178(3):363–9.

ELSEVIER
SAUNDERS

Endocrinol Metab Clin N Am
37 (2008) 753–768

ENDOCRINOLOGY
AND METABOLISM
CLINICS
OF NORTH AMERICA

The Adipocyte as an Endocrine Cell

Nils Halberg, PhD[a,b],
Ingrid Wernstedt-Asterholm, PhD[a],
Philipp E. Scherer, PhD[a,*]

[a]*Touchstone Diabetes Center, Department of Internal Medicine, University of Texas
Southwestern Medical Center, 5323 Harry Hines Boulevard, Dallas, TX 75390-8549, USA*
[b]*Department of Biomedical Sciences, University of Copenhagen,
Blegdamsvej 3B, 2200 Copenhagen N, Denmark*

Adipose tissue has important endocrine functions under physiologic and pathophysiologic conditions [1–4]. This article focuses on areas of adipokine biology that have so far received little attention but, at the same time, represent areas the authors believe have great implication in our understanding of adipocytes and adipokine physiology. In particular, a comprehensive "meta-analysis" of proteomics efforts on adipocytes is lacking to date. Here, the authors summarize what they consider to be the key findings in the area of secretion of adipocyte-derived factors.

The adipocyte secretome

So far, much attention in the study of adipocyte-derived factors (so-called "adipokines") has been devoted to the study of a few proteins with important physiologic functions. Notably, these include leptin, adiponectin, resistin, interleukin 6 (IL-6), monocyte chemotractant protein 1, and tumor necrosis factor alpha (TNF-α). On the other hand, several proteomic approaches in primary and tissue culture–derived 3T3-L1 adipocytes have emphasized the complex nature of the adipocyte secretome, highlighting that the adipocyte secretes many different proteins [5–12]. Although the analyses of primary adipocyte isolates and tissue culture–derived adipocytes have limitations because of the nonphysiologic nature of the culture conditions, they help us elucidate aspects of the adipocyte secretome that are

* Corresponding author.
E-mail address: Philipp.Scherer@utsouthwestern.edu (P.E. Scherer).

0889-8529/08/$ - see front matter © 2008 Elsevier Inc. All rights reserved.
doi:10.1016/j.ecl.2008.07.002
endo.theclinics.com

underappreciated and define functional clusters of adipokines that have not yet been the focus of a systematic analysis.

The authors have collected information from all available published studies and generated a list of proteins that have been reported to be secreted from adipocytes (Table 1). These proteins have been clustered according to their postulated function or functions. These adipokines fall into several groups, including adipokines contributing to the extracellular matrix, those involved in metabolism, those involved in the immune response, and other categories, which highlights the important regulatory role of the adipocyte with respect to extracellular matrix components, inflammatory pathways, and angiogenesis. The total number of confirmed proteins identified as secretory components of the adipocyte approaches 100 distinct proteins, and that list is likely to grow as the methods for the analysis of supernatants become more sensitive (see Table 1).

The extracellular matrix of adipose tissue

During the progression from the lean to the obese state, adipose tissue undergoes hyperplasia and hypertrophy in an attempt to cope with the increased demand for triglyceride storage. Therefore, the extracellular matrix of adipose tissue faces unique challenges with respect to adjusting to the need for remodeling and expansion.

The changes in cell morphology seen during differentiation in cell culture of preadipocytes to adipocytes and the accompanying impact on the expression of various extracellular matrix proteins have been appreciated for some time. For instance, a decrease in the key extracellular matrix protein fibronectin is an absolute prerequisite for differentiation [13,14]. In the extracellular matrix compartment, fibronectin can be degraded by another adipokine, cathepsin S. This cysteine protease is secreted at increasing levels in the obese state and is able to drive the differentiation of primary human preadipocytes [15].

Another protease, cathepsin K, is also up-regulated in the obese state and is required for the induction of lipid storage during 3T3-L1 differentiation [16]. Cathepsin K can degrade several matrix constituents, such as collagens type 1 and 2, but its primary target is the secreted protein acidic and rich in cysteine (SPARC). SPARC does not serve as a structural extracellular matrix protein, but as a mediator of cell–matrix interactions [17]. Mice with a genetic deletion at the SPARC locus display an interesting phenotype. Even though no difference in body weight is apparent, these mice have a significant increase in adipose tissue volume, associated with an increased number of adipocytes and accompanied by an altered composition of other extracellular matrix components, such as a decrease in the levels of collagen 1 relative to the wild-type controls [18]. SPARC expression is dysregulated in adipocytes from ob/ob mice that have higher expression and secretion of SPARC [19].

Matrix metalloproteases (MMPs) are a family of proteins that carry a zinc-dependent protease domain, with specificity to several extracellular matrix proteins. The activity of these MMPs is controlled by another family of regulatory proteins, the tissue inhibitors of matrix metalloproteinases (TIMPs) that neutralize MMP activity in a 1:1 stoichiometric manner. Several MMPs and TIMPs are secreted from the adipocyte (see Table 1). This large array of proteases and protease inhibitors is a reflection of the critical need of the adipose tissue extracellular matrix to undergo remodeling during times of expansion. In obese mouse models (eg, ob/ob and db/db mice), many MMPs, including MMP-2, -3, -12, -14, and -19 are up-regulated, whereas MMP-7 is down-regulated, and the expression of MMP-9, -11, and -13 are maintained at similar levels in lean and obese mice [20].

To date, it is not known whether the modulation of extracellular matrix constituents is a primary player in the development of obesity or whether changes in these proteins are simply downstream effectors that respond secondarily to changes in adipocyte size and number. However, in at least one example, the activity of an MMP has been shown to be critical. The membrane type 1 (MT1)-MMP has been critically implicated in adipocyte differentiation in vivo. A mouse model with a genetic disruption of the MT1-MMP locus shows a significant impairment in white adipose tissue differentiation, resulting in adipose tissue that is populated with small adipocytes, giving rise to a lipodystrophic animal. Also, the proteolytic activity of MMP-2 and -9, two of the most abundant MMPs, is induced further during differentiation. This up-regulation is significant because direct inhibition of these MMPs by neutralizing antibodies prevents differentiation [21]. Similar to cathepsin S, a critical MMP-2 substrate is fibronectin. When the action of MMP-2 is blocked, cathepsin S fails to compensate fully for the loss of MMP-2 activity, and adipogenesis is inhibited because of a failure to degrade the fibronectin network surrounding the adipocyte while leaving unaffected the expression of other critical adipogenesis factors such as peroxisome proliferator–activated receptor gamma (PPAR-γ) and CCAAT/enhancer binding protein beta [22].

Given the importance of these factors, it is not surprising that MMPs and TIMPs are tightly and differentially regulated in the obese state. TIMP-1 is strongly induced, whereas TIMP-3 is down-regulated in the expanding adipose tissue [20]. After exposure to a high-fat diet, TIMP-1$-/-$ mice have smaller adipocytes, less subcutaneous fat, and a lower body weight than their wild-type littermates [23]. Indeed, TIMP-1 expression decreases with adipogenesis, and in vivo overexpression leads to adipocyte hypertrophy and accelerated adipogenesis [24]. TIMP-1 is circulating in plasma in the ng/mL range, and has been postulated to be a predictor of adiposity (but not insulin resistance) in humans [25].

Although our insight into the physiologic relevance of the extracellular matrix of adipose tissue during obesity remains rather rudimentary, all the studies discussed above clearly highlight that a partial breakdown of

Table 1
Proteins secreted from adipocytes clustered according to postulated fuction

Extracellular matrix	Metabolism	Immune system	Others
Alpha 2 Macroglobulin [1]	Adipsin	Alpha 1 acid glycoprotein	Angiopoietin 1
Cathepsin B	Adiponectin	Colony-stimulating factor-1	Angiopoietin 2
Cathepsin D	Apelin	Complement component	Angiotensinogen
Cathepsin L	Apolipoprotein E	inhibitor C1	Calcitonin
Cathepsin S	Cortisol	Complement C1	Chemerin
Collagen alpha 1 (I)	Insulin like growth factor-1	Complement C2	Cyclophilin A
Collagen alpha 1 (III)	Insulin like growth factor	Complement C3	Cyclophilin C
Collagen alpha 1 (IV)	bindihg protein 7	Complement C4	Extracellular superoxide dismutase
Collagen alpha 1 (VI)	Lipoprotein lipase	Complement C7	Galectin 1
Collagen alpha 1 (XV)	Leptin	Complement factor B	Firbroblast growth factor
Collagen alpha 1 (XIV)	Fasting-induced adipose factor	Complement factor C	Hepatic growth factor
Collagen alpha 1 (XVII)	Plasminogen activated	Complement factor D	Mineralocorticoid-releasing factor
Collagen alpha 2 (I)	inhibitor-1	C reactive protein	Nerve growth factor
Collagen alpha 2 (IV)	Resistin	Haptoglobin	Pigment epithelium-derived factor
Collagen alpha 2 (VI)	Retinol binding protein 4	Interukin 1 beat	Prostaglandin E2
Collagen alpha 3 (VI)	Vaspin	Interukin 4	Prostaglandin I2
Dystroglycan	Visfatin	Interukin 6	Prostaglandin 2alpha
Entactin		Interukin 7	Serum transferrin
Fibulin-2		Interukin 8	Stromal derived factor 1
Fibulin-3		Interukin 10	TGF beta
Fibronectin		Interukin 12	Tissue Factor
Galectin-3-binding protein		Interukin 18	Vascular endothelial growth factor
Gelsolin		Lipocalin 24p3	
Laminin alpha 4		Macrophage migration inhibitory factor 1	
Liaminin beta 1		Serum Amyloid A3	
Liminin gamma		TNF-α	
Lysyl oxidase			
Matrilin-2			

MMP-1
MMP-2
MMP-3
MMP-7
MMP-9
MMP-10
MMP-11
MMP-12
MMP-13
MMP-14
MMP-15
MMP-16
MMP-17
MMP-19
MMP-23
MMP-24
TIMP-1
TIMP-2
TIMP-3
TIMP-4
Osteonection (SPARC)
Perlecan
Procollagen C-proteinase enhancer protein
Protein-lysine 6-oxidase
Spondin-1
Tenacin
Thrombospondin-1
Thrombospondin-2

Abbreviations: MMP, matrix metalloproteinase; TIMP, tissue inhibitor of matrix metalloproteinase.

the extracellular matrix is required for adipocyte differentiation, both in vitro and in vivo. As such, the expanding adipose tissue needs to modulate/degrade some of the extracellular matrix constituents to prevent the extracellular matrix from restraining the expanding adipocytes. Failure to do so may cause stress at the level of the individual adipocyte, leading to local inflammation and a significant impairment in accommodating the increased triglyceride load (Fig. 1). As a result of these local problems in adipose tissue, systemic effects occur, such as ectopic lipid deposition in organs such as the liver, muscle, and pancreas, triggering a significant degree of lipotoxicity [26]. In a recent study by Kim and colleagues [27], a modest overexpression of adiponectin enabled ob/ob mice to expand their fat pad further, relieving other tissues of triglyceride deposition and resulting in a normalization of the metabolic phenotype. One of the notable differences reported in these mice was that a host of extracellular matrix proteins were down-regulated, including a number of collagens, MMPs, and TIMPs, which strongly suggests that the dysregulation of extracellular matrix components in adipose tissue goes hand in hand with a systemic dysregulation of metabolism. Whether this is cause or effect will need to be shown on a case-by-case basis for the major components of the extracellular matrix in adipose tissue.

The immune-regulatory role of the adipocyte

Many adipocyte-derived factors play an intricate role in various aspects of the innate and adaptive immune response (see Table 1). They may be

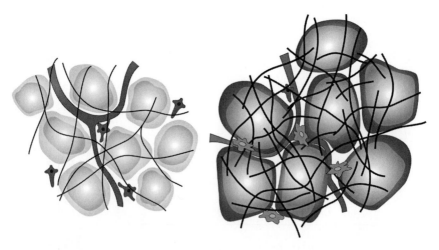

Fig. 1. White adipose tissue in the lean (*left*) versus obese (*right*) state. Adipocytes are shown with yellow triglyceride droplets and blue cytoplasm. In the lean state, the light blue cytoplasm represents a state of normoxia, whereas the dark blue in the obese state represents a hypoxic state. Preadipocytes are shown in brown, macrophages in green, blood vessels/endothelial cells in red, and the extracellular matrix in black.

directly involved as chemokines or cytokines, or they may play a regulatory role [28]. It is therefore not surprising that local, obesity-driven changes in adipokine secretion have a systemic impact on several branches of the immune system. The best described phenomenon relates to changes in the inflammatory status. Many aspects of the interactions between the immune system and metabolic function have been intensely studied, and many manifestations of the metabolic syndrome have been blamed on macrophage infiltration and chronic low-grade inflammation in adipose tissue as it is expanding. These phenomena remain under intense study in many laboratories and have been revisited in numerous reviews, and are not discussed further here (see Fig. 1) [29–34].

In contrast to the chronic subclinical inflammatory state, the role of adipokines in regular sepsis remains vastly unexplored. The liver is traditionally thought of as the major site for the release of most mediators of the innate immune response. But because the adipocyte expresses and secretes many acute-phase reactants at high levels [35], it is highly likely that the adipocyte also plays a role in the acute septic state. The adipocyte expresses the lipopolysaccharide (LPS)-activated toll-like receptor 4 and it reacts to LPS exposure by increasing the expression and activity of nuclear factor kappa B, which, in turn, induces the high-level production of serum amyloid A3 (SAA3), IL-6, and the lipocalin 24p3 [35–37]. The important systemic role that the adipocyte plays in the context of proinflammatory signals is evidenced in mice, where the adipocytes undergo a triggered, rapid adipocyte apoptosis through activation of a caspase-8 construct provided through transgenic expression in adipose tissue. When these fatless mice are challenged with LPS, they have a significantly reduced systemic level of SAA3 and IL-6 relative to their control mice, which have normal adipocytes [38]. These observations, along with reports from several other laboratories, suggest that the adipocyte can contribute to the systemic LPS-induced immune response, in part on its own, or, more significantly, in concert with local paracrine interactions with adipose tissue macrophages.

The PPAR-γ agonists serve as potent antidiabetic drugs. Much needs to be learned about the complex set of responses triggered by PPAR-γ activation in various tissues. The adipocyte and the macrophage serve as important targets for the antidiabetic effects of PPAR-γ agonists, but additional cell types are clearly also affected. Adipocytes respond to PPAR-γ agonist treatment by initiating an anti-inflammatory program with increased secretion of the anti-inflammatory adipokine adiponectin and decreased secretion of proinflammatory adipokines, such as TNF-α and haptoglobin [39–41]. A similar response is seen in the macrophages, where PPAR-γ activation suppresses the LPS-induced production of nitric oxide, IL-6, and TNF-α [42]. Anti-inflammatory properties have been reported for PPAR-γ agonists under additional conditions (eg, an impairment colonic inflammation in models of colitis [43] and an attenuation of local liver inflammation in models of nonalcoholic liver disease [44]).

Aside from the direct inflammatory aspects of sepsis, septic patients also experience profound insulin resistance. Insulin not only can control hyperglycemia but also has anti-inflammatory roles under some circumstances. In fact, insulin treatment of patients undergoing sepsis is now widely used [45]. Whether adipose tissue constitutes a major target for the anti-inflammatory actions of insulin under these conditions remains to be seen.

Another area where the adipocyte may play a major role in local inflammatory processes is in the context of rheumatoid arthritis and osteoarthritis. Adipocytes not only serve as a storage depot for energy but can also provide mechanical support within joints. These adipocytes and their pathophysiologic changes in arthritis remain extremely poorly characterized but, given their potent proinflammatory potential, it is possible that they make a significant contribution to the local inflammation in the context of an arthritic joint. Adipokines such as leptin, adiponectin, and resistin can be measured in the synovial fluid of arthritic patients [46]. Other investigators have suggested that adiponectin, in particular, plays a protective role in synovial fluid and may modulate cartilage destruction in chondrocytes [47]. These structural fat pads deserve further investigation and it remains to be seen whether strategies specifically targeting the anti-inflammatory aspects of these cells will contribute productively toward a reduction in the degenerative aspects of the disease.

Angiogenesis

Although adipocytes occupy the bulk of the volume of adipose tissue, the adipose tissue stroma contains many more cell types that at least equal the adipocytes in number. Nonadipocytic cell types in adipose tissue include fibroblastic preadipocytes that can be triggered to embark on the adipogenic differentiation pathway. Other cell types include immune cells and, importantly, endothelial cells. New endothelium may sprout from existing endothelial cells or it may occur through maturation of new endothelial cells from circulating endothelial progenitor cells. Although the latter does not seem to play as prominent a role, the sprouting of the endothelium seems to be a highly active and coordinated event; sprouting is especially active in the vicinity of differentiating adipocytes [48–50]. In fact, adipose tissue development has a critical dependency on angiogenesis. Ongoing neovascularization is required for healthy adipose tissue because exposure to angiogenesis inhibitors triggers a reduction in fat mass [51–53]. Evidence even suggests that the vascular network forms before the mature lipid-carrying adipocytes reside in the area [50].

The adipocyte secretes several factors that modulate the production of new blood vessels (eg, angiopoietin-1, angiopoietin-2, vascular endothelial growth factor [VEGF], transforming growth factor beta, hepatic growth factor, stromal-derived factor 1, TNF-α, resistin, leptin, tissue factor, placental growth factor, insulin-like growth factor, and lower molecular weight lipid factor monobutyrin) (reviewed in [54]). Despite this great angiogenic potential, a rapidly expanding fat pad still experiences hypoxia, whereas other tissues in the same animal (such as muscle) do not [55–57]. As a consequence, the master regulator of hypoxia, hypoxia-induced factor alpha, and several of its downstream targets are induced (eg, glucose transporter [GLUT] 1, VEGF, pyruvate dehydrogenase-1, and hemeoxygenase-1). Besides VEGF, hypoxic isolated adipocytes secrete higher levels of several proangiogenic factors, such as leptin, IL-6, migration inhibitory factor, leptin, and plasminogen activator inhibitor 1 [11]. The obese state is associated with increased levels of plasma levels of TNF-α, resistin, angiopoietin-1, and hepatic growth factor [58]. Even though the adipocyte remains at the center of these proangiogenic processes, much evidence points toward the macrophage as another extremely important source for angiogenic factors. The macrophages that reside in the adipose tissue in the lean state increase sharply in number as an individual becomes more obese. These macrophages are active players in the course of the new vascularization associated with postnatal outgrowth of epididymal adipose tissue [50] and have a potent proangiogenic profile under normoxic conditions, and are even more active when subjected to hypoxia [57]. The adipose tissue macrophages polarize into two populations. M1 is involved in the killing of intracellular parasites and is characterized by a type 1 inflammatory response, releasing factors such as IL6 and TNF-α. M2 macrophages, on the other hand, are recruited for tissue remodeling, with a proangiogenic potential, and a type 2 inflammatory response [59]. Recently, it has become apparent that obesity induces a phenotypic switch from the M2 to the M1 macrophages [60], thereby seemingly decreasing the angiogenic potential of the residing macrophages.

The extracellular matrix and angiogenesis also have an important connection. Hypoxia induces MMP-2 and -9 in adipocytes [61]. MMP-9 especially deserves attention in this sense, in that it is a known tumor angiogenic factor that works through extracellular matrix-bound VEGF [62]. Anti-VEGF treatment of rodents demonstrates that VEGF is an important player not only in adipose tissue vascularization but also in the development of new adipocytes [49,50].

Despite the seemingly massive induction of a proangiogenic response, it is apparently not sufficient to prevent the development of hypoxia in the expanding adipose tissue, which could be partly because of the synthesis of additional signals that send a rather ambivalent message; the increase in proangiogenic factors may be accompanied by an even larger increase in inhibitors of neovascularization. For instance, circulating levels of angiopoietin-2 and endostatin correlate well with body mass index [58]. The underlying reasons for the up-regulation of these antiangiogenic factors are unknown. Another factor may be that although many proangiogenic factors may be induced, some critical downstream mediators of these signals may fail to be produced at appropriate levels.

TNP-470 is an angiogenesis inhibitor that has also been tested in the context of obesity. Ablation of the vasculature in the adipose tissue with this compound leads to a significant loss of body weight and fat mass, even though it is difficult to interpret because TNP-470 may also have effects on satiety [63]. However, these results have certainly raised speculation as to whether angiogenesis inhibitors may be used as antiobesity drugs. The results presented by Koloni and colleagues [52] are certainly intriguing. In this case, the targeted disruption of the adipose tissue vasculature through the use of a phage peptide–directed toxin destroying the adipose tissue endothelium leads to a reduction of adipose tissue, a phenotype reminiscent of other lipodystrophic mice models. In contrast to most lipodystrophic models, partial loss of fat leads to a decreased accumulation of liver lipids and lower fasting glucose and fasting insulin levels. Presumably, this result is due to a lower energy intake and higher energy expenditure. Given what we know about this model to date, it is difficult to speculate about the underlying mechanisms of this phenotype.

An important question could be raised in this context. Although it is clear that obese adipose tissue suffers from hypoxia, is this hypoxia truly rate limiting for further expansion of fat mass? Is it the hypoxia that is at the source of local inflammation in adipose tissue? We do not yet know the answers to these questions, but they can clearly be addressed with mouse models that display a constitutive activation of the hypoxia-associated factors in adipose tissue.

Posttranslational regulation of adipokine secretion

The authors have described the tremendous versatility of the adipose tissue proteome and have focused their summary mostly on the local effects of adipokines in adipose tissue proper. These effects, of course, also translate into systemic physiologic changes that, in turn, are further modified by adipokines that have endocrine functions and exert their effects on target cells not directly exposed to adipose tissue. A wealth of information is available on the transcriptional regulation of many of these adipokines. However, the adipocyte also seems to be remarkably versatile when it comes to posttranslational ways of controlling protein export. A good example can be seen in the context of adiponectin. PPAR-γ agonist treatment increases circulating levels of adiponectin up to fourfold while leaving the mRNA levels relatively unchanged [64], suggesting that potent mechanisms are in place to regulate the release of adiponectin at the posttranslational level. Research on trafficking through the endoplasmic reticulum and Golgi in adipocytes has for many years been biased toward studying the movements of the insulin-responsive GLUT4 transporter [65]. GLUT4 vesicles are indeed fusing with the plasma membrane at an increased rate in the presence of insulin. However, these GLUT4 vesicles are not well suited to carry soluble cargo molecules because the cycling of these vesicles to and from the plasma membrane is extensive, even in the unstimulated state. Therefore, other mechanisms must be in place in the adipocyte that regulate the release of adiponectin. This finding is even more relevant in light of the fact that the adipocyte releases several different forms of adiponectin, and the processing of each of these forms seems to be differentially regulated. A novel mechanism has been suggested in two recent studies that demonstrate that adiponectin is assembled and processed in a manner similar to IgM molecules. Adiponectin is retained in the ER by the chaperone ERp44 and released by the action of the oxidoreductase Ero-Lα [66,67]. This process is highly regulated, particularly at the level of these chaperones. It is, in fact, these chaperones that are the primary transcriptional target for PPAR-γ agonists, leading to a more efficient release of the high–molecular-weight form of adiponectin from the adipocyte.

The adipocyte secretory pathway

Is this ERp44/Ero1-mediated pathway a widely used mechanism to shunt proteins through later stages of the secretory pathway? Is it also used by other adipokines? At least one other adipokine, resistin, does not get retained in the ER by ERp44 [67], arguing that this mechanism is at least partially specific for adiponectin. However, we still know little about the mechanisms by which the adipocyte handles the differential release of factors to the extracellular environment. Is a triggered release of factors from the adipocyte a possibility? Little evidence suggests that a rapidly releasable pool of proteins exists similar to that which can be seen in neuroendocrine cells. The exposure of adipocytes to b3 adrenergic agonists can trigger a rapid release of insulin from b cells [68]. However, conventional wisdom holds that this process is primarily caused by lipolysis, resulting in the release of free fatty acids rather than a triggered release of a protein constituent. Other than the insulin-induced translocation of GLUT4 vesicles, little additional evidence indicates that the adipocyte can release proteins in a shorter time scale. Lipoprotein lipase may be another example of a protein whose release from the ER is regulated [69]. Insulin triggers a profound reshuffling of intracellular membranes, but with limited consequences on the release of soluble proteins [70].

However, the adipocyte is a tremendously active secretory cell whose mechanisms have yet to be revealed. The high-level production of abundant secretory constituents, such as adiponectin that is present at high levels in plasma and turns over rapidly, requires secretory machinery that can keep up with the high demands on the production of these proteins. Complement factor C3 is another component that is highly abundantly produced. Exposure to proinflammatory stimuli such as cytokines and LPS can rapidly transform the adipocyte into a cell devoted to the massive production of acute-phase reactants, such as SAA3 and many others, while maintaining the production and release of the conventional adipokines. Under these conditions, factors such as macrophage migration inhibitory factor are also produced a high levels. This protein's mechanism of release is still not yet well defined and it is unlikely to involve the conventional secretory pathway [71].

An additional unusual feature of the adipocyte is the abundance of caveolar structures throughout the entire cell. The presence of the flask-shaped structures gives the adipocyte plasma membrane its characteristic structure, where up to 25% of the cell surface is occupied by these raft structures [70] that display a unique lipid composition compared with the remainder of the plasma membrane. Although these caveolae are involved in signaling events [72–74], they also play a critical role in lipolysis. However, to date, we do not know whether these structures or their structural components, caveolin-1 and caveolin-2, are involved in vesicular trafficking of proteins. The abundant presence of these proteins throughout the secretory pathway, with high levels in the ER and Golgi, makes these proteins prime candidates as mediators for additional trafficking events within the realm of the classic secretory pathway or as mediators of trafficking of lipids and proteins directly from the ER to other subcellular compartments. Future efforts will have to be directed toward probing the existence and potential relevance of these additional trafficking events once appropriate cargo molecules have been identified whose secretion is critically affected by these pathways.

Summary

The role of adipose tissue as an important source of local mediators in the stroma of a host of organs and its role as an endocrine gland are now widely appreciated. As a whole, adipose tissue can make up a significant proportion of total body weight. So by sheer mass action, it is difficult to ignore the contribution it makes to plasma protein. In addition, because fat pads are interspersed in many different places systemically, they constitute different "miniorgans" with unique characteristics depending on their location, and a differential proteomics fingerprint. The authors have attempted to provide a comprehensive overview of protein factors that have been described in the literature. They have devoted much of the discussion to aspects of the adipocyte secretome that usually get less attention. It is not clear in all instances to what extent it is the adipocyte that serves as the primary site of production or whether another adipose tissue cell type in concert with the adipocyte is the major production site. In either case, one must treat the whole tissue as an entity. Thus, much remains to be understood about the cross talk between the different cell types within the adipose tissue and the secretory pathway.

Acknowledgments

The authors would like to thank Nancy Heard for help with the cartoon.

References

[1] Ahima RS. Adipose tissue as an endocrine organ. Obesity (Silver Spring) 2006;14(Suppl 5): 242S–9S.

[2] Nawrocki AR, Scherer PE. Keynote review: the adipocyte as a drug discovery target. Drug Discov Today 2005;10:1219–30.

[3] Scherer PE. Adipose tissue: from lipid storage compartment to endocrine organ. Diabetes 2006;55:1537–45.

[4] Trayhurn P. Endocrine and signalling role of adipose tissue: new perspectives on fat. Acta Physiol Scand 2005;184:285–93.

[5] Alvarez-Llamas G, Szalowska E, de Vries MP, et al. Characterization of the human visceral adipose tissue secretome. Mol Cell Proteomics 2007;6:589–600.

[6] Chen X, Cushman SW, Pannell LK, et al. Quantitative proteomic analysis of the secretory proteins from rat adipose cells using a 2D liquid chromatography-MS/MS approach. J Proteome Res 2005;4:570–7.

[7] Klimcakova E, Moro C, Mazzucotelli A, et al. Profiling of adipokines secreted from human subcutaneous adipose tissue in response to PPAR agonists. Biochem Biophys Res Commun 2007;358:897–902.

[8] Kratchmarova I, Kalume DE, Blagoev B, et al. A proteomic approach for identification of secreted proteins during the differentiation of 3T3-L1 preadipocytes to adipocytes. Mol Cell Proteomics 2002;1:213–22.

[9] Scherer PE, Bickel PE, Kotler M, et al. Cloning of cell-specific secreted and surface proteins by subtractive antibody screening. Nat Biotechnol 1998;16:581–6.

[10] Tsuruga H, Kumagai H, Kojima T, et al. Identification of novel membrane and secreted proteins upregulated during adipocyte differentiation. Biochem Biophys Res Commun 2000;272:293–7.

[11] Wang P, Mariman E, Keijer J, et al. Profiling of the secreted proteins during 3T3-L1 adipocyte differentiation leads to the identification of novel adipokines. Cell Mol Life Sci 2004;61: 2405–17.

[12] Zhang Y, Proenca R, Maffei M, et al. Positional cloning of the mouse obese gene and its human homologue. Nature 1994;372:425–32.

[13] Antras J, Hilliou F, Redziniak G, et al. Decreased biosynthesis of actin and cellular fibronectin during adipose conversion of 3T3-F442A cells. Reorganization of the cytoarchitecture and extracellular matrix fibronectin. Biol Cell 1989;66:247–54.

[14] Spiegelman BM, Ginty CA. Fibronectin modulation of cell shape and lipogenic gene expression in 3t3-adipocytes. Cell 1983;35:657–66.

[15] Taleb S, Cancello R, Clement K, et al. Cathepsin S promotes human preadipocyte differentiation: possible involvement of fibronectin degradation. Endocrinology 2006;147:4950–9.

[16] Xiao Y, Junfeng H, Tianhong L, et al. Cathepsin K in adipocyte differentiation and its potential role in the pathogenesis of obesity. J Clin Endocrinol Metab 2006;91:4520–7.

[17] Brekken RA, Sage EH. SPARC, a matricellular protein: at the crossroads of cell-matrix communication. Matrix Biol 2001;19:816–27.

[18] Bradshaw AD, Graves DC, Motamed K, et al. SPARC-null mice exhibit increased adiposity without significant differences in overall body weight. Proc Natl Acad Sci U S A 2003;100: 6045–50.

[19] Tartare-Deckert S, Chavey C, Monthouel MN, et al. The matricellular protein SPARC/ osteonectin as a newly identified factor up-regulated in obesity. J Biol Chem 2001;276: 22231–7.

[20] Chavey C, Mari B, Monthouel MN, et al. Matrix metalloproteinases are differentially expressed in adipose tissue during obesity and modulate adipocyte differentiation. J Biol Chem 2003;278:11888–96.

[21] Bouloumie A, Sengenes C, Portolan G, et al. Adipocyte produces matrix metalloproteinases 2 and 9: involvement in adipose differentiation. Diabetes 2001;50:2080–6.

[22] Croissandeau G, Chretien M, Mbikay M. Involvement of matrix metalloproteinases in the adipose conversion of 3T3-L1 preadipocytes. Biochem J 2002;364:739–46.

[23] Lijnen HR, Demeulemeester D, Van Hoef B, et al. Deficiency of tissue inhibitor of matrix metalloproteinase-1 (TIMP-1) impairs nutritionally induced obesity in mice. Thromb Haemost 2003;89:249–55.

[24] Alexander CM, Selvarajan S, Mudgett J, et al. Stromelysin-1 regulates adipogenesis during mammary gland involution. J Cell Biol 2001;152:693–703.

[25] Kralisch S, Bluher M, Tonjes A, et al. Tissue inhibitor of metalloproteinase-1 predicts adiposity in humans. Eur J Endocrinol 2007;156:257–61.

[26] Unger RH. Lipotoxic diseases. Annu Rev Med 2002;53:319–36.

[27] Kim JY, van de Wall E, Laplante M, et al. Obesity-associated improvements in metabolic profile through expansion of adipose tissue. J Clin Invest 2007;117:2621–37.

[28] Tataranni PA, Ortega E. A burning question: does an adipokine-induced activation of the immune system mediate the effect of overnutrition on type 2 diabetes? Diabetes 2005;54: 917–27.

[29] Kim JK, Kim YJ, Fillmore JJ, et al. Prevention of fat-induced insulin resistance by salicylate. J Clin Invest 2001;108:437–46.

[30] Visser M, Bouter LM, McQuillan GM, et al. Elevated C-reactive protein levels in overweight and obese adults. JAMA 1999;282:2131–5.

[31] Weisberg SP, McCann D, Desai M, et al. Obesity is associated with macrophage accumulation in adipose tissue. J Clin Invest 2003;112:1796–808.

[32] Xu H, Barnes GT, Yang Q, et al. Chronic inflammation in fat plays a crucial role in the development of obesity-related insulin resistance. J Clin Invest 2003;112:1821–30.

[33] Hotamisligil GS, Shargill NS, Spiegelman BM. Adipose expression of tumor necrosis factor-alpha: direct role in obesity-linked insulin resistance. Science 1993;259:87–91.

[34] Pickup JC, Crook MA. Is type II diabetes mellitus a disease of the innate immune system? Diabetologia 1998;41:1241–8.

[35] Lin Y, Rajala MW, Berger JP, et al. Hyperglycemia-induced production of acute phase reactants in adipose tissue. J Biol Chem 2001;276:42077–83.

[36] Ajuwon KM, Jacobi SK, Kuske JL, et al. Interleukin-6 and interleukin-15 are selectively regulated by lipopolysaccharide and interferon-gamma in primary pig adipocytes. Am J Physiol Regul Integr Comp Physiol 2004;286:R547–53.

[37] Berg AH, Lin Y, Lisanti MP, et al. Adipocyte differentiation induces dynamic changes in NF-kappaB expression and activity. Am J Physiol Endocrinol Metab 2004;287:E1178–88.

[38] Pajvani UB, Trujillo ME, Combs TP, et al. Fat apoptosis through targeted activation of caspase 8: a new mouse model of inducible and reversible lipoatrophy. Nat Med 2005;11: 797–803.

[39] Tsuchida A, Yamauchi T, Takekawa S, et al. Peroxisome proliferator-activated receptor (PPAR)alpha activation increases adiponectin receptors and reduces obesity-related inflammation in adipose tissue: comparison of activation of PPARalpha, PPARgamma, and their combination. Diabetes 2005;54:3358–70.

[40] Moller DE, Berger JP. Role of PPARs in the regulation of obesity-related insulin sensitivity and inflammation. Int J Obes Relat Metab Disord 2003;27(Suppl 3):S17–21.

[41] do Nascimento CO, Hunter L, Trayhurn P. Regulation of haptoglobin gene expression in 3T3-L1 adipocytes by cytokines, catecholamines, and PPARgamma. Biochem Biophys Res Commun 2004;313:702–8.

[42] Alleva DG, Johnson EB, Lio FM, et al. Regulation of murine macrophage proinflammatory and anti-inflammatory cytokines by ligands for peroxisome proliferator-activated receptor-gamma: counter-regulatory activity by IFN-gamma. J Leukoc Biol 2002;71:677–85.

[43] Ramakers JD, Verstege MI, Thuijls G, et al. The PPARgamma agonist rosiglitazone impairs colonic inflammation in mice with experimental colitis. J Clin Immunol 2007;27:275–83.

[44] Tahan V, Eren F, Avsar E, et al. Rosiglitazone attenuates liver inflammation in a rat model of nonalcoholic steatohepatitis. Dig Dis Sci 2007;52(12):3465–72.

[45] Russell JA. Management of sepsis. N Engl J Med 2006;355:1699–713.

[46] Toussirot E, Streit G, Wendling D. The contribution of adipose tissue and adipokines to inflammation in joint diseases. Curr Med Chem 2007;14:1095–100.

[47] Chen TH, Chen L, Hsieh MS, et al. Evidence for a protective role for adiponectin in osteo-arthritis. Biochim Biophys Acta 2006;1762:711–8.

[48] Neels JG, Thinnes T, Loskutoff DJ. Angiogenesis in an in vivo model of adipose tissue development. FASEB J 2004;18:983–5.

[49] Nishimura S, Manabe I, Nagasaki M, et al. Adipogenesis in obesity requires close interplay between differentiating adipocytes, stromal cells, and blood vessels. Diabetes 2007;56: 1517–26.

[50] Cho CH, Koh YJ, Han J, et al. Angiogenic role of LYVE-1-positive macrophages in adipose tissue. Circ Res 2007;100:e47–57.

[51] Brakenhielm E, Cao R, Gao B, et al. Angiogenesis inhibitor, TNP-470, prevents diet-induced and genetic obesity in mice. Circ Res 2004;94:1579–88.

[52] Kolonin MG, Saha PK, Chan L, et al. Reversal of obesity by targeted ablation of adipose tissue. Nat Med 2004;10:625–32.

[53] Rupnick MA, Panigrahy D, Zhang CY, et al. Adipose tissue mass can be regulated through the vasculature. Proc Natl Acad Sci U S A 2002;99:10730–5.

[54] Cao Y. Angiogenesis modulates adipogenesis and obesity. J Clin Invest 2007;117:2362–8.

[55] Hosogai N, Fukuhara A, Oshima K, et al. Adipose tissue hypoxia in obesity and its impact on adipocytokine dysregulation. Diabetes 2007;56:901–11.

[56] Rausch ME, Weisberg S, Vardhana P, et al. Obesity in C57BL/6J mice is characterized by adipose tissue hypoxia and cytotoxic T-cell infiltration. Int J Obes (Lond) 2008;32(3):451–63.

[57] Ye J, Gao Z, Yin J, et al. Hypoxia is a potential risk factor for chronic inflammation and adiponectin reduction in adipose tissue of ob/ob and dietary obese mice. Am J Physiol Endocrinol Metab 2007;293:E1118–28.

[58] Silha JV, Krsek M, Sucharda P, et al. Angiogenic factors are elevated in overweight and obese individuals. Int J Obes (Lond) 2005;29:1308–14.

[59] Mantovani A, Sica A, Locati M. New vistas on macrophage differentiation and activation. Eur J Immunol 2007;37:14–6.

[60] Lumeng CN, Bodzin JL, Saltiel AR. Obesity induces a phenotypic switch in adipose tissue macrophage polarization. J Clin Invest 2007;117:175–84.

[61] Lolmede K, Durand de Saint Front V, Galitzky J, et al. Effects of hypoxia on the expression of proangiogenic factors in differentiated 3T3-F442A adipocytes. Int J Obes Relat Metab Disord 2003;27:1187–95.

[62] Bergers G, Brekken R, McMahon G, et al. Matrix metalloproteinase-9 triggers the angio-genic switch during carcinogenesis. Nat Cell Biol 2000;2:737–44.

[63] Kim YM, An JJ, Jin YJ, et al. Assessment of the anti-obesity effects of the TNP-470 analog, CKD-732. J Mol Endocrinol 2007;38:455–65.

[64] Combs TP, Wagner JA, Berger J, et al. Induction of adipocyte complement-related protein of 30 kilodaltons by PPARgamma agonists: a potential mechanism of insulin sensitization. Endocrinology 2002;143:998–1007.

[65] Watson RT, Kanzaki M, Pessin JE. Regulated membrane trafficking of the insulin-responsive glucose transporter 4 in adipocytes. Endocr Rev 2004;25:177–204.

[66] Qiang L, Wang H, Farmer SR. Adiponectin secretion is regulated by SIRT1 and the endo-plasmic reticulum oxidoreductase Ero1-L alpha. Mol Cell Biol 2007;27:4698–707.

[67] Wang ZV, Schraw TD, Kim JY, et al. Secretion of the adipocyte-specific secretory protein adiponectin critically depends on thiol-mediated protein retention. Mol Cell Biol 2007;27: 3716–31.

[68] Grujic D, Susulic VS, Harper ME, et al. Beta3-adrenergic receptors on white and brown adipocytes mediate beta3-selective agonist-induced effects on energy expenditure, insulin secretion, and food intake. A study using transgenic and gene knockout mice. J Biol Chem 1997;272:17686–93.

[69] Roh C, Roduit R, Thorens B, et al. Lipoprotein lipase and leptin are accumulated in different secretory compartments in rat adipocytes. J Biol Chem 2001;276:35990–4.

[70] Scherer PE, Lisanti MP, Baldini G, et al. Induction of caveolin during adipogenesis and association of GLUT4 with caveolin-rich vesicles. J Cell Biol 1994;127:1233–43.

[71] Flieger O, Engling A, Bucala R, et al. Regulated secretion of macrophage migration inhibitory factor is mediated by a non-classical pathway involving an ABC transporter. FEBS Lett 2003;551:78–86.

[72] Anderson RG. Caveolae: where incoming and outgoing messengers meet. Proc Natl Acad Sci U S A 1993;90:10909–13.

[73] Okamoto T, Schlegel A, Scherer PE, et al. Caveolins, a family of scaffolding proteins for organizing "preassembled signaling complexes" at the plasma membrane. J Biol Chem 1998;273:5419–22.

[74] Shaul PW, Anderson RG. Role of plasmalemmal caveolae in signal transduction. Am J Physiol 1998;275:L843–51.

ELSEVIER
SAUNDERS

Endocrinol Metab Clin N Am
37 (2008) 769–787

ENDOCRINOLOGY
AND METABOLISM
CLINICS
OF NORTH AMERICA

Role of Gut Hormones in Obesity

Channa N. Jayasena, MA, MB BChir, MRCP,
Steve R. Bloom, MA, MD, DSc, FRCPath, FRCP, FMedSci*

*Department of Investigative Medicine, Imperial College London, Hammersmith Hospital,
6th Floor, Commonwealth Building, Du Cane Road, W12 0NN, London, UK*

Obesity is one of the major challenges to human health in the developed world, and the need to develop new treatments has never been more imperative. In pursuit of this goal, researchers have attempted to dissect the mechanisms through which satiety and hunger manifest. Consequently, a critical role for the gut in energy homeostasis has emerged. The gut is ideally placed to be receptive to the availability of nutrients, to signal such information to the brain, and then to regulate the ingestion of food according to the energy requirements of the body. In keeping with this notion, several gut hormones have been found not only to regulate digestion but also to modulate appetite in animals and humans [1–9]. Thus, the gut may be viewed as an endocrine organ, which functions not only to mediate but also to control energy intake.

Current nonendocrine pharmacologic therapies for obesity are limited by their modest efficacies. Bariatric surgery remains by far the most effective weight-loss therapy for morbidly obese individuals [10]; however, its use is confined to severe cases. Although the mechanisms by which bariatric surgery induces anorexia have for years remained elusive, we now realize that manipulation of gut hormone secretion may be partially responsible. Furthermore, the discovery of important signaling pathways from the gut to the brain has led to the emergence of several gut hormone–derived drugs that are currently being investigated for clinical use [11].

This article aims to summarize the physiology of the major gut hormones implicated in appetite regulation, and to review clinical studies that give us insight into their potential as clinical treatments for obesity.

C.N. Jayasena is supported by a Wellcome Trust Clinical Training Research Fellowship.

* Corresponding author.

E-mail address: s.bloom@imperial.ac.uk (S.R. Bloom).

doi:10.1016/j.ecl.2008.07.001

Pancreatic polypeptide-fold peptides

The pancreatic polypeptide (PP)-fold family of peptide hormones comprises the central nervous system (CNS) peptide, the neuropeptide Y (NPY), and the two gut hormones, pancreatic polypeptide (PP), and peptide tyrosine-tyrosine (PYY). Each of these hormones is thought to have an important but distinct role in appetite regulation. The genes encoding each hormone are thought to have arisen from successive duplications of a common ancestral gene [12].

The general structure of a PP-fold hormone is a chain of 36 amino acid residues, which is α-amidated at the C-terminal to display biologic activity [13]. Furthermore, the three-dimensional structure possesses a hairpin-like PP-fold motif, which is vital for receptor binding. Signaling of PP-fold peptides is mediated by a family of G protein–coupled receptors named Y1, Y2, Y4, Y5, and Y6. Repeated attempts to clone a receptor with the pharmacologic profile assigned "Y3" have failed, and Y5 encodes a nonfunctional, truncated receptor in almost all mammal studies. It is important to consider that although the NPY, PYY, and PP have distinctive relative binding affinities to each functional Y receptor, considerable receptor–ligand binding promiscuity exists. Thus, the PP-fold peptides may have overlapping domains of biologic activity.

Peptide tyrosine-tyrosine

PYY is coreleased from L cells of the gastrointestinal tract with two other gut hormones, glucagon-like peptide (GLP)-1 and oxyntomodulin (OXM) [14]. PYY immunoreactivity is at its highest level in the rectum, and diminishes proximally to low levels in the duodenum and jejunum. PYY immunoreactivity is also distributed in the human adrenal medulla and in regions of the rat CNS such as the hypothalamus, medulla, pons, and spinal cord [15]. Two endogenous circulating forms of PYY are synthesized within the gut, PYY_{1-36} and PYY_{3-36}. Of these, PYY_{3-36} is produced by cleavage of the Tyr-Pro amino terminal residues of PYY_{1-36} by the ubiquitous enzyme, dipeptidyl peptidase (DPP-IV).

The pattern of PYY secretion suggests a role in satiety. PYY is released into the circulation following the ingestion of food, in proportion to calorie intake [14]. In a canine model using fistulas to isolate sections of the gut, PYY release (predominantly from the distal gut) was equivalent, whether or not fat was placed within the proximal or distal gut [16]. Thus, factors must exist that signal the distal gut to release PYY in response to nutrients within the proximal gut. Indeed, humoral factors (such as gastrin and cholecystokinin [CCK]) or a vagal reflex, are thought to mediate this rapid release of PYY, which occurs before the transit of food to the distal gut [17].

Evidence from pathologic and iatrogenic human models of anorexia also supports a role for PYY in satiety. Anorectic conditions such as inflammatory bowel disease, tropical sprue, and cardiac cachexia, are characterized by elevated circulating levels of PYY_{3-36} [18]. Furthermore, gastric bypass surgery is associated with elevated basal and postprandial levels of PYY_{3-36}. It is possible that the postsurgical diversion of nutrients beyond most of the stomach and proximal intestine, toward the PYY-secreting distal gut, might explain this phenomenon [19].

In keeping with its putative role as a hormone of satiety, peripheral administration of PYY_{3-36} has been shown to inhibit food intake in fasted rats when compared with saline-injected controls [2,20]. Some investigators failed to demonstrate an anorectic action of PYY, but this may have been because of inadequate acclimatization of control and treated animals [21]. As a result, increased stress (a potently anorectic state) may have masked the anorectic effect of PYY [22].

How might PYY act to suppress appetite? PYY seems to act on the hypothalamus as a satiety signal. The arcuate nucleus (ARC) of the hypothalamus is in close proximity to the deficient blood–brain barrier (BBB) of the median eminence, so it is well placed to respond to circulating PYY. Injection of PYY into rodents increased c-fos expression (a marker of neuronal activity) in the ARC. It also reduced expression of the orexigenic peptide, NPY, and up-regulated expression of the anorexigenic peptide, pro-opiomelanocortin (POMC), within the ARC [2,20]. PYY might also act on the brainstem, because peripherally injected ^{125}iodine (^{125}I)-PYY_{3-36} accumulates not only in the median eminence but also in the area postrema (AP) [23]. PYY has multiple effects that slow the passage of nutrients through the gut, such that it is regarded as a component of the functional mechanism known as the "ileal brake." PYY delays gastric emptying and inhibits gallbladder contraction, pancreatic exocrine secretions, and gastric acid secretion [18]. Therefore, PYY inhibits feeding by modulation of hypothalamic appetite control circuits and the delayed transit of food through the gut.

Disturbance in the release of PYY might play a role in the development of obesity. This possibility is suggested by the blunted PYY_{3-36} response to feeding in obese human subjects, when compared with lean controls [24,25]. Mice with diet-induced obesity have impairment of postprandial levels circulating PYY_{3-36}, but raised immunoreactivity and normal expression of PYY_{3-36} in the ascending colon [25]. These data suggest that, at least in mice, impaired secretion from the gut might explain the relative deficiency of PYY in diet-induced obesity. However, other factors, such as reduced posttranslational processing or increased plasma clearance of PYY, cannot be excluded.

Interest exists as to whether a satiety factor such as PYY could be used therapeutically to treat obesity. Intravenous infusion of PYY_{3-36} to healthy lean humans was associated with a 36% reduction in calorie intake during a free-choice buffet meal 2 hours postinfusion [2]. Furthermore, in a follow-up study, PYY_{3-36} infusion was shown to reduce calorie intake in obese individuals to an extent similar to that of lean controls (30% versus 31%) [24], which demonstrates that sensitivity to the anorectic action of peripheral PYY is preserved in obese individuals, in contrast to leptin resistance, which characterizes most cases of obesity [26]. PYY, therefore, offers promise as a future therapy for obesity. Accordingly, several analogs of PYY are being investigated for clinical use.

Uncertainty surrounds the physiologic role of PYY in the central regulation of appetite, stemming from its opposing actions within different regions of the CNS. Administration of PYY to the lateral ventricle of rodents has been shown to stimulate appetite [27]. However, direct injection to the ARC actually suppresses appetite, which is consistent with its peripheral effect [2]. Sense may be made from such seemingly confusing actions by considering that PYY_{3-36} has binding affinity not only to the anorexigenic Y2 receptor but also to the orexigenic Y1 and Y5 receptors [13]. Inhibitory presynaptic Y2 receptors are expressed abundantly on NPY neurons within the ARC, and PYY_{3-36} fails to reduce food intake in Y2 knockout mice [2,28]. Hence, Y2 might mediate the anorexia seen by local injection of PYY_{3-36}. In addition, the increased food intake seen after intracerebroventricular (ICV) administration of PYY_{3-36} is attenuated in Y1 and Y5 knockout mice [27]. Therefore, PYY_{3-36} may act within the brain to stimulate appetite by way of Y1 and Y5 receptors. But in the ARC, an area with a deficient BBB, exposure to circulating PYY_{3-36} may cause Y2-mediated appetite inhibition. Clearly, a more complete understanding of the distribution of individual Y receptor species, and their interactions with each PP-fold peptide, is needed to determine the true physiologic action of PYY.

Pancreatic polypeptide

Being the first PP-fold peptide hormone to be identified, PP was originally isolated as an impurity of insulin extracted from chicken pancreas [29]. Subsequent work found its source to be type F (PP) cells within the periphery of pancreatic islets [15].

The major stimulus of PP secretion is the ingestion of food [30]. Indeed, circulating levels reflect calorie intake and remain elevated for approximately 6 hours postprandially. Various humoral factors have also been found to stimulate PP release (CCK, ghrelin, motilin, and secretin) and inhibit its release (somatostatin). Furthermore, adrenergic stimulation secondary to hypoglycemia or exercise increases circulating levels of PP [31].

PP is considered a component of the "ileal brake" because it acts in various ways to slow the transit of food through the gut; PP delays gastric emptying, attenuates pancreatic exocrine secretion, and inhibits gallbladder contraction [31].

An inverse correlation of PP release with body weight implies a role in satiety. Reduced postprandial secretion is associated with human obesity, and elevated postprandial levels are found in those with anorexia nervosa [32,33]. Although levels of circulating PP have been shown to be reduced after some forms of gastric surgery for morbid obesity, jejunoileal bypass actually increases levels of PP [34]. Hence, part of the weight loss secondary to jejunoileal bypass may be the result of elevated PP levels.

PP may have an additional role in the pathogenesis of Prader-Willi syndrome (PWS), a genetic syndrome characterized by hyperphagia, short stature, and intellectual impairment. Subjects who have PWS have reduced basal and postprandial PP release, even when compared with age- and weight-matched controls with nonsyndromic obesity [35].

In rodents and humans, peripheral injection inhibits food intake. In mice, repeated intraperitoneal injection of PP reduced food intake and body weight [1,36]. A similarly anorectic state was displayed by transgenic mice overexpressing PP, and this phenotype was partially reversed by antiserum to PP [37]. In lean human volunteers, PP infusion reduced food intake by 25% over 24 hours [3]. Although the efficacy of PP in nonsyndromic obesity remains undetermined, twice-daily infusion of PP into subjects who have PWS leads to a 12% reduction in food intake [38].

PP is thought to induce anorexia principally through an action on the brainstem and vagus, mediated by the Y4 receptor. Electrophysiologic studies show that PP reduces activity within afferent and efferent vagal neurons. In addition, the anorectic action of intraperitoneal PP is abolished by vagotomy in rodents [36]. PP may also exert a direct action on the dorsal vagal complex of the brainstem, by way of the incomplete BBB of the AP. Consistent with this, the Y4 receptor to which PP binds with greatest affinity is highly expressed in the AP and various hypothalamic regions, including the ARC [39,40]. Furthermore, the nucleus tractus solitarius (NTS) is in close proximity to the AP. It receives afferent chemosensory and mechanosensory vagal fibers from in the viscera, and projects vagal efferents to the viscera. Therefore, PP may act on vagal afferents within the gut and, by way of Y4 receptors within the AP, modify the vagovagal reflex arc at the NTS, thus inhibiting food intake.

Although the principal site of action of PP is thought to be the brainstem, PP may also act on the hypothalamus. The Y4 receptor is distributed within the ARC and paraventricular nucleus (PVN), and peripheral injection of PP into mice reduced the hypothalamic expression of the orexigenic neuropeptides, NPY and orexin [36]. However, it is not known whether such an action is mediated by way of the brainstem, or is a direct action through exposure to circulating PP at the median eminence.

Peripheral PP may also inhibit feeding through the reduction of ghrelin release. Peripheral PP injection into mice leads to reduced expression of the orexigenic hormone, ghrelin, within the stomach [36]. Similarly, PP infusion into subjects who have PWS reduces its circulating levels [38].

Although the overwhelming source of circulating PP within the body is the pancreas, it is far from clear whether or not PP is additionally synthesized in the CNS. Reverse-transcriptase PCR has identified PP mRNA, but in situ hybridization has failed to do so. Although immunoreactivity for PP has been identified within the brainstem and spinal cord, it is possible that antibody cross-reactivity might have misidentified neurons that actually contained actual PYY or NPY [41]. Hence, the existence of any

PP-expressing neurons within the brain remains unresolved. It is also curious that contrary to its peripheral action, centrally injected PP actually increases food intake, a phenomenon that resembles the paradoxical actions of PYY [1]. Whether such an observation represents a physiologic action of PP, or merely demonstrates an effect of NPY that has been experimentally induced by virtue of receptor-ligand promiscuity, remains to be determined.

Products of cleavage of preproglucagon

Zunz and LeBarre [42] first postulated the existence of an insulinotropic gastrointestinal factor, referred to as "incretin," in 1929. Subsequent work by McIntyre and colleagues [43] in 1964 validated this theory by demonstrating that oral glucose administration induced a much greater insulin response than intravenous glucose. Of the various candidate peptides having been examined for incretin activity, GLP-1 and OXM are cleavage products of preproglucagon, which both have an additional putative role in energy homeostasis.

Preproglucagon is a 160–amino acid peptide expressed in the α cells of the pancreas, the L cells of the intestine, and within the CNS [44]. The differential cleavage of preproglucagon by the prohormone convertases 1 and 2 results in the production of several hormones, the combination of which is specific to each individual tissue. Alongside the cleavage fragments of preproglucagon implicated in appetite regulation (GLP-1 and OXM), other products include glucagon, GLP-2, and glicentin.

Glucagon-like peptide–1

GLP-1 is secreted and released by the L cells of the intestine, together with PYY and another fragment of preproglucagon, OXM. Differential cleavage from preproglucagon results in a 36– or 37–amino acid peptide, differing by one C-terminal glycine residue [44]. However, further cleavage is required to produce the bioactive fragments, GLP-$1_{7\text{-}36amide}$ and GLP-$1_{7\text{-}37}$. Although both active isoforms of GLP-1 have equivalent potency, GLP-$1_{7\text{-}36amide}$ is the major circulating species found. The GLP-1 receptor is G protein–coupled and is the only currently identified receptor to bind GLP-1 [45].

Although not itself an endogenous mammalian peptide, exendin-4, discovered to be an agonist of GLP-1 receptor, has proved an invaluable experimental tool in the investigation of the physiologic role of GLP-1 [44]. Exendin-4, a 39–amino acid peptide originally isolated from the venom of a lizard named the Gila monster, *Heloderma suspectum*, is much more resistant to degradation DPP-IV than GLP-1. Because the half-life of GLP-1 in the circulation is only approximately 2 minutes, exendin-4 offers a useful means of investigating the long-acting effects of GLP-1 receptor activation [46]. In addition, whereas the full-length exendin-4 peptide is a long-acting agonist of GLP-1, its truncated form, extendin$_{9-39}$, is actually a competitive antagonist of GLP-1 [44].

In general terms, GLP-1 is best thought of as a component of the "ileal brake," with an additional role in the metabolism of ingested carbohydrate. Accordingly, GLP-1 inhibits gastric acid secretion and delays gastric emptying. Furthermore, it has potent incretin activity because it up-regulates various stages of the production and release of insulin, together with attenuation of glucagon release [47]. GLP-1 is released from the gut in response to ingestion of food, and its release is in proportion to the calorific value of the meal [48,49].

In addition to its secretion within the gut, GLP-1$_{7-36amide}$ is distributed within the CNS. Immunoreactive neurons for GLP-1$_{7-36amide}$ are located in the PVN and dorsomedial hypothalamus regions of the hypothalamus, and in the dorsovagal complex, thalamus, and pituitary [50]. Further support for a central action of GLP-1 within the CNS comes from the observation that GLP-1 receptor mRNA is distributed throughout the rostrocaudal hypothalamus, with dense accumulation in the ARC, PVN, and supraoptic nucleus [51].

GLP-1$_{7-36amide}$ has been shown to inhibit food intake in various species, whether administered peripherally or centrally. Turton and colleagues [7] first demonstrated the anorectic action of GLP-1 by central injection of GLP-1$_{7-36amide}$ to fasted rats; a potent inhibition of food intake was observed when compared with saline injection, and extendin$_{9-39}$ completely abolished this effect. Furthermore, extendin$_{9-39}$ doubled food intake in satiated rats, and potentiated the feeding response to the orexigenic peptide, NPY. The suggestion that blockade of endogenous GLP-1 signaling by extendin$_{9-39}$ actually increases food intake implicates GLP-1 in the physiologic regulation of appetite.

In addition to its acute effects, chronic administration of GLP-1 leads to weight loss in rodents [52]. Repeated ICV injection of GLP-1$_{7-36amide}$ for 6 days resulted in significant weight loss, a phenomenon that was also inhibited by extendin$_{9-39}$. Although knockout mice for the GLP-1 receptor are predictably glucose intolerant, they have normal food intake and body weight [53]. This observation serves to illustrate the compensatory mechanisms that evidently exist to preserve feeding behavior, and thus sustain life.

The brainstem is thought to be an important site of action for the effects of peripheral GLP-1. Although peripheral and central injection of GLP-1$_{7-36amide}$ induces c-fos expression in the PVN, up-regulation in the brainstem only occurs after peripheral injection [7,54]. Furthermore, vagotomy or lesioning of the brainstem–hypothalamic connections reduces the appetite suppression induced by peripheral GLP-1$_{7-36amide}$ injection [55]. Therefore, peripheral GLP-1 may owe part of its activity to a direct action on the brainstem and vagal afferents, which subsequently relay signals to the hypothalamus by neuronal projections.

In agreement with animal data, GLP-1 has been shown to dose-dependently reduce appetite and calorie intake in humans. This effect is seen in lean, obese, and diabetic subjects. Across a range of studies, GLP-1$_{7\text{-}36\text{amide}}$ acutely reduced food intake by an average of 11.7% without adverse effects, most notably nausea [8]. In addition, prandial injections of GLP-1$_{7\text{-}36\text{amide}}$ to obese subjects for 5 days led to 0.55 kg weight loss [56].

The rapid degradation of native forms of GLP-1 by the enzyme DPP-IV makes them unsuitable for the clinical treatment of obesity; in fact, GLP-1$_{7\text{-}36\text{amide}}$ has a half-life of only 2 minutes [46]. However, the recognition of exendin-4 as a long-acting analog of GLP-1 has provided one method of overcoming this problem. Indeed, in April 2005, the US Food and Drug Administration (FDA) licensed the exendin-4 analog, exenatide, as the first incretin mimetic for use as adjunctive therapy in type 2 diabetes. In addition to its lowering effect on fasting glycemia, postprandial glycemia, and hemoglobin A1c (HbA1c), a recent meta-analysis of five studies (with durations of 15 to 52 weeks) revealed exenatide to reduce weight by an average of 1.44 kg (-2.13 to -0.75 kg, 95% confidence interval) compared with placebo, and 4.76 kg (-6.03 to 3.49 kg, 95% confidence interval) when compared with insulin treatment [11]. However, exenatide posed an increased risk for gastrointestinal side effects such as nausea, vomiting, and diarrhea (risk ratios 2.9, 3.3, and 2.2, respectively), when it was compared with either placebo or insulin. Such effects were generally mild to moderate, most frequent during the first 8 weeks of therapy, and attenuated by dose titration.

Liraglutide is a GLP-1 analog that owes part of its extended half-life to being albumin bound. Two studies have demonstrated that 12 weeks of once-daily subcutaneous liraglutide injection led to weight loss of 1.2 kg, when compared with placebo, in addition to improvements in HbA1c [57,58]. However, similar gastrointestinal side effects were observed when compared with exenatide. Liraglutide is currently undergoing phase 3 clinical trials for use in type 2 diabetes.

A third strategy to overcome the short half-life of native GLP-1 is to pharmacologically inhibit the enzyme DPP-IV; oral DPP-IV antagonists such as sitagliptin and vildagliptin are being introduced as treatments for type 2 diabetes (sitagliptin received FDA approval in 2006). However, a meta-analysis of 13 studies revealed that they actually increase weight by a mean of 0.48 kg when compared with placebo (0.30–0.66 kg, 95% confidence interval) [11]. Whether such weight gain results from actions on peptide hormones other than GLP-1 remains to be determined.

Administration of GLP-1 or its analogs is associated with gastrointestinal side effects. It is therefore important to consider whether the induction of visceral illness is, in fact, integral to their anorectic mode of action. Indeed, evidence implicates GLP-1 in the mediation of conditioned taste aversion (CTA). The pattern of *c-fos* induction by GLP-1$_{7\text{-}36\text{amide}}$ injection in rodents resembles that following administration of the toxin lithium chloride, a potent inducer of visceral illness in rodents. Furthermore, ICV extendin$_{9\text{-}39}$ to rodents attenuates the induction of CTA by lithium chloride [59]. However, one could argue that extendin$_{9\text{-}39}$ attenuates CTA by opposition of the actions of a GLP-1 receptor ligand, other than GLP-1. CTA may also be mediated ·by signaling pathways other than the GLP-1 receptor, because its targeted disruption in mice abolishes CTA induced by GLP-1$_{7\text{-}36amide}$, but not by lithium chloride [60]. On the other hand, disruption of GLP-1 receptor signaling may unmask minor pathways that do not physiologically play a major role in the mediation of CTA behavior. Although its relative importance in CTA remains ill defined, GLP-1 does appear to play a role in its mediation.

One view to reconcile a role for GLP-1 in ingestion-mediated appetite suppression and CTA is that they are merely different points on the same spectrum of satiety. According to this theory, low levels of stimulation of appetite-suppressing pathways give rise only to satiety; however, high levels of stimulation also produce nausea. An alternative view is that GLP-1 mediates satiety and CTA through two separate pathways. In support of this latter theory, injection of GLP-1 $_{7\text{-}36amide}$ into the lateral ventricle of rodents induces anorexia and nausea; however, injection into the fourth ventricle induces anorexia without nausea [61]. Furthermore, direct injection of GLP-1$_{7\text{-}36amide}$ into the central nucleus of the amygdala induces CTA but has no effect on food intake. Hence, GLP-1 signaling in the PVN and brainstem may mediate anorexia but its action within the amygdala may mediate CTA.

Oxyntomodulin

OXM is a 37–amino acid peptide originally isolated from porcine jejunoileal cells, found to display glucagon-like activity in the liver [62]. In fact, OXM contains the entire sequence of glucagon, with the addition of a basic octapeptide C-terminal extension referred to as spacer peptide-1 [44]. It is coreleased with GLP-1 and PYY from L cells, particularly those of more distal sections of the gastrointestinal tract. Similarities between OXM and GLP-1 extend beyond the route of synthesis to their biologic actions. Furthermore, the only receptor to date identified to mediate the signal of OXM is the GLP-1 receptor [63]. Although OXM does possess incretin activity, it stimulates insulin release with a much lower potency than that of GLP-1 [64].

OXM appears to function as a hormone of satiety. In keeping with this, it is released into the circulation following ingestion of food, with plasma levels reflecting the calorific value of the meal [65]. OXM is also a powerful inhibitor of pentagastrin-induced gastric acid secretion and gastric emptying, which both delay the transit of nutrients through the gut [64,66].

Circulating levels of OXM are raised after gastric bypass surgery [67]. Such a procedure artificially diverts nutrients away from the stomach and proximal small intestine, toward regions of higher OXM expression, such as the distal small intestine and colon, which clearly raises the possibility that OXM plays a role in the weight loss secondary to gastric bypass surgery. Plasma levels of OXM are also raised in small bowel disorders such as tropical sprue, which are characterized by weight loss [68].

Injections of OXM result in appetite suppression and weight loss. Central administration (ICV or directly into the PVN) or intraperitoneal injection of OXM inhibits fasting and nonfasted dark phase food intake in rodents, with a similar potency to that of GLP-1$_{7\text{-}36\text{amide}}$ [5,69]. Furthermore, repeated intraperitoneal administration over 7 days reduces weight gain and adiposity. Rodents given OXM lose more weight than saline-treated controls given the same amount of food (pair-fed controls), which suggests that OXM may, in part, reduce body weight by way of increased energy expenditure [70]. One of the key functions of OXM as an appetite-suppressing hormone may be to suppress endogenous release of the appetite-stimulating hormone, ghrelin; peripheral OXM reduced plasma ghrelin levels in rodents by 20%. This finding could go some way to explaining the fall in plasma ghrelin, which occurs postprandially.

OXM also appears to function as a satiety hormone in humans. Healthy, fasted volunteers experienced significantly reduced hunger scores and plasma ghrelin levels during an intravenous infusion of OXM when compared with placebo [4]. Furthermore, energy intake during a postinfusion buffet meal was markedly reduced (19.3%) compared with placebo, and 12-hour energy intake also remained significantly reduced. Volunteers reported no nausea or adverse effects with regard to meal palatability, which is an important observation considering the side effect profile of GLP-1.

Chronic OXM administration leads to weight loss in humans. Chronic preprandial subcutaneous injections of OXM to obese subjects over 4 weeks produced 2.3 kg weight loss compared with 0.5 kg in the saline-treated group [71]. The observed weight loss was progressive (approximately 0.45 kg per week), and energy intake for a meal during the final study day was reduced (by an average of 250 kcal). These two observations are important because they suggest that OXM has a sustained action on food intake, therefore making it an attractive therapeutic target.

It is noteworthy that although the anorectic potency of OXM is equivalent to that of GLP-1$_{7\text{-}36\text{amide}}$ in rodents, the binding affinity to GLP-1 receptor is approximately two orders of magnitude weaker than that of GLP-1$_{7\text{-}36\text{amide}}$ (IC$_{50}$ 8.2 nM versus 0.16 nM) [63]. Furthermore, patterns of c-fos activation differ subtly; OXM, but not GLP-1, increases c-fos expression in the ARC [5]. In addition, extendin$_{9\text{-}39}$ administered directly to the ARC fails to inhibit the anorectic effect of OXM but does indeed inhibit that of GLP-1 [5], which suggests that the action of OXM on the ARC may be mediated by an unidentified receptor other than GLP-1. On the other hand, evidence indicates that the GLP-1 receptor is important in mediating the anorectic action of OXM; OXM injection loses its anorectic action in mice with targeted disruption of the GLP-1 receptor [54]. Also, neither ICV injection of GLP-1 nor of OXM inhibits food intake with coadministration of extendin$_{9\text{-}39}$ [69].

Unanswered questions clearly remain about OXM, including its anatomic sites of action and whether signaling is mediated by another receptor, in addition to GLP-1. Nevertheless, the much milder incretin activity of OXM in comparison to GLP-1 makes it an appealing therapeutic target for the treatment of obese individuals, particularly those who do not have diabetes.

Ghrelin

Growth hormone secretagogues (GHS) such as growth hormone (GH)–releasing peptide-6 and hexarelin, are a family of synthetic peptide and nonpeptide molecules that have, for a number of years, been distinguished by their GH-releasing properties in various species [72]. Subsequent work identified the GHS receptor (GHR-R) as an endogenous seven transmembrane G protein–coupled receptor able to bind and mediate the effects of such secretagogues. The discovery of GHS-R was significant because it logically implied the existence of an endogenous ligand, which was later identified by Kojima and colleagues [73] as being ghrelin. Ghrelin was named in accordance with its GH stimulating action; "ghre" is the Proto-Indo-European root of the word "grow."

Ghrelin consists of a chain of 28 amino acids, with esterification of the hydroxyl group of the third serine residue by octanoic acid [73]. This side chain is essential for binding to GHS-R and bioactivity of ghrelin. Ghrelin, originally identified as an extract from rat stomach, is principally secreted from X/A–like cells within gastric oxyntic glands [74]. In keeping with this, gastrectomy reduces plasma ghrelin levels by 80%; the remainder is secreted from the intestine, pancreas, pituitary, and colon [75]. Ghrelin has an additional role as a neurotransmitter, being expressed within the ARC and periventricular area of the hypothalamus [73,76]. GHR-R has a wide distribution within the body, including the gastrointestinal tract, hypothalamus, pituitary, myocardium, pancreas, adipose tissue, liver, kidney, and placenta [75].

The actions of ghrelin are not restricted to GH secretion; strong evidence implicates ghrelin as a hormone of hunger. Plasma levels of ghrelin correlate inversely with body weight; levels are significantly higher in lean than in obese human subjects [77,78]. Furthermore, diet-induced weight loss increases circulating levels of ghrelin in obese individuals [77]. The view of ghrelin as a hunger hormone is strengthened by its prandial rise and postprandial fall in lean humans and sheep [79–81]. Furthermore, the observation that food intake fails to suppress plasma ghrelin in obese subjects suggests that dysregulation of ghrelin secretion may play a role in the pathogenesis of obesity [82]. In addition to stimulating appetite, ghrelin promotes gastric motility, up-regulates the hypothalamo-pituitary-adrenal axis, and has cardiovascular effects such as vasodilatation and increased cardiac contractility [75].

Ghrelin is unique because it is the only identified circulating gut hormone to stimulate food intake. Peripheral or central injection of ghrelin to rats stimulated acute food intake [83]. Furthermore, repeated peripheral or central injection for 7 days induced weight gain [84].

The effect of intravenous infusion of ghrelin to healthy human volunteers is dramatic. Wren and colleagues [9] observed a 28% increase in energy consumption during a buffet meal, which led to the question of whether such a potent appetite stimulant might be used to antagonize pathologic states of cachexia therapeutically. Early results have been promising because ghrelin infusion to subjects with cancer-induced weight loss led to a 31% increase in energy intake during unrestricted feeding [85]. A similar picture was seen in patients who had mild-to-moderate malnutrition from chronic renal failure; subcutaneous ghrelin injection doubled acute energy intake [86]. Cardiac and chronic obstructive pulmonary disease–induced cachexia may also benefit from ghrelin injection [87,88].

Circulating levels of ghrelin are reduced in obese subjects who have undergone gastric bypass surgery, maybe as a consequence of the permanent diversion of food past all but a small pouch of the stomach [19,77]. One may therefore postulate that the anorexia that has long been observed from such established operative procedures is partially explained by attenuation of ghrelin release.

Patients who have PWS present a unique profile of ghrelin secretion; they have markedly increased circulating levels of ghrelin, which is in contrast to the abnormally low levels observed in individuals with nonsyndromic forms of obesity [89]. This finding suggests that part of the hyperphagic phenotype of PWS may be accounted for by excessive circulating levels of ghrelin. Attempts to test this hypothesis, by suppressing ghrelin release with an infusion of somatostatin, unexpectedly led to unaltered food intake in PWS patients [90]. However, interpretation of such an experiment is difficult because reduction in the orexigenic hormone ghrelin may have been masked by the concomitant reduction in anorectic circulating factors such as PYY, PP, and insulin, by somatostatin.

The question of how ghrelin mediates its orexigenic action is an important one because its blockade might provide a means to treat obesity. The ARC of the hypothalamus appears pivotal to the orexigenic action of ghrelin. First, the ARC is well situated to be receptive to the fluxes in circulating ghrelin by virtue of its deficient BBB and expression of GHS-R. In addition, specific ablation of the ARC with monosodium glutamate is sufficient to abolish ghrelin-stimulated food intake [91]. Indeed, it seems to be the orexigenic population of NPY/agouti-related protein (AgRP) coexpressing neurons within the ARC that mediate the orexigenic action of ghrelin. Centrally administered ghrelin up-regulates expression of NPY and AgRP, and induces *c-fos* expression in NPY/AgRP neurons within the ARC [92]. Furthermore, mice with targeted disruption of NPY and AgRP similarly fail to respond to exogenous ghrelin [93]. In addition to the ARC, the brainstem may play a role in mediating the actions of ghrelin; *c-fos* expression within the NTS and area postrema increase following peripheral ghrelin administration [92]. As with other gut hormones, the actions of ghrelin on the brainstem may be partially mediated by way of

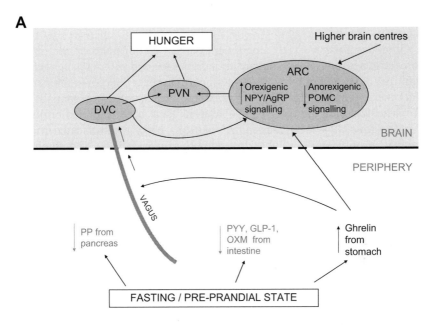

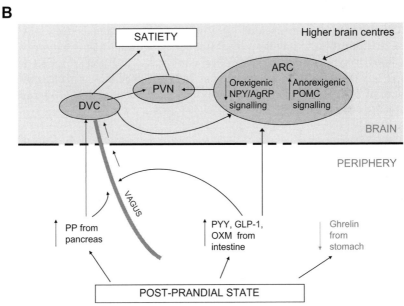

Fig. 1. Gut hormone signaling to the brain under fasted and fed states. (*A*) During the fasting/preprandial state, ghrelin release from the stomach acts on the ARC and vagus to stimulate hunger. (*B*) In the postprandial state, intestinal release of anorectic hormones PYY, GLP-1, OXM, and PP act on the ARC, brainstem, and vagus as signals of satiety. DVC, dorsal vagal complex.

the vagus; it fails to stimulate food intake in either humans or rodents after vagotomy [94,95].

Ghrelin is not exclusively a peripherally released hormone; ghrelin-immunoreactive neuronal cell bodies are abundantly located within the periventricular area of the hypothalamus and terminate in several hypothalamic nuclei and other regions, such as the amygdala and nucleus of stria terminalis [76]. In particular, these ghrelin-positive neurons have been found to project to hypothalamic NPY/AgRP and POMC neurons, which are implicated in appetite regulation. Hence, peripherally and perhaps centrally derived ghrelin act on multiple sites within the brain to stimulate hunger and feeding behavior.

Cholecystokinin

CCK is notable for being the first gut hormone to be implicated in appetite regulation, by Gibbs and colleagues in 1973 [96]. However, its physiologic role in appetite regulation still remains unclear. It is a peptide hormone expressed within the small intestine and is released rapidly in response to feeding. CCK stimulates pancreatic and gallbladder exocrine secretions, inhibits gastric emptying, and increases intestinal motility. CCK is also expressed as a neurotransmitter in the CNS and has been implicated in reward behavior, anxiety, and memory. It acts by way of two G protein–coupled receptors, CCK-1 and CCK-2 [6]. Although repeated injection of CCK in animals decreases meal size and duration, it increases meal frequency, without any resultant change in body weight [97,98]. Furthermore, continuous infusion of CCK fails to have any effect on food intake beyond 24 hours. The lack of a clear role for CCK in appetite regulation currently makes it unsuitable as a therapeutic target for obesity.

Summary

Our view of the gut has shifted fundamentally, such that it is now recognized as a means of feeding and as a regulator of feeding. The gut uses an array of humoral factors, together with the vagus nerve, to signal the availability of nutrients to the brain, thus influencing appetite (Fig. 1).

Although bariatric surgery is the most effective means of weight loss, its invasive nature limits its application to severe cases. Hence, the need for novel therapies to treat the milder and more prevalent forms of obesity is pressing. The potential of gut hormones to treat obesity is illustrated by their likely contribution to the anorexia associated with some forms of bariatric surgery. Furthermore, drugs based on gut hormones (such as GLP-1 analogs) are already emerging in clinical use, and others are likely to follow. The gut–brain axis is indeed a complex endocrine system, a further understanding of which will aid the development of more effective drugs to treat obesity.

References

[1] Asakawa A, Inui A, Ueno N, et al. Mouse pancreatic polypeptide modulates food intake, while not influencing anxiety in mice. Peptides 1999;20:1445–8.

[2] Batterham RL, Cowley MA, Small CJ, et al. Gut hormone PYY(3-36) physiologically inhibits food intake. Nature 2002;418:650–4.

[3] Batterham RL, Le Roux CW, Cohen MA, et al. Pancreatic polypeptide reduces appetite and food intake in humans. J Clin Endocrinol Metab 2003;88:3989–92.

[4] Cohen MA, Ellis SM, Le Roux CW, et al. Oxyntomodulin suppresses appetite and reduces food intake in humans. J Clin Endocrinol Metab 2003;88:4696–701.

[5] Dakin CL, Gunn I, Small CJ, et al. Oxyntomodulin inhibits food intake in the rat. Endocrinology 2001;142:4244–50.

[6] Little TJ, Horowitz M, Feinle-Bisset C. Role of cholecystokinin in appetite control and body weight regulation. Obes Rev 2005;6:297–306.

[7] Turton MD, O'Shea D, Gunn I, et al. A role for glucagon-like peptide-1 in the central regulation of feeding. Nature 1996;379:69–72.

[8] Verdich C, Flint A, Gutzwiller JP, et al. A meta-analysis of the effect of glucagon-like peptide-1 (7-36) amide on ad libitum energy intake in humans. J Clin Endocrinol Metab 2001;86:4382–9.

[9] Wren AM, Seal LJ, Cohen MA, et al. Ghrelin enhances appetite and increases food intake in humans. J Clin Endocrinol Metab 2001;86:5992–5.

[10] Kral JG, Naslund E. Surgical treatment of obesity. Nat Clin Pract Endocrinol Metab 2007;3: 574–83.

[11] Amori RE, Lau J, Pittas AG. Efficacy and safety of incretin therapy in type 2 diabetes: systematic review and meta-analysis. J Am Med Assoc 2007;298:194–206.

[12] Conlon JM. The origin and evolution of peptide YY (PYY) and pancreatic polypeptide (PP). Peptides 2002;23:269–78.

[13] Berglund MM, Hipskind PA, Gehlert DR. Recent developments in our understanding of the physiological role of PP-fold peptide receptor subtypes. Exp Biol Med (Maywood) 2003;228: 217–44.

[14] Adrian TE, Ferri GL, Bacarese-Hamilton AJ, et al. Human distribution and release of a putative new gut hormone, peptide YY. Gastroenterology 1985;89:1070–7.

[15] Ekblad E, Sundler F. Distribution of pancreatic polypeptide and peptide YY. Peptides 2002; 23:251–61.

[16] Lin HC, Chey WY. Cholecystokinin, peptide YY are released by fat in either proximal or distal small intestine in dogs. Regul Pept 2003;114:131–5.

[17] Onaga T, Zabielski R, Kato S. Multiple regulation of peptide YY secretion in the digestive tract. Peptides 2002;23:279–90.

[18] Le Roux CW, Bloom SR. Peptide YY, appetite and food intake. Proc Nutr Soc 2005;64: 213–6.

[19] Korner J, Inabnet W, Conwell IM, et al. Differential effects of gastric bypass and banding on circulating gut hormone and leptin levels. Obesity (Silver Spring) 2006;14:1553–61.

[20] Challis BG, Pinnock SB, Coll AP, et al. Acute effects of PYY3-36 on food intake and hypothalamic neuropeptide expression in the mouse. Biochem Biophys Res Commun 2003;311: 915–9.

[21] Tschop M, Castaneda TR, Joost HG, et al. Physiology: does gut hormone PYY3-36 decrease food intake in rodents? Nature 2004;430:1–3.

[22] Halatchev IG, Ellacott KL, Fan W, et al. Peptide YY3-36 inhibits food intake in mice through a melanocortin-4 receptor-independent mechanism. Endocrinology 2004;145: 2585–90.

[23] Dumont Y, Moyse E, Fournier A, et al. Distribution of peripherally injected peptide YY (((125)I) PYY (3-36)) and pancreatic polypeptide (((125)I) hPP) in the CNS: enrichment in the area postrema. J Mol Neurosci 2007;33:294–304.

[24] Batterham RL, Cohen MA, Ellis SM, et al. Inhibition of food intake in obese subjects by peptide YY3-36. N Engl J Med 2003;349:941–8.

[25] Le Roux CW, Batterham RL, Aylwin SJ, et al. Attenuated peptide YY release in obese subjects is associated with reduced satiety. Endocrinology 2006;147:3–8.

[26] Enriori PJ, Evans AE, Sinnayah P, et al. Leptin resistance and obesity. Obesity (Silver Spring) 2006;14(Suppl 5):254S–8S.

[27] Kanatani A, Mashiko S, Murai N, et al. Role of the Y1 receptor in the regulation of neuropeptide Y-mediated feeding: comparison of wild-type, Y1 receptor-deficient, and Y5 receptor-deficient mice. Endocrinology 2000;141:1011–6.

[28] Broberger C, Landry M, Wong H, et al. Subtypes Y1 and Y2 of the neuropeptide Y receptor are respectively expressed in pro-opiomelanocortin- and neuropeptide-Y-containing neurons of the rat hypothalamic arcuate nucleus. Neuroendocrinology 1997;66:393–408.

[29] Kimmel JR, Pollock HG, Hazelwood RL. Isolation and characterization of chicken insulin. Endocrinology 1968;83:1323–30.

[30] Track NS, McLeod RS, Mee AV. Human pancreatic polypeptide: studies of fasting and postprandial plasma concentrations. Can J Physiol Pharmacol 1980;58:1484–9.

[31] Kojima S, Ueno N, Asakawa A, et al. A role for pancreatic polypeptide in feeding and body weight regulation. Peptides 2007;28:459–63.

[32] Lassmann V, Vague P, Vialettes B, et al. Low plasma levels of pancreatic polypeptide in obesity. Diabetes 1980;29:428–30.

[33] Uhe AM, Szmukler GI, Collier GR, et al. Potential regulators of feeding behavior in anorexia nervosa. Am J Clin Nutr 1992;55:28–32.

[34] Meryn S, Stein D, Straus EW. Fasting- and meal-stimulated peptide hormone concentrations before and after gastric surgery for morbid obesity. Metabolism 1986;35:798–802.

[35] Zipf WB, O'Dorisio TM, Cataland S, et al. Pancreatic polypeptide responses to protein meal challenges in obese but otherwise normal children and obese children with Prader-Willi syndrome. J Clin Endocrinol Metab 1983;57:1074–80.

[36] Asakawa A, Inui A, Yuzuriha H, et al. Characterization of the effects of pancreatic polypeptide in the regulation of energy balance. Gastroenterology 2003;124:1325–36.

[37] Ueno N, Inui A, Iwamoto M, et al. Decreased food intake and body weight in pancreatic polypeptide-overexpressing mice. Gastroenterology 1999;117:1427–32.

[38] Berntson GG, Zipf WB, O'Dorisio TM, et al. Pancreatic polypeptide infusions reduce food intake in Prader-Willi syndrome. Peptides 1993;14:497–503.

[39] Larsen PJ, Kristensen P. The neuropeptide Y (Y4) receptor is highly expressed in neurones of the rat dorsal vagal complex. Brain Res Mol Brain Res 1997;48:1–6.

[40] Whitcomb DC, Puccio AM, Vigna SR, et al. Distribution of pancreatic polypeptide receptors in the rat brain. Brain Res 1997;760:137–49.

[41] Katsuura G, Asakawa A, Inui A. Roles of pancreatic polypeptide in regulation of food intake. Peptides 2002;23:323–9.

[42] Zunz E, LaBarre J. [Contributions a l'etude des variations physiologiques de la secretion interne du pancreas: realations entre les secretions externe et interne du pancreas]. Arch Int Physiol Biochim 1929;31:20–44 [in French].

[43] McIntyre N, Holdsworth CD, Turner DS. New interpretation of oral glucose tolerance. Lancet 1964;2:20–1.

[44] Kieffer TJ, Habener JF. The glucagon-like peptides. Endocr Rev 1999;20:876–913.

[45] Thorens B, Porret A, Buhler L, et al. Cloning and functional expression of the human islet GLP-1 receptor. Demonstration that exendin-4 is an agonist and exendin-(9-39) an antagonist of the receptor. Diabetes 1993;42:1678–82.

[46] Kieffer TJ, McIntosh CH, Pederson RA. Degradation of glucose-dependent insulinotropic polypeptide and truncated glucagon-like peptide 1 in vitro and in vivo by dipeptidyl peptidase IV. Endocrinology 1995;136:3585–96.

[47] Holst JJ. The physiology of glucagon-like peptide 1. Physiol Rev 2007;87:1409–39.

[48] Ghatei MA, Uttenthal LO, Christofides ND, et al. Molecular forms of human enteroglucagon in tissue and plasma: plasma responses to nutrient stimuli in health and in disorders of the upper gastrointestinal tract. J Clin Endocrinol Metab 1983;57:488–95.

[49] Orskov C, Rabenhoj L, Wettergren A, et al. Tissue and plasma concentrations of amidated and glycine-extended glucagon-like peptide I in humans. Diabetes 1994;43:535–9.

[50] Larsen PJ, Tang-Christensen M, Holst JJ, et al. Distribution of glucagon-like peptide-1 and other preproglucagon-derived peptides in the rat hypothalamus and brainstem. Neuroscience 1997;77:257–70.

[51] Shughrue PJ, Lane MV, Merchenthaler I. Glucagon-like peptide-1 receptor (GLP1-R) mRNA in the rat hypothalamus. Endocrinology 1996;137:5159–62.

[52] Meeran K, O'Shea D, Edwards CM, et al. Repeated intracerebroventricular administration of glucagon-like peptide-1-(7-36) amide or exendin-(9-39) alters body weight in the rat. Endocrinology 1999;140:244–50.

[53] Gallwitz B, Schmidt WE. GLP-1 receptor gene "knock out" causes glucose intolerance, but no alterations of eating behavior. Z Gastroenterol 1997;35:655–8.

[54] Baggio LL, Huang Q, Brown TJ, et al. Oxyntomodulin and glucagon-like peptide-1 differentially regulate murine food intake and energy expenditure. Gastroenterology 2004;127: 546–58.

[55] Abbott CR, Monteiro M, Small CJ, et al. The inhibitory effects of peripheral administration of peptide YY(3-36) and glucagon-like peptide-1 on food intake are attenuated by ablation of the vagal-brainstem-hypothalamic pathway. Brain Res 2005;1044:127–31.

[56] Naslund E, King N, Mansten S, et al. Prandial subcutaneous injections of glucagon-like peptide-1 cause weight loss in obese human subjects. Br J Nutr 2004;91:439–46.

[57] Madsbad S, Schmitz O, Ranstam J, et al. Improved glycemic control with no weight increase in patients with type 2 diabetes after once-daily treatment with the long-acting glucagon-like peptide 1 analog liraglutide (NN2211): a 12-week, double-blind, randomized, controlled trial. Diabetes Care 2004;27:1335–42.

[58] Vilsboll T, Zdravkovic M, Le-Thi T, et al. Liraglutide, a long-acting human glucagon-like peptide-1 analog, given as monotherapy significantly improves glycemic control and lowers body weight without risk of hypoglycemia in patients with type 2 diabetes. Diabetes Care 2007;30:1608–10.

[59] Seeley RJ, Blake K, Rushing PA, et al. The role of CNS glucagon-like peptide-1 (7-36) amide receptors in mediating the visceral illness effects of lithium chloride. J Neurosci 2000;20: 1616–21.

[60] Lachey JL, D'Alessio DA, Rinaman L, et al. The role of central glucagon-like peptide-1 in mediating the effects of visceral illness: differential effects in rats and mice. Endocrinology 2005;146:458–62.

[61] Kinzig KP, D'Alessio DA, Seeley RJ. The diverse roles of specific GLP-1 receptors in the control of food intake and the response to visceral illness. J Neurosci 2002;22:10470–6.

[62] Bataille D, Gespach C, Tatemoto K, et al. Bioactive enteroglucagon (oxyntomodulin): present knowledge on its chemical structure and its biological activities. Peptides 1981; 2(Suppl 2):41–4.

[63] Fehmann HC, Jiang J, Schweinfurth J, et al. Stable expression of the rat GLP-I receptor in CHO cells: activation and binding characteristics utilizing GLP-I (7-36)-amide, oxyntomodulin, exendin-4, and exendin(9-39). Peptides 1994;15:453–6.

[64] Schjoldager BT, Baldissera FG, Mortensen PE, et al. Oxyntomodulin: a potential hormone from the distal gut. Pharmacokinetics and effects on gastric acid and insulin secretion in man. Eur J Clin Invest 1988;18:499–503.

[65] Le QA, Kervran A, Blache P, et al. Oxyntomodulin-like immunoreactivity: diurnal profile of a new potential enterogastrone. J Clin Endocrinol Metab 1992;74:1405–9.

[66] Schjoldager B, Mortensen PE, Myhre J, et al. Oxyntomodulin from distal gut. Role in regulation of gastric and pancreatic functions. Dig Dis Sci 1989;34:1411–9.

[67] Holst JJ, Sorensen TI, Andersen AN, et al. Plasma enteroglucagon after jejunoileal bypass with 3:1 or 1:3 jejunoileal ratio. Scand J Gastroenterol 1979;14:205–7.

[68] Besterman HS, Cook GC, Sarson DL, et al. Gut hormones in tropical malabsorption. Br Med J 1979;2:1252–5.

[69] Dakin CL, Small CJ, Batterham RL, et al. Peripheral oxyntomodulin reduces food intake and body weight gain in rats. Endocrinology 2004;145:2687–95.

[70] Dakin CL, Small CJ, Park AJ, et al. Repeated ICV administration of oxyntomodulin causes a greater reduction in body weight gain than in pair-fed rats. Am J Physiol Endocrinol Metab 2002;283:E1173–7.

[71] Wynne K, Park AJ, Small CJ, et al. Subcutaneous oxyntomodulin reduces body weight in overweight and obese subjects: a double-blind, randomized, controlled trial. Diabetes 2005;54:2390–5.

[72] Smith RG, Palyha OC, Feighner SD, et al. Growth hormone releasing substances: types and their receptors. Horm Res 1999;51(Suppl 3):1–8.

[73] Kojima M, Hosoda H, Date Y, et al. Ghrelin is a growth-hormone-releasing acylated peptide from stomach. Nature 1999;402:656–60.

[74] Date Y, Kojima M, Hosoda H, et al. Ghrelin, a novel growth hormone-releasing acylated peptide, is synthesized in a distinct endocrine cell type in the gastrointestinal tracts of rats and humans. Endocrinology 2000;141:4255–61.

[75] Hosoda H, Kojima M, Kangawa K. Biological, physiological, and pharmacological aspects of ghrelin. J Pharm Sci 2006;100:398–410.

[76] Cowley MA, Smith RG, Diano S, et al. The distribution and mechanism of action of ghrelin in the CNS demonstrates a novel hypothalamic circuit regulating energy homeostasis. Neuron 2003;37:649–61.

[77] Cummings DE, Weigle DS, Frayo RS, et al. Plasma ghrelin levels after diet-induced weight loss or gastric bypass surgery. N Engl J Med 2002;346:1623–30.

[78] Tschop M, Weyer C, Tataranni PA, et al. Circulating ghrelin levels are decreased in human obesity. Diabetes 2001;50:707–9.

[79] Cummings DE, Purnell JQ, Frayo RS, et al. A preprandial rise in plasma ghrelin levels suggests a role in meal initiation in humans. Diabetes 2001;50:1714–9.

[80] Sugino T, Hasegawa Y, Kikkawa Y, et al. A transient ghrelin surge occurs just before feeding in a scheduled meal-fed sheep. Biochem Biophys Res Commun 2002;295:255–60.

[81] Tschop M, Wawarta R, Riepl RL, et al. Post-prandial decrease of circulating human ghrelin levels. J Endocrinol Invest 2001;24:RC19–21.

[82] English PJ, Ghatei MA, Malik IA, et al. Food fails to suppress ghrelin levels in obese humans. J Clin Endocrinol Metab 2002;87:2984–7.

[83] Wren AM, Small CJ, Ward HL, et al. The novel hypothalamic peptide ghrelin stimulates food intake and growth hormone secretion. Endocrinology 2000;141:4325–8.

[84] Tschop M, Smiley DL, Heiman ML. Ghrelin induces adiposity in rodents. Nature 2000;407:908–13.

[85] Neary NM, Small CJ, Wren AM, et al. Ghrelin increases energy intake in cancer patients with impaired appetite: acute, randomized, placebo-controlled trial. J Clin Endocrinol Metab 2004;89:2832–6.

[86] Wynne K, Giannitsopoulou K, Small CJ, et al. Subcutaneous ghrelin enhances acute food intake in malnourished patients who receive maintenance peritoneal dialysis: a randomized, placebo-controlled trial. J Am Soc Nephrol 2005;16:2111–8.

[87] Nagaya N, Itoh T, Murakami S, et al. Treatment of cachexia with ghrelin in patients with COPD. Chest 2005;128:1187–93.

[88] Nagaya N, Kangawa K. Therapeutic potential of ghrelin in the treatment of heart failure. Drugs 2006;66:439–48.

[89] Cummings DE, Clement K, Purnell JQ, et al. Elevated plasma ghrelin levels in Prader Willi syndrome. Nat Med 2002;8:643–4.

[90] Tan TM, Vanderpump M, Khoo B, et al. Somatostatin infusion lowers plasma ghrelin without reducing appetite in adults with Prader-Willi syndrome. J Clin Endocrinol Metab 2004; 89:4162–5.

[91] Tamura H, Kamegai J, Shimizu T, et al. Ghrelin stimulates GH but not food intake in arcuate nucleus ablated rats. Endocrinology 2002;143:3268–75.

[92] Nakazato M, Murakami N, Date Y, et al. A role for ghrelin in the central regulation of feeding. Nature 2001;409:194–8.

[93] Chen HY, Trumbauer ME, Chen AS, et al. Orexigenic action of peripheral ghrelin is mediated by neuropeptide Y and agouti-related protein. Endocrinology 2004;145:2607–12.

[94] Le Roux CW, Neary NM, Halsey TJ, et al. Ghrelin does not stimulate food intake in patients with surgical procedures involving vagotomy. J Clin Endocrinol Metab 2005;90:4521–4.

[95] Williams DL, Grill HJ, Cummings DE, et al. Vagotomy dissociates short- and long-term controls of circulating ghrelin. Endocrinology 2003;144:5184–7.

[96] Gibbs J, Young RC, Smith GP. Cholecystokinin decreases food intake in rats. J Comp Physiol Psychol 1973;84:488–95.

[97] Gibbs J, Young RC, Smith GP. Cholecystokinin decreases food intake in rats. 1973. Obes Res 1997;5:284–90.

[98] Kissileff HR, Carretta JC, Geliebter A, et al. Cholecystokinin and stomach distension combine to reduce food intake in humans. Am J Physiol Regul Integr Comp Physiol 2003; 285:R992–8.

ELSEVIER
SAUNDERS

Endocrinol Metab Clin N Am
37 (2008) 789–810

ENDOCRINOLOGY
AND METABOLISM
CLINICS
OF NORTH AMERICA

Index

Note: Page numbers of article titles are in **boldface** type.

A

Abdominal obesity. See also *Waist circumference (WC); Waist-to-hip ratio.*
    definition of, 665
    ethnicity and, 561, 623
    insulin resistance and, 584–588
        as cardiovascular disease risk predictor, 590–592
        variability of, 592–593
    metabolic syndrome and, 560, 562

Acipimox, for free fatty acids, in obesity, 642

Activity level. See also *Physical entries.*
    adiposity variation vs., as cardiovascular disease risk, 583

Adaptive immune response, adipocyte role in, 759–761

Adhesion molecules, as cardiovascular disease risk, 676
    vascular cell, in insulin resistance, endothelial dysfunction and, 686, 688–689, 691

Adipocyte fatty acid binding protein (A-FABP), in metabolic syndrome, 569–570

Adipocyte-binding protein aP2, cardiovascular disease risk factors and, adiposity variations vs. activity level as, 583
    in insulin resistance, atherogenesis and, 613

Adipocytes, as endocrine cell, **753–769.** See also *Adipose tissue.*
    angiogenesis role of, 761–763
    extracellular matrix of, 754, 758–759
    immune-regulatory role of, 759–761
    posttranslational adipokine secretion regulation and, 763–764
    secretome functions of, 753–754

proteins clustered according to postulated function, 755–757
    secretory pathway of, 764–765
    secretory products of, free fatty acids as, insulin resistance and, 636, 654
        in hypertension with obesity, 653–656
        adiponectin as, 656
        endothelin as, 654
        free fatty acids as, 654
        glucocorticoid excess as, 655
        leptin as, 655–656
        resistin as, 653–654
    summary overview of, 753, 765

Adipogenesis, 758

Adipokines, adipocyte secretion of, 753–754
    clustered according to postulated function, 755–757
    posttranslational regulation of, 763–764
    in insulin resistance, 608
        endothelial dysfunction and, 694–695
    in obesity and dyslipidemia, 628–629
    proinflammatory, 760–761

Adiponectin, adipocyte secretion of, 753
    as proinflammatory, 761
    in metabolic syndrome, 569–571
    in mitochondrial dysfunction, with T2D and obesity, 725
    in obesity, dyslipidemia and, 628–629
        hypertension and, 656
    PPAR-γ agonists effect on, 763–764

Adipose tissue, angiogenesis reduction of, 761
    dysfunction of, in obesity and dyslipidemia, 628–629
    extracellular matrix of, 754, 758–759
        angiogenesis connection in, 762
    in hypertension with obesity, 650–652
    in insulin resistance, atherogenesis and, 613

doi:10.1016/S0889-8529(08)00052-2   *endo.theclinics.com*

Moving?

Make sure your subscription moves with you!

To notify us of your new address, find your **Clinics Account Number** (located on your mailing label above your name), and contact customer service at:

E-mail: elspcs@elsevier.com

800-654-2452 (subscribers in the U.S. & Canada)
1-407-563-6020 (subscribers outside of the U.S. & Canada)

Fax number: 407-363-9661

Elsevier Periodicals Customer Service
6277 Sea Harbor Drive
Orlando, FL 32887-4800

*To ensure uninterrupted delivery of your subscription, please notify us at least 4 weeks in advance of move.